NOSOCOMIAL
PNEUMONIA

LUNG BIOLOGY IN HEALTH AND DISEASE

Executive Editor

Claude Lenfant
Director, National Heart, Lung and Blood Institute
National Institutes of Health
Bethesda, Maryland

1. Immunologic and Infectious Reactions in the Lung, *edited by C. H. Kirkpatrick and H. Y. Reynolds*
2. The Biochemical Basis of Pulmonary Function, *edited by R. G. Crystal*
3. Bioengineering Aspects of the Lung, *edited by J. B. West*
4. Metabolic Functions of the Lung, *edited by Y. S. Bakhle and J. R. Vane*
5. Respiratory Defense Mechanisms (in two parts), *edited by J. D. Brain, D. F. Proctor, and L. M. Reid*
6. Development of the Lung, *edited by W. A. Hodson*
7. Lung Water and Solute Exchange, *edited by N. C. Staub*
8. Extrapulmonary Manifestations of Respiratory Disease, *edited by E. D. Robin*
9. Chronic Obstructive Pulmonary Disease, *edited by T. L. Petty*
10. Pathogenesis and Therapy of Lung Cancer, *edited by C. C. Harris*
11. Genetic Determinants of Pulmonary Disease, *edited by S. D. Litwin*
12. The Lung in the Transition Between Health and Disease, *edited by P. T. Macklem and S. Permutt*
13. Evolution of Respiratory Processes: A Comparative Approach, *edited by S. C. Wood and C. Lenfant*
14. Pulmonary Vascular Diseases, *edited by K. M. Moser*
15. Physiology and Pharmacology of the Airways, *edited by J. A. Nadel*
16. Diagnostic Techniques in Pulmonary Disease (in two parts), *edited by M. A. Sackner*
17. Regulation of Breathing (in two parts), *edited by T. F. Hornbein*
18. Occupational Lung Diseases: Research Approaches and Methods, *edited by H. Weill and M. Turner-Warwick*
19. Immunopharmacology of the Lung, *edited by H. H. Newball*
20. Sarcoidosis and Other Granulomatous Diseases of the Lung, *edited by B. L. Fanburg*
21. Sleep and Breathing, *edited by N. A. Saunders and C. E. Sullivan*
22. *Pneumocystis carinii* Pneumonia: Pathogenesis, Diagnosis, and Treatment, *edited by L. S. Young*
23. Pulmonary Nuclear Medicine: Techniques in Diagnosis of Lung Disease, *edited by H. L. Atkins*
24. Acute Respiratory Failure, *edited by W. M. Zapol and K. J. Falke*
25. Gas Mixing and Distribution in the Lung, *edited by L. A. Engel and M. Paiva*

56. Physiological Adaptations in Vertebrates: Respiration, Circulation, and Metabolism, *edited by S. C. Wood, R. E. Weber, A. R. Hargens, and R. W. Millard*
57. The Bronchial Circulation, *edited by J. Butler*
58. Lung Cancer Differentiation: Implications for Diagnosis and Treatment, *edited by S. D. Bernal and P. J. Hesketh*
59. Pulmonary Complications of Systemic Disease, *edited by J. F. Murray*
60. Lung Vascular Injury: Molecular and Cellular Response, *edited by A. Johnson and T. J. Ferro*
61. Cytokines of the Lung, *edited by J. Kelley*
62. The Mast Cell in Health and Disease, *edited by M. A. Kaliner and D. D. Metcalfe*
63. Pulmonary Disease in the Elderly Patient, *edited by D. A. Mahler*
64. Cystic Fibrosis, *edited by P. B. Davis*
65. Signal Transduction in Lung Cells, *edited by J. S. Brody, D. M. Center, and V. A. Tkachuk*
66. Tuberculosis: A Comprehensive International Approach, *edited by L. B. Reichman and E. S. Hershfield*
67. Pharmacology of the Respiratory Tract: Experimental and Clinical Research, *edited by K. F. Chung and P. J. Barnes*
68. Prevention of Respiratory Diseases, *edited by A. Hirsch, M. Goldberg, J.-P. Martin, and R. Masse*
69. *Pneumocystis carinii* Pneumonia: Second Edition, *edited by P. D. Walzer*
70. Fluid and Solute Transport in the Airspaces of the Lungs, *edited by R. M. Effros and H. K. Chang*
71. Sleep and Breathing: Second Edition, *edited by N. A. Saunders and C. E. Sullivan*
72. Airway Secretion: Physiological Bases for the Control of Mucous Hypersecretion, *edited by T. Takishima and S. Shimura*
73. Sarcoidosis and Other Granulomatous Disorders, *edited by D. G. James*
74. Epidemiology of Lung Cancer, *edited by J. M. Samet*
75. Pulmonary Embolism, *edited by M. Morpurgo*
76. Sports and Exercise Medicine, *edited by S. C. Wood and R. C. Roach*
77. Endotoxin and the Lungs, *edited by K. L. Brigham*
78. The Mesothelial Cell and Mesothelioma, *edited by M.-C. Jaurand and J. Bignon*
79. Regulation of Breathing: Second Edition, *edited by J. A. Dempsey and A. I. Pack*
80. Pulmonary Fibrosis, *edited by S. Hin. Phan and R. S. Thrall*
81. Long-Term Oxygen Therapy: Scientific Basis and Clinical Application, *edited by W. J. O'Donohue, Jr.*
82. Ventral Brainstem Mechanisms and Control of Respiration and Blood Pressure, *edited by C. O. Trouth, R. M. Millis, H. F. Kiwull-Schöne, and M. E. Schläfke*
83. A History of Breathing Physiology, *edited by D. F. Proctor*
84. Surfactant Therapy for Lung Disease, *edited by B. Robertson and H. W. Taeusch*
85. The Thorax: Second Edition, Revised and Expanded (in three parts), *edited by C. Roussos*

ADDITIONAL VOLUMES IN PREPARATION

The opinions expressed in these volumes do not necessarily represent the views of the National Institutes of Health.

NOSOCOMIAL PNEUMONIA

Edited by

William R. Jarvis

Centers for Disease Control and Prevention
Atlanta, Georgia

MARCEL DEKKER, INC.   NEW YORK · BASEL

ISBN: 0-8247-0384-7

This book is printed on acid-free paper.

Headquarters
Marcel Dekker, Inc.
270 Madison Avenue, New York, NY 10016
tel: 212-696-9000; fax: 212-685-4540

Eastern Hemisphere Distribution
Marcel Dekker AG
Hutgasse 4, Postfach 812, CH-4001 Basel, Switzerland
tel: 41-61-261-8482; fax: 41-61-261-8896

World Wide Web
http://www.dekker.com

The publisher offers discounts on this book when ordered in bulk quantities. For more information, write to Special Sales/Professional Marketing at the headquarters address above.

INTRODUCTION

Infections have plagued mankind for centuries and for this reason, all issues relevant to infection have been studied and debated for a very long time. In 1584, Hieronymus Fracastoreus Veronensis published the *Theory of Infection* and chapter one addressed "What is contagion?" Although the presentation was limited to the passing of infection from one individual to another, there is no doubt that the broader concept of transmissibility was introduced at this time.

Centuries later, in 1921, Theobold Smith, from Princeton, presented a paper titled "Discussion on the Causation or Etiology of Infectious and Parasitic Diseases" at the meeting of the Association of American Physicians. He said: "Modern medicine has made the concept of causation its own. On it is founded all rational progress in prophylaxis and therapy. First to comprehend the cause, then to intercept and suppress it, and thereby to prevent the next step is the kernel of medical science and practice."

That was 1921! Undoubtedly the application of this dictum should have led to the elimination of a number of infectious manifestations, not the least of which is nosocomial pneumonia. Surely, this should have been greatly helped by the development of anti-infectious compounds and by the antibiotic revolution from which the later half of the twentieth century has greatly benefited. However, during the same period of time, we have witnessed the emergence and the greater use of devices such as ventilators and bronchoscopes and of intensive care facilities—all of which are often related to development of nosocomial infection. Although everyone knows about prevention and understands what needs to be done, hospital acquired pneumonia remains a huge public health problem.

As the editor, William R. Jarvis, says in his preface, this book is "a comprehensive reference on *prevention* and *management*." These are the two key words that all those coming close to hospitalized patients must keep in mind . . . prevention and management.

Dr. Jarvis brings to this volume his own expertise coming from years of research and clinical work at the U.S. Centers for Disease Control and Prevention. He has also assembled a remarkable group of contributors whose international reputations are well established.

The series of monographs, *Lung Biology in Health and Disease*, has presented volumes in all areas and aspects of lung disease. This book is among those that can be expected to have the most impact on public health. It is, indeed, a very valuable addition to the series.

Claude Lenfant, M.D.
Bethesda, Maryland

PREFACE

Nosocomial pneumonia continues to be a significant cause of morbidity and mortality among hospitalized patients. In recent years, nosocomial pneumonia has become the second most frequently occurring nosocomial infection (after that of the urinary tract) in U.S. hospitals. Factors contributing to the increased occurrence of nosocomial pneumonia include increased severity of illness in hospitalized patients and the rapidly increasing complexity of medical technology.

A number of publications about nosocomial pneumonia are available; most focus primarily on the diagnosis and treatment of the infection. However, unlike other publications, this book will emphasize the importance of *prevention* as a healthcare worker's primary goal in the approach to a patient at risk of pneumonia. This means increasing one's awareness of the risk factors for development of pneumonia in a patient admitted to the hospital, and practicing appropriate preventive measures.

Because prevention and management of a disease require an understanding of the pathogenesis and methods of controlling the disease progression, this book includes sections on the diagnosis, epidemiology, and pathogenesis of nosocomial pneumonia.

The book will serve as a comprehensive reference on prevention and management of patients with nosocomial pneumonia. It is intended for use by a cross-section of the medical and paramedical community, including physicians (general practitioners, family doctors, internists, surgeons, pediatricians, epidemiologists, etc.); nurses; medical, nursing, and paramedical students; respiratory therapists; and those involved in infection control and hospital epidemiology.

To facilitate the understanding of some of the complex and controversial areas of the prevention and control of nosocomial pneumonia, this book provides point–counterpoint sections that address particularly difficult issues at the end of selected chapters.

William R. Jarvis

CONTRIBUTORS

Nancy H. Arden, R.N. Professor, Department of Virology, Baylor University School of Medicine, Houston, Texas

Arnold J. Berry, M.D., M.P.H. Professor, Department of Anesthesiology, Emory University School of Medicine, Atlanta, Georgia

Marc J. M. Bonten, M.D., Ph.D. Internist, Department of Internal Medicine, University Hospital Utrecht, Utrecht, The Netherlands

Michael T. Brady, M.D. Vice Chair for Clinical Affairs, Children's Hospital, and Professor, Department of Pediatrics, The Ohio State University, Columbus, Ohio

Jay C. Butler, M.D. Director, Arctic Investigations Program, Centers for Disease Control and Prevention, Anchorage, Alaska

Jean Chastre, M.D.   Professor, Medical Intensive Care Unit, Bichat Hospital, Paris, France

Raymond Chinn, M.D., F.A.C.P.   Hospital Epidemiologist, Department of Infectious Disease, Sharp Memorial Hospital, San Diego, California

Donald E. Craven, M.D.   Professor, Department of Infectious Diseases, Boston University School of Medicine, Boston Medical Center, Boston, Massachusetts

Jean-Yves Fagon, M.D.   Professor and Department Head, Medical Intensive Care Unit, Broussais Hospital, Paris, France

Catherine A. Fleming, M.B., M.P.H.   Instructor, Department of Medicine, Boston University School of Medicine, Boston Medical Center, Boston, Massachusetts

Robert P. Gaynes, M.D.   Chief, Nosocomial Infections Surveillance Activity, Hospital Infections Program, Centers for Disease Control and Prevention, Atlanta, Georgia

Olivia Keita-Perse, M.D.   Nosocomial Infections Surveillance Activity, Hospital Infections Program, Centers for Disease Control and Prevention, Atlanta, Georgia

Kathleen A. Steger, R.N., M.P.H.   Assistant Professor, Boston University School of Medicine, and Associate Director, Clinical AIDS Program, Boston Medical Center, Boston, Massachusetts

Jean-Louis Trouillet, M.D.   Medical Intensive Care Unit, Bichat Hospital, Paris, France

Robert A. Weinstein, M.D., F.A.C.P., F.I.D.S.A.   Chairman, Division of Infectious Diseases, Cook County Hospital, and Professor, Department of Medicine, Rush Medical College, Chicago, Illinois

Richard P. Wenzel, M.D., M.Sc.   Professor and Chairman, Department of Internal Medicine, Medical College of Virginia, Virginia Commonwealth University, Richmond, Virginia

Walter W. Williams National Immunizations Program, Respiratory Diseases Branch, Centers for Disease Control and Prevention, Atlanta, Georgia

Alice H. M. Wong, M.D. Assistant Professor, Division of Infectious Diseases, Department of Medicine, Royal University Hospital, Saskatoon, Saskatchewan, Canada

CONTENTS

1

Diagnosis of Nosocomial Pneumonia
Ventilator-Associated Pneumonia (VAP) Versus Non-VAP

**JEAN CHASTRE and
JEAN-LOUIS TROUILLET**

Bichat Hospital
Paris, France

JEAN-YVES FAGON

Broussais Hospital
Paris, France

I. INTRODUCTION

Nosocomial pneumonia is thought to be the second most common nosocomial infection in the United States (1–3). At least 5% of patients hospitalized in acute care institutions acquire a pulmonary infection that was neither present nor incubating on admission. In intensive care units (ICUs), patients have nosocomial pulmonary infection rates that are as much as 5 to 10 times higher than those in the general wards (4–16). The incidence ranges from 20% in general medical ICUs to ≥50% in patients with the adult respiratory distress syndrome (ARDS). Such nosocomially acquired pneumonias are known to add significant morbidity, mortality, and economic burden to the outcome expected from the patient's overal clinicall status alone (17–23). Because several studies have shown that appropriate antimicrobial treatment of patients with nosocomial pulmonary infection significantly improves outcome, more rapid identification of infected patients and accurate selection of antimicrobial agents represent important clinical goals.

Because it may be difficult to determine whether pneumonia has developed in some patients, especially those who are receiving mechanical ventilation in the ICU, using common clinical criteria (e.g., fever, pulmonary infiltrates, and purulent sputum), the role of flexible bronchoscopy as an aid in the diagnosis of bacterial parenchymal lung infection has been expanded in recent years (5). Various techniques, including bronchoalveolar lavage (BAL), protected specimen brush (PSB), plugged telescoping catheter, and protected BAL, applied by way of bronchoscopy, have been shown in small, well-defined groups of patients to be useful in establishing the diagnosis of nosocomial pneumonia. However, despite broad clinical experience with these techniques, the optimal management strategy remains controversial for patients in whom symptoms suggestive of lung infection develop (24,25). Many investigators continue to state that bronchoscopy is an invasive, time-consuming, and expensive procedure that is not readily available on a 24-hour basis in all institutions (24). They insist that these techniques may be exposed to some false-negative results and that they should first be validated in prospective, randomized trials demonstrating that they improve survival rate or other meaningful endpoints, such as antimicrobial resistance, antibiotic complications, or costs compared with clinical diagnosis. Consequently, many experts prefer to treat fever and a new pulmonary infiltrate by using one or more antibiotics, even if it may be difficult to determine whether pneumonia has really developed. In case of infection, this approach may also render difficult to identify precisely the responsible microorganisms and thereby select the optimal antimicrobial treatment. Finally, in patients without true infection, this approach may lead to unnecessary broad-spectrum drug coverage with its risk of facilitating the emergence of resistant pathogens.

The appropriateness of diagnostic tools may also differ depending on whether the goal is to prevent the spread of resistant organisms, compare incidence rates of pneumonia, or prescribe treatment for a patient. For example, for calculating incidence rates, one should use a definition that is applicable to all patients over prolonged time periods. Infection control personnel should be able to make the diagnosis based on common clinical and laboratory findings. Definitions that require the performance of specialized diagnostic tests are not universal enough to produce comparable rates in most health care settings. However, specialized tests may provide the most accurate diagnosis for patient care. They may allow physicians to make the most appropriate decisions to initiate or withhold antimicrobial treatment for an individual patient.

Based on our personal experience and recent literature, this chapter reviews the potential advantages and drawbacks of using bronchoscopic techniques compared with using noninvasive modalities or clinical evaluation alone for the diagnosis of nosocomial pneumonia in different settings.

II. CLINICAL EVALUATION

The diagnosis of nosocomial pneumonia is usually based on three components: (1) systemic signs of infection, (2) new or worsening infiltrates seen on the chest roentgenogram, and (3) bacteriological evidence of pulmonary parenchymal infection (26). The systemic signs of infection such as fever, tachycardia, and leukocystosis are nonspecific findings and can be caused by any condition that releases cytokines (27). Hemorrhage, soft tissue trauma, and thermal injury are among the noninfectious conditions that are associated with elevated circulating levels of cytokines. In trauma and other surgical patients, fever and leukocytosis should prompt the physician to suspect infection, but in the early posttraumatic or postoperative period (i.e., during the first 72 hours), these findings usually are not helpful. Later in the course, fever and leukocytosis are more likely to be caused by infection, but even then, other problems associated with an inflammatory response (e.g., devitalized tissue, open wounds) can underlie these findings.

The plain (usually portable) chest roentgenogram remains an important component in the evaluation of hospitalized patients with suspected pneumonia, although it is most helpful when findings are normal, ruling out pneumonia. When infiltrates are evident, the particular pattern is of limited value for differentiating cardiogenic pulmonary edema, noncardiogenic pulmonary edema, pulmonary contusion, atelectasis (or collapse), and pneumonia (Table 1). Atelectasis is common in surgical patients. Caplan and colleagues empha-

Table 1 Noninfectious Conditions Causing Lung Infiltrate in Hospitalized Patients

Cancer
Connective tissue disease
Vascularitis syndrome
Alveolar hemorrhage
Drug-induced pneumonitis
Atelectasis
Thromboembolic disease
Aspiration of gastric content
Nonresolving community-acquired pneumonia
Congestive heart failure

sized the value of repeating the chest roentgenogram after vigorous pulmonary physiotherapy to differentiate infiltrates caused by atelectasis from infiltrates caused by infection (28). Recognizing that atelectasis or cardiogenic pulmonary edema often confounds the identification of pneumonic infiltrates, Mock and colleagues devised an objective scoring system evaluating chest roentgenograms in critically ill surgical patients (29). In this system, 1 point is awarded for each of 10 criteria; the radiograph is scored for being highly suggestive of pneumonia (8–10 points), moderately suggestive of pneumonia (4–7 points), or minimally suggestive of pneumonia (0–3 points) (Table 2). Very few studies have examined the accuracy of the portable chest radiograph in the ICU. In a review of 24 patients with autopsy-proven pneumonia who were receiving mechanical ventilation, no single radiographic sign had a diagnostic accuracy greater than 68% (30). The presence of air bronchograms was the only sign that correlated well with pneumonia, correctly predicting 64% of pneumonias in the entire group. When the group was divided into patients with and without ARDS, however, a significant difference was noted. In patients without ARDS, the presence of air bronchograms or alveolar opacities correlated with pneumonia; in patients with ARDS, no such correlation was found. A variety of causes other than pneumonia can explain asymmetrical consolidation in patients with ARDS (e.g., atelectasis, emphysema, pulmonary edema, thromboembolic disease). Marked asymmetry of radiographical abnormalities have also been reported in patients with uncomplicated ARDS (31).

Table 2 Criteria for Diagnosing Pneumonia in Surgical Patients in the Intensive Care Unit

Presence of
   New infiltrate
   Acinar shadows
   Air bronchograms
   Segmental infiltrates
   Asymmetric infiltrates
   Infiltrates in nondependent regions of the lung
   Infiltrate with ipsilateral pleural effusion
Absence of
   Volume loss
   Cardiomegaly
   Hilar enlargement

From Ref. 29.

Microscopic evaluation and culture of tracheal secretions or expectorated sputum are also frequently inconclusive in patients with a clinical suspicion of pneumonia, because the upper respiratory tract of most ICU patients is colonized with potential pulmonary pathogens, whether or not deep pulmonary infection is present (32). Studies evaluating the usefulness of clinical parameters or tracheal secretions in identifying ICU patients with nosocomial pneumonia have generally been disappointing (33–35). In one study conducted in 84 ventilated patients suspected of having lung infection, Fagon et al. prospectively compared the diagnostic predictions independently formulated by a team of physicians aware of all clinical, radiological, and laboratory data, including the results of gram-stained bronchial aspirates with those resulting from a complete workup including quantitative culture results of PSB specimens (33). The results showed that only 27 of the 84 clinically suspected patients actually had pneumonia and that the presence of pneumonia was accurately diagnosed in only 62% of the predictions. The mean value of temperature, blood leukocytes and blood lymphocytes, Pao_2/Fio_2, radiological score, and changes in temperature, blood leukocytes, and radiological score in the 3 preceding days were not different in patients who had pneumonia and those who did not, confirming previous data (26,34,35) and the fact that no objective clinical criteria exist for differentiating patients who have pneumonia from those who do not. Recently, however, Pugin et al. described a composite clinical score based on six variables (temperature, blood leukocyte count, volume and purulence of tracheal secretions, oxygenation, pulmonary radiography, and semiquantitative culture of tracheal aspirate) (36). In their study of 28 patients requiring prolonged mechanical ventilation, a good correlation was observed between this clinical score and quantitative bacteriology of BAL samples, with a cutoff of six enabling identification of patients with infection.

III. MICROBIOLOGICAL DIAGNOSIS OF PNEUMONIA USING NONBRONCHOSCOPIC TECHNIQUES

A. Expectorated Sputum and Endotracheal Aspirates

Expectorated sputum and tracheal aspirate specimens obtained by direct suctioning through the endotracheal tube in mechanically ventilated patients are easily obtained but notoriously nonspecific in the diagnosis of nosocomial pneumonia. Bartlett et al. prospectively evaluated cultures of expectorated sputum in 67 patients with nosocomial pneumonia whose final diagnosis was based on bacterial studies from uncontamined specimens (blood, transtracheal aspirates, or pleural fluid) (37). Sputum cultures of 80% of the patients with infections involving *Staphylococcus aureus* and gram-negative bacilli yielded the same microorganism. The incidence of false-positive results for *S. aureus* was only 10%. Aerobic gram-negative bacilli, however, were recovered in the expectorated sputum from 45% of patients who did not have these organisms growing in the uncontaminated specimen. In a large study of bacteremic nosocomial bacterial pneumonia, only 49% of the sputum samples had the identical microorganism recovered by blood cultures (38). Pollock et al. determined that only 33% of expectorated sputum cultures recovered the same isolates that grew in significant growth in protected specimen brushing quantitative cultures (39).

Similarly, when compared to culture results of open lung biopsy or results from other specimens such as protected specimen brushings, cultural analysis of tracheal aspirate specimens obtained from patients receiving mechanical ventilation showed moderate to high sensitivity but generally low specificity. Endotracheal aspirate cultures are rarely negative in ventilated patients with a clinical suspicion of pneumonia, and the great number of false-positive results may lead to overdiagnosis of pneumonia and misdiagnosis of its cause (32). Hill et al. obtained simultaneous cultures of the deep trachea and lung in 48 patients with respiratory failure subjected to open lung biopsy (40). Culture results agreed in only 40% of these paired samples. In 56% of patients, cultures were positive only in the trachea (false-positive); in 4%, cultures were positive only in the lung (false-negative). In patients with pneumonia documented by histology, endotracheal aspirated sensitivity was 82%, but specificity was only 27% (40). Microscopic analysis of tracheal aspirates may be, however, of some potential value in the empirical selection of antimicrobial therapy. Salata et al. reported that specimens from intubated patients with pneumonia showed higher semiquantitative grading of neutrophils and bacteria, including intra-alveolar organisms, than in patients without pneumonia (41). In the same study, elastin fibers seen on KOH preparation of endotracheal aspirates had a sensitivity of 52% and a specificity of 100% for detecting pneumonia. Interestingly, the demonstration of elastin fibers preceded the radiographical evidence of pulmonary infiltrates by a mean of 1.8 ± 1.3 days. However, in patients with ARDS, elastin fibers have only a 50% positive predictive value for pneumonia because noninfectious lung necrosis is a common occurrence in this setting (41).

Even when the clinical diagnosis of pneumonia is accurate, results of Gram's stain examination and culture of tracheal aspirates could be misleading when choosing the appropriate antibiotics. In the study by Fagon et al., only

33% of the treatments proposed for patients who were subsequently given the diagnosis of pneumonia proved to be effective, even though the physicians who were questioned in this study usually used combination antibiotic regimens that are currently considered to be standard therapy for nosocomial pneumonia (33). These results confirm the difficulty in selecting an initial antibiotic regimen for treatment of suspected pneumonia in hospitalized patients. Because of the emergence of multiresistant extended-spectrum beta-lactamase–producing gram-negative pathogens in many institutions and the increasing role played by gram-positive bacteria such as methicillin-resistant *S. aureus*, even a protocol combining amikacin and imipenem would not ensure adequate coverage of all cases of nosocomial pneumonia in these ICUs (42–44).

Routine culture of the endotracheal aspirate also cannot be used to monitor response to antibiotic treatment in patients with nosocomial pneumonia. Finally, the only undisputable value of this diagnostic test is when results are completely negative in a patient with no modification of prior antimicrobial treatment. In that case, the negative predictive value is very high and the probability for the patient to have pneumonia is close to zero (45).

The antibody-coated bacteria test is another microscopic procedure that has been applied to tracheal aspirates from intubated patients. The results from one study were similar to those reported for sputa from patients not receiving ventilation, with low sensitivity in detection of pneumonia (48%–73%) but excellent specificity (98%–100%) (46). In another study, however, specificity was only 56% when compared to quantitative PSB cultures (47). It has also been suggested that a positive antibody-coated test (1) may precede a subsequent infection, (2) may be positive when quantitative culture results are low because of prior antimicrobial treatment or poor specimen handling or processing, and (3) may show antibiotic effectiveness by conversion to a negative test after treatment.

B. Quantitative Cultures of Endotracheal Aspirates

While the simple qualitative culture of endotracheal aspirates (EA) is a technique with a high percentage of false-positive results owing to the bacterial colonization of the proximal airways observed in most ICU patients, some recent studies using quantitative culture techniques suggest that EA cultures may have a reasonable overall diagnostic accuracy, similar to that of several other more invasive techniques (48–51). In the study by Marquette et al., the operating characteristics of EA quantitative cultures, using 10^6 cfu/mL of respiratory secretions as the interpretative cutoff point, compared favorably with those of the protected specimen brush technique, with a slightly higher sensitivity (82% versus 64%) and a lower specificity (83% versus 96%) (48). Similarly, when using 10^5 cfu/mL as a cutoff point for interpreting EA quantitative cultures in 54 patients suspected of having pneumonia, El-Ebiary et al. found that this technique represented a relatively sensitive (70%) and relatively specific (72%) method to diagnose patients with true pneumonia (49). To assess the reliability of this technique, Jourdain et al. used fiberoptic bronchoscopy with PSB and BAL to study 57 episodes of suspected lung infection in 39 ventilator-dependent patients with no recent changes in antimicrobial therapy (51). The operating characteristics of EA cultures were calculated over a range of cutoff values (from 10^3 to 10^7 cfu/mL) and the threshold of 10^6 cfu/mL appeared to be the most accurate with a sensitivity of 68% and a specificity of 84% (Fig. 1). However, when this threshold was applied, almost one-third of the patients with pneumonia were not identified. Furthermore, only 40% of microorganisms cultured in EA samples coincided with those obtained from PSB specimens (Fig. 2). Other studies have emphasized that, although EA quantitative cultures can correctly identify patients with pneumo-

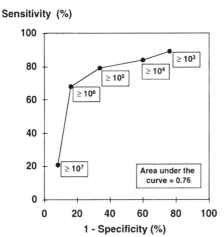

Figure 1   Receiver operating curve obtained with quantitative cultures of endotracheal aspirates (EA) for the diagnosis of pneumonia in 57 ventilator-dependent patients in whom pulmonary infection is clinically thought to have developed. (From Ref. 51, with permission.)

Log$_{10}$ cfu/ml (EA)

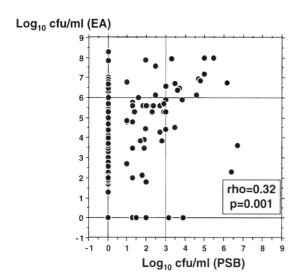

Log$_{10}$ cfu/ml (PSB)

Figure 2 Correlation between quantitative cultures of endotracheal aspirate and protected specimen brush specimens in 57 ventilator-dependent patients in whom pulmonary infection is clinically thought to have developed. Each point represents a single microorganism. (From Ref. 51, with permission).

nia, microbiological results cannot be used to infer which microorganisms present in the trachea are really present in the lung. In the study by Borderon et al., in which EA quantitative culture results were compared with postmortem lung biopsy quantitative cultures, only 53% of the microorganisms isolated in EA samples in concentrations $>10^7$ cfu/mL were also found in lung tissue cultures (52).

Therefore, EA quantitative cultures may be an acceptable tool for diagnosing pneumonia when no fiberoptic techniques are available. But, this technique has several potential disadvantages. First, many patients may not be identified by this technique using the cutoff value of 10^6 cfu/mL. Second, as soon as a lower threshold is used, specificity sharply decreases and overtreatment becomes a problem. Third, selecting antimicrobial therapy solely on the basis of EA culture results can lead to either unnecessary antibiotic therapy or overtreatment with broad-spectrum antimicrobial agents. Given the potential risk of these practices in an intensive care unit, a more rigorous diagnostic approach in such patients seems warranted whenever possible.

C. Sampling of Distal Airways Using Nonbronchoscopic Techniques

Collection of secretions in the distal airways can be performed through a bronchoscope or by blindly using an endobronchial catheter that is wedged in the tracheobronchial tree. The nonbronchoscopic techniques are essentially used in mechanically ventilated patients because the endotracheal tube, which bypasses the proximal airways, permits an easy access to the lower airways. At least 10 studies have described a variety of nonbronchoscopic techniques for sampling lower respiratory tract secretions (5,36,53–56). Inherent advantages of these techniques are less invasiveness, availability to nonbronchoscopists, lower initial cost than bronchoscopy, lack of contamination presented by the bronchoscopic channel, less compromise of patient gas exchange during the procedure, and availability to patients with small endotracheal tubes. Disadvantages include the potential sampling errors inherent in a blind technique and the lack of airway visualization.

Apparently acceptable results were, however, obtained by several investigators using nonbronchoscopic methods. For example, in a study of 78 suspected episodes of nosocomial pneumonia in 55 patients, Pham et al. found that a protected telescoping catheter (PTC) gave results similar to those obtained with the PSB technique in 74 percent of cases (54). A major discrepancy was observed between the two techniques in only 20 episodes, including 6 false-negatives of PSB in episodes of proven pneumonia, 4 possible false-positives of PSB, and 10 possible false-positives of PTC. Furthermore, blind or directed PTC samples showed a similar concordance with PSB samples obtained by way of bronchoscopy. Similar results were obtained by Kollef et al. in a study of 42 patients suspected of having ventilator-associated pneumonia on the basis of clinical evidence (53). Using 10^3 cfu/mL as the threshold to define a positive minibronchoalveolar lavage, a good diagnostic agreement was shown for quantitative cultures obtained with the protected specimen brush and minibronchoalveolar lavage technique (Kappa statistic, 0.63; concordance, 83.3%).

Although autopsy studies indicate that pneumonia in ventilator-dependent patients has often spread into every pulmonary lobe and predominantly involves the posterior portion of the lower lobes (57,58), two clinical studies of ventilated patients with pneumonia contradict these findings, in that some patients had sterile PSB specimen cultures of the noninvolved lung (59,60). Furthermore, in most studies that concluded on the comparable sensitivities of nonbronchoscopic and bronchoscopic techniques, the overall concordance was, in fact, only approximately 80%, emphasizing the fact that, in some patients, the diagnosis could be missed by this technique, especially in the case of pneumonia involving the upper lobes or the left lung, as demonstrated by Jorda et al. (56).

IV. MICROBIOLOGICAL DIAGNOSIS OF PNEUMONIA USING BRONCHOSCOPIC TECHNIQUES

A. Procedure

Bronchoscopy provides direct access to the lower airways for sampling bronchial and parenchymal tissues directly at the site of lung inflammation. To reach the bronchial tree, however, the bronchoscope must traverse the endotracheal tube and proximal airways where contamination is likely to occur. Therefore, distal secretions directly aspirated through the bronchoscope suction channel are frequently contaminated, thereby limiting their clinical specificity. In a study of 16 nonventilated patients without lung infection who underwent flexible fiberoptic bronchoscopy (FOB), Bartlett et al. found that all bronchoscopic aspirates were contaminated by bacteria, with an average of five bacterial species per aspirate (61). Modifications of specimen retrieval (discussed later) and quantitative cultures are used to control for this contamination. However, poor technique during bronchoscopy can negate the benefit of these modifications. Therefore, to obtain meaningful results with FOB, it is very important to follow a very precise methodology, as summarized in a recent International Consensus Conference (62).

Because suctioning through the working channel before retrieval of specimens for bacterial culture increases the likelihood of contamination, aggressive suctioning of the proximal airways using a separate suction catheter before beginning bronchoscopy must be systematically performed in patients requiring mechanical ventilation. The use of topical anesthetic agents such as lidocaine may also lead to contamination of the specimen and, potentially, to suppression of growth of some bacteria (63). Because the concentration of lidocaine in specimens is below the minimal inhibitory threshold of most infectious agents, the major risk appears to be contamination by injection of lidocaine through the working channel with expulsion of secretions that had accumulated in the channel. This is a particular problem in nonintubated patients because of the need to pass the tube past the vocal cords. Aerosolization of lidocaine into the oropharynx and proximal airways provides adequate anesthesia in many such patients. In patients undergoing mechanical ventilation, use of intravenously administered sedatives and neuromuscular blocker agents completely alleviates the need to use topical anesthesics (62).

One major technical problem with all bronchoscopic techniques is proper selection of the sampling area in the tracheobronchial tree. Almost all intubated patients have purulent-looking secretions and the secretions first seen may represent those aspirated from another site into gravity-dependent airways or from upper-airway secretions aspirated around the endotracheal tube. Usually, the sampling area is selected based on the location of infiltrate on chest radiograph or the segment visualized during bronchoscopy as having purulent secretions (62). Collection of secretions in the lower trachea or mainstem bronchi, which may represent recently aspirated secretions around the endotracheal tube cuff, should be avoided. In patients with diffuse pulmonary infiltrates or minimal changes in a previously abnormal chest radiograph, determining the correct airway to sample may be difficult. In these case, sampling should be directed to the area where endobronchial abnormalities are maximal. In case of doubt, and because autopsy studies indicate that ventilator-associated pneumonia frequently involves the posterior portion of the right lower lobe, this area should probably be sampled in priority (57,58,64). Even though bilateral sampling has been advocated in the immunosuppressed host with diffuse infiltrates, there is no convincing evidence that multiple specimens are more accurate than single specimens for diagnosing nosocomial bacterial pneumonia in patients requiring mechanical ventilation (31).

B. Complications

Fiberoptic bronchoscopy is generally regarded as safe, based on surveys of endoscopists. The risk inherent in such an examination appears slight, even in critically ill patients requiring mechanical ventilation, although the associated occurrence of cardiac arrhythmias, hypoxemia, or bronchospasm is not unusual. A study conducted by Trouillet et al. in 107 ventilated patients has shown that fiberoptic bronchoscopy under midazolam sedation is practicable in this setting (65). No death or cardiac arrest occurred during or within the 2 hours immediately following the procedure. However, patients in the ICU are at risk of relative hypoxemia during fiberoptic bronchoscopy, even when high levels of oxygen are provided to the ventilator and gas leaks around the endoscope are minimized by a special adaptor. An average decline in mean arterial oxygen tension of 26% was observed at the end of the procedure, compared to the baseline value, and this was associated with a mild increase in $Paco_2$. The degree of hypoxemia induced by fiberoptic bronchoscopy in this study was linked to the severity of pulmonary dysfunction and the decrease in alveolar ventilation. Clinical hypoxemia, as defined by Pao_2 lower that 60 mmHg, was more frequent in patients with ARDS and in those who "fought" the ventilator during the procedure, as shown by multivariate analysis. Careful, methodical attention to the anesthetic protocol, with addition of a short-acting neuromuscular blocking agent, and monitoring of patients during bronchoscopy should probably permit rapid correction and more frequent prevention of hypoxemia in this setting, and therefore should further decrease the morbidity associated with this procedure. In a recent study that was conducted in a large series of patients with ARDS, only 5% of patients had arterial oxygen desaturation to <90% during bronchoscopy despite severe hypoxemia in many patients before bronchoscopy (66). Certain procedures, however, increase the risk of complications, particularly in some subsets of patients. The bleeding risk observed with the PSB technique is thus particularly significant in patients with thrombocytopenia or a coagulopathy (62). Pneumothorax is also principally a complication of PSB, although it can occur after BAL alone in mechanically ventilated patients. In fact, the risk of FOB is paradoxically more important in nonventilated patients than in patients receiving mechanical ventilation, because performance of bronchoscopy in a critically ill patient with impending respiratory failure may lead to profound hypoxemia and rapid decompensation. Although bacteremia does not appear to occur after PSB, release of tumor necrosis factor-alpha has been documented in patients undergoing BAL (67). Transbronchial spread of infection is also an extremely remote possibility (62).

C. Specimen Types and Laboratory Methods

There are a variety of bronchoscopic techniques that can be used for the diagnosis of bacterial pneumonia, but of these various techniques, two have been suggested as of particular value in establishing a specific diagnosis of bacterial pneumonia in hospitalized patients: (1) the use of a double lumen catheter with a protected specimen brush (PSB) to collect uncontaminated culture specimens directly from the affected area in the lower respiratory tract, and (2) the use of bronchoalveolar lavage (BAL), because this technique is a safe and practical method for obtaining cells and secretions from a large area of the lung that can be examined microscopically immediately after the procedure and is also suitable for culture using quantitative techniques.

The Protected Specimen Brush Technique

The methodology for PSB sampling was described originally by Wimberley et al. (68) and is summarized in Table 3. This method is based on the combina-

Table 3 Methodology of the Protected Specimen Brush Technique

1. In intubated patients, sedation and a short-acting paralytic agent are recommended.
2. Do not inject lidocaine through the suction channel of the fiberoptic bronchoscope (FOB) and avoid suction of upper airway secretions.
3. Position the FOB close to the orifice of the bronchus, draining the subsegment with new or increased infiltrate on chest radiograph.
4. Advance the protected specimen brush (PSB) catheter 3 cm out of the FOB into the desired subsegment and eject the distal plug.
5. Advance the brush and wedge it into a peripheral position to sample distal secretions.
6. Retract the brush into the inner cannula, the inner into the outer cannula, and remove from the FOB.
7. Separately and sequentially, wipe the distal portions of the outer and inner cannulae clean with 70% alcohol, cut and discard.
8. Extrude the brush and sever it into a recipient containing 1 mL of saline or Ringer's solution.
9. Submit the sample for quantitative culture within 15 minutes.

From Ref. 62.

tion of four different techniques: (1) the use of FOB to directly sample the site of inflammation in the lung, (2) the use of a double-lumen catheter brush system with a distal occluding plug to prevent secretions from entering the catheter during passage through the bronchoscope channel, (3) the use of a brush to calibrate the volume of secretions retrieved, and (4) the use of quantitative culture techniques to aid in distinguishing between airway colonization and serious underlying infection, with a cutoff point of 10^3 cfu/mL for making this distinction. In an in vitro study, this system proved to be the most effective among seven different types of brush catheters passed through an FOB heavily contaminated with saliva to sample a number of organisms at the distal end (68). Single-sheathed catheter brushes and telescoping plugged catheter tips with or without distal plugs are, however, also available and have been used for the diagnosis of pneumonia, even if neither has been subjected to the rigorous evaluation reported for the PSB.

Bronchoalveolar Lavage

BAL requires careful wedging of the tip of the bronchoscope into an airway lumen, isolating that airway from the rest of the central airways. Infusion of at least 120 mL of saline in several (3–6) aliquots is needed to sample fluids and secretions in the distal respiratory bronchioles and alveoli (62,69,70). It is estimated that the alveolar surface area distal to the wedged bronchoscope is 100 times greater than that of the peripheral airway and that approximately 1 million alveoli (1% of the lung surface) are sampled, with approximately 1 mL of actual lung secretions retrieved in the total lavage fluid (69). The fluid return on BAL varies greatly and may affect the validity of results. In patients with emphysema, collapse of airways with the negative pressure needed to aspirate fluid may limit the amount of fluid retrieved. A very small return may contain only diluted material from the bronchial rather than alveolar level and result in false-negative results.

Specimen Handling

Whatever the bronchoscopic technique used, rapid processing of specimens for culture is desirable to prevent loss of viability of pathogens or overgrowth of contaminants in these unpreserved specimen types. For PSB, it is recommended that the brush be aseptically cut into a measured volume (1 mL) of sterile diluent, most commonly, nonbacteriostatic saline or lactated Ringer's solution (62,68,70). For BAL, transport in a sterile, leak-proof, nonadherent glass container is recommended to avoid loss of cells for cytological assessment. The initial aliquot, which is usually considered to be essentially representative of distal bronchi, should be either discarded or transported separately from the remaining pooled fractions (71). Excessive delays in transport to the laboratory should be avoided. Quantitative cultures of freshly collected sputa versus samples transported at room temperature over an approximately 4-hour period showed selective decreases in *Streptococcus pneumoniae* and *Haemophilus influenzae* isolation rates and fewer bacterial species overall in delayed specimens but higher counts of some other organisms, particularly gram-negative bacilli (72). Similar results using bronchoscopic specimens were obtained by Moser et al. in an experimental canine model of pneumonia resulting from infection with *S. pneumoniae* (73). Although no absolute guideline exists, it is generally accepted that a delay of 30 minutes should not be exceeded for transport and holding of respiratory specimens before they are processed for microbiological analysis (62,70). According to some investigators, refrigeration to prolong transport time may be used, but this technique remains controversial (70).

Once bronchoscopic specimens are received in the laboratory, they should be handled according to clearly defined procedures (see Ref. 70 for complete description). Because of the inevitable oropharyngeal bacterial contamination that occurs in the collection of all bronchoscopic samples, quantitative culture techniques are always needed to differentiate oropharyngeal contaminants present at low counts from higher count infecting organisms. Several investigators have confirmed that, in case of pneumonia, pathogens are present in lower respiratory tract inflammatory secretions at a concentration of at least 10^5 to 10^6 cfu/mL, and contaminants generally are present at $<10^4$ cfu/mL (37,58,72–75). The diagnostic thresholds proposed for PSB and BAL are an extension of this concept (Table 4). Since PSB collects between 0.001 to 0.01 mL of secretions, the presence of more than 10^3 bacteria in the originally diluted sample (1 mL) actually represents 10^5 to 10^6 cfu/mL of pulmonary secretions. Similarly, 10^4 cfu/mL for BAL, which collects 1 mL of secretions in 10 to 100 mL of effluent, represents 10^5 to 10^6 cfu/mL (see Table 4).

Direct microscopic analysis of PSB may be performed, but the optimal method for smear preparation has not been established. Methods used include direct smearing of the secretions retrieved by the brush and cytocentrifugation of the material suspended in the diluent used to perform quantitative cultures. Although more sensitive, the former method has the disadvantages of decreasing the amount of secretions available for quantitative cultures and possibly contaminating the specimen. Sensitivy and specificity for PSB Gram's stain have ranged from 20% to 100% and from 95% to 100% (70).

For BAL, it is recommended that a total cell count be performed to assess adequacy and a differential count be performed to assess cellularity. For quality assessment, the percentage of squamous and bronchial epithelial cells may be used to predict heavy upper respiratory contamination. A level of $>1\%$ of the total cells has been suggested as a rejection criterion (76). The

Table 4 Interpretation of Quantitative Culture Results from Lower Respiratory Tract Secretions

Specimen type	Quantity collected	Dilution factor	Diagnostic threshold (cfu/mL)
Sputum, bronchoscopic aspirates, endotracheal aspirates	Several ml	1	10^5–10^6
Protected specimen brush	0.01–0.001 mL in 1 mL of diluent	1/100–1/1000	10^3
Bronchoalveolar lavage	1 mL in 10–100 mL of BAL effluent	1/10–1/100	10^4

From Ref. 70.

recommended staining method is a modified Giemsa stain (e.g., Diff-Quik, Scientific Products, McGaw Park, IL) (70,77). This stain offers a number of advantages over a Gram's stain, including better host cell morphology, improved detection of bacteria, particularly intracellular ones, and detection of some protozoan and fungal pathogens (e.g., *Histoplasma*, *Pneumocystis*, *Toxoplasma*, and *Candida* species).

D. Usefulness of the PSB Technique

The potential value of the PSB technique to evaluate hospitalized patients in whom pneumonia is suspected of having developed has been extensively investigated in both human and animal studies, including seven investigations in which the cultural accuracy of this technique was determined by comparison with both histological features and quantitative cultures from the same area of the lung (57,58,64,73,74,77,79). Many investigators have confirmed that secretions obtained using this technique can ensure optimal antimicrobial treatment for most patients with pneumonia without resorting to broad-spectrum drugs in all patients clinically suspected of having pneumonia (5,33,34,39,47–51,54,55,58,59,62,63,70,73–75,77–82). Nevertheless, some controversy persists in the literature concerning the sensitivity of this technique, especially for detecting some cases of pneumonia in patients already receiving antimicrobial treatment (24).

Four recent studies using a protocol based on postmortem lung biopsies have suggested that, in the presence of prior antibiotic treatment, many patients with histopathological signs of pneumonia have no or only minimal growth from lung and bronchoscopic specimen cultures (57,64,78,83). In one study, lesions of bronchopneumonia were characterized by bacterial concentrations $>10^3$ cfu/mL of lung tissue in only 55% of lobes and one-third of lung segments with histological bronchopneumonia even remained negative when cultured (57). Similarly, in a study of 30 patients who died under mechanical ventilation after having received prior antibiotic treatment, Torres et al. found that quantitative bacterial cultures of lung biopsies using 10^3 cfu/g of tissue as a cutoff point had low sensitivity (40%) and low specificity (45%), and could not differentiate the histological absence or presence of pneumonia (78). Interestingly, in this study, the operating characteristics of the PSB technique were very similar to those obtained with lung cultures.

However, several constraints specific to the evaluation of any procedure used in the diagnosis of bacterial pneumonia must be respected even when using a model in which the gold standard includes both histological features and quantitative cultures of lung tissue. First, diagnostic methods based on microbiological techniques can only document, both qualitatively and quantitatively, the bacterial burden present in lung tissue. By no means can these techniques retrospectively identify a resolving pneumonia, at a time when antimicrobial treatment and lung antibacterial defenses might have been successful in suppressing microbial growth in lung tissue. Second, although several studies have shown that, once bacterial infection of the lung is clinically apparent, there are at least 10^4 microorganisms per gram of tissue, this assumption is valid only when patients have not received appropriate antimicrobial treatment after the onset of lung infection before obtaining lung cultures. Therefore, to evaluate the cultural accuracy of any microbiological technique using lung cultures as the ''gold standard,'' it is imperative that no new antibiotics have been introduced during this time interval. Third, using histological criteria as a reference implies that lung infection had not developed before the episode to be evaluated; otherwise, it would be difficult, if not impossible, to distinguish a recent infection from the sequelae of the previous one, and thus to correctly interpret the results of the diagnostic tools being evaluated. Fourth, lesions of bronchopneumonia in patients with ventilator-associated pneumonia (VAP) may be limited to some foci of infection in the lungs (57,58,64,79). Therefore, if postmortem tissue samples are too small, the histological diagnosis of pneumonia can be underestimated using this technique. But, because a diagnostic technique based on peripheral samplings can provide information only on the lung segment from which specimens are taken, so-called ''false-negative'' results of PSB or BAL, as defined by entire examination of the lung, can be explained by the absence of pneumonia at the very level of the sampling area.

Unfortunately, in the studies by Papazian et al. (83), Torres et al. (78), and Marquette et al. (64), pneumonia had developed in many patients several days before their death and lung cultures were in fact obtained during the recovery phase of the infection, at a time when antimicrobial therapy and lung antibacterial defenses might have been successful in suppressing microbial growth in lung tissue and therefore in pulmonary secretions. Even a few doses of an effective antimicrobial agent can rapidly decrease or even transiently eliminate bacterial counts in the lung and thereby invalidate all comparisons between microbiological and histological features of the lung (84). Interestingly, when analyses in these studies were restrained to patients with no prior antibiotics or when only lung tissue cultures were used as gold standard, results obtained using bronchoscopic techniques for diagnosing nosocomial pneumonia were much better, with a sensitivity always greater than 80%.

Other studies have confirmed the accuracy of bronchoscopic techniques for diagnosing nosocomial pneumonia (58,79). In a study evaluating spontaneous lung infections occurring in baboons with permeability pulmonary edema and undergoing mechanical ventilation, Johanson et al. found an excellent correlation between the bacterial content of lung tissue and results of quantitative culture of lavage fluid and PSB specimens (58). The BAL recovered 74% of all species present in lung tissue, including 100% of those present at a concentration $\geq 10^4$ cfu/g of tissue. In this study, PSB specimens identified only 41% of all species recovered from lung tissue, but only microorganisms present at low concentrations in the lung were missed; 78% of species present at concentrations $> 10^4$ cfu/g of tissue were correctly isolated (Table 5). Similarly, in a study of 20 ventilated patients in whom pneumonia had not developed before the terminal phase of their disease and who had no recent changes in antimicrobial therapy, Chastre et al. found that bronchoscopic PSB specimens obtained just after death were able to identify 80% of all species present in the lung, with a strong correlation between the results of quantitative cultures of both specimens (Fig. 3) (79). Using a discriminative value of $\geq 10^3$ cfu/mL to define positive PSB cultures, this technique identified lung segments yielding $\geq 10^4$ bacteria/g of tissue with a sensitivity of 82% and a specificity of 89%. These findings confirm that bronchoscopic PSB samples reliably identify, both qualitatively and quantitatively, microorganisms present in lung segments with bacterial pneumonia, even when the infection develops as a superinfection in a patient already receiving antimicrobial treatment for several days.

Table 5 Results of Quantitative PSB and BAL Cultures in 19 Baboons Using Tissue Cultures as Gold Standard

Lung tissue concentration ($\log_{10}$ cfu/mL)	No. of species isolated		
	Lung tissue	Protected specimen brush	Bronchoalveolar lavage
<4	18	4	11
≥4	9	7	9
Total	27	11	20
Organisms not found in tissue	—	4	3

From Ref. 58.

PSB sample cultures
(log$_{10}$ cfu/ml)

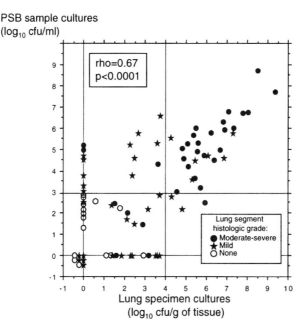

Lung specimen cultures
(log$_{10}$ cfu/g of tissue)

Figure 3   Scatter plot of the relationship between the quantitative culture results for
all bacterial species recovered from protected specimen brush (PSB) and lung specimens in 39 lung segments obtained from 20 patients who died under mechanical ventilation. Each symbol represents a single microorganism. *Closed circles* correspond to
microorganisms present in the 11 lung segments that demonstrated ''moderate'' or
''severe'' pneumonia by histological criteria, *stars* to microorganisms present in the
17 lung segments with ''mild'' signs of pneumonia, and *open circles* to microorganisms present in the 11 lung segments with no histological signs of pneumonia. The
PSB and lung specimen cultures were negative in eight cases and are shown at the
origin of the log–log plot. (From Ref. 79, adapted with permission.)

However, three major drawbacks are still inherent in this technique.
First, even using the most accurate threshold of 10^3 cfu/mL to distinguish
patients with airway colonization from those with deep lung infection, a small
number of false-positive results may be observed (85). Second, results of such
cultures require 24 to 48 hours, and, therefore, no information is available to
guide initial decisions concerning the appropriateness of antimicrobial therapy
and which antibiotics should be used. Third, the PSB technique can yield
negative results in patients with pneumonia in the following situations: (1)

bronchoscopy performed at an early stage of infection with a bacterial burden below the concentration necessary to reach diagnostic significance, (2) specimens obtained from an unaffected segment (this problem is probably very important in patients with diffuse lung injury, in whom it is sometimes difficult to be sure to have selected the proper site of sampling), (3) specimens incorrectly processed, and (4) specimens obtained after initiation of a new antimicrobial therapy. Values within 1 $\log_{10}$ of the cutoff must therefore be interpreted cautiously, and fiberoptic bronchoscopy should be repeated in symptomatic patients with a negative ($<10^3$ cfu/mL) result (86). Many technical factors, including medium and adequacy of incubation and antibiotic or other toxic components, may influence results. The reproducibility of PSB sampling has been recently evaluated (87,88). Two groups have concluded that, although in vitro repeatability is excellent and in vivo qualitative recovery is 100%, quantitative results are more variable. In 14% to 17% of patients, results of replicate samples fell on both sides of the 10^3 cfu/mL threshold, and results varied by more than 1 $\log_{10}$ in 59% to 67% of samples. This variability is presumably related to both irregular distribution of organisms in secretions and the very small volume actually sampled by PSB. The conclusion is that, as with all diagnostic tests, borderline PSB quantitative culture results should be interpreted cautiously and the clinical circumstances considered before drawing any therapeutic conclusion.

E. Usefulness of Bronchoalveolar Lavage

Although BAL provides a broader reflection of lung content than PSB, BAL is subject to the same risk of contamination as bronchoscopic aspirates. Many studies have investigated the value of BAL quantitative culture in the diagnosis of pneumonia in mechanically ventilated patients (see Refs. 5, 62, and 70). Although some investigators have concluded that BAL provides the best reflection of the lung's bacterial burden, both quantitatively and qualitatively, others have reported mixed results with poor specificity of BAL fluid cultures in patients with high tracheobronchial colonization. In one recent study from Chastre et al., using a protocol based on postmortem lung biopsies, the results obtained by quantitative cultures of BAL fluid proved to be as useful as those of PSB cultures (79). Although a few more microorganisms that were not present in lung tissue were grown from lavage specimens as compared with PSB specimens, there was a strong correlation between the concentrations of organisms grown in cultures of BAL fluid and lung tissue specimens (see Fig.

4). Using $\geq 10^4$ bacteria/mL of lavage fluid as the discriminative value for differentiating between infected lung segments with at least 10^4 cfu/g of tissue (n = 11) and noninfected lung segments (n = 9), only one false-negative and two false-positive results were observed, giving a sensitivity of 91% and a specificity of 78%. To further evaluate the role of quantitative cultures of BAL for diagnosing nosocomial pneumonia in mechanically ventilated patients,

BAL specimen cultures
($\log_{10}$ cfu/ml)

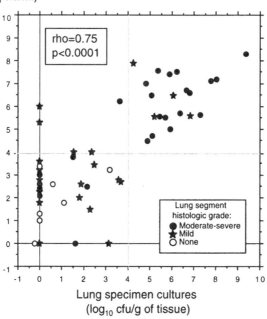

Lung specimen cultures
($\log_{10}$ cfu/g of tissue)

Figure 4 Scatter plot of the relationship between the quantitative culture results for all bacterial species recovered from bronchoalveolar lavage (BAL) and lung specimens in 20 lung segments obtained from patients who died under mechanical ventilation. Each symbol represents a single microorganism. *Closed circles* correspond to microorganisms present in the eight lung segments that demonstrated "moderate" or "severe" pneumonia by histological criteria, *stars* to microorganisms present in the seven lung segments with "mild" signs of pneumonia, and *open circles* to microorganisms present in the five lung segments with no histological signs of pneumonia. The BAL and lung specimen cultures were negative in two cases and are shown at the origin of the log–log plot. (From Ref. 79, adapted with permission).

Jourdain et al. recently studied a total of 141 episodes of suspected lung infection in 84 consecutive patients (89). Microbiological findings obtained using BAL were compared with those obtained with PSB samples, and their operating characteristics were determined. The level of qualitative agreement between BAL and PSB specimen cultures was high, with 83% of the organisms isolated in PSB specimens being recovered simultaneously from BAL fluid. In addition, the results of quantitative BAL and PSB cultures were significantly correlated. Using a cutoff point of 10^4 cfu/mL to define a positive result, 47 of 57 diagnosed cases of pneumonia were identified by BAL, for a sensitivity of 82% and a specificity of 85%.

Because BAL allows harvesting of cells and secretions from a large area of the lung, which can be microscopically examined immediately after the procedure to detect the presence of intracellular or extracellular bacteria in the lower respiratory tract, this technique is particularly well adapted to provide rapid identification of patients with pneumonia. Several studies have confirmed the diagnostic value of this approach (36,77,79,88,89). In each study, either the Giemsa or Gram's stain was positive (more than 2% or 5% of BAL cells containing intracellular bacteria) in most patients with pneumonia and negative in patients without pneumonia. Furthermore, in patients with pneumonia, the morphology and Gram's staining of these bacteria were closely correlated with the result of bacterial cultures, enabling early formulation of a specific antimicrobial therapy before the results of cultures were available. In one study in which the diagnostic accuracy of direct microscopic examination of BAL cells could be directly assessed with both histological and microbiological postmortem lung features in the same segment, Chastre et al. could demonstrate a very high correlation between the percentage of BAL cells containing intracellular bacteria and the total number of bacteria recovered from the corresponding lung samples and with the histological grades of pneumonia (Fig. 5) (79). In 10 of 11 lung segments with $\geq 10^4$ bacteria/g lung tissue cultured, $\geq 5\%$ of the cells recovered by lavage contained intracellular organisms. In contrast, <1% of cells recovered by lavage contained intracellular bacteria in eight of nine noninfected lung segments, and >5% of the cells contained intracellular organisms in only one lung segment in which the diagnosis of infection in the same lung segment was excluded. In this study, the morphology of intracellular and extracellular bacteria observed in BAL fluid preparations obtained from infected lung segments was consistent with the types of organisms ultimately cultured at high concentrations from lung tissue samples, confirming the potential usefulness of this technique for selecting an effective antimicrobial treatment before culture results are available.

% BAL cells containing
intracellular bacteria

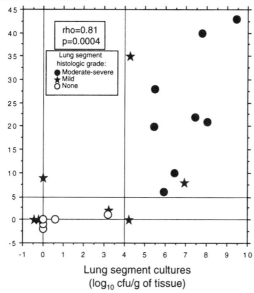

Lung segment cultures
($\log_{10}$ cfu/g of tissue)

Figure 5   Relationship between the percentage of bronchoalveolar lavage cells containing intracellular bacteria and the total numbers of bacteria recovered from lung cultures in 20 lung segments. Each symbol represents one single lung segment from which histological examination demonstrated moderate or severe (*closed circles*), mild (*stars*), and no signs of pneumonia (*open circles*). (From Ref. 79, with permission.)

One technique was recently proposed by Meduri et al. to circumvent the problem of contamination of BAL fluid by the flora present in proximal airway (90). This technique uses a protected transbronchoscopic balloon-tipped catheter designed to avoid exposing the instilled and aspirated BAL solution to the contaminants present in the working lumen of the broncho-scope. The samples obtained with this device in 33 patients without pneumonia and in 13 patients with pneumonia had ≤1 squamous epithelial cell in 91% of specimens and an absence of bacterial growth in 59% of patients without pneumonia. Using a threshold of 10^4 cfu/mL, only one false-positive result and one false-negative result were observed for a diagnostic sensitivity of 97% and a specificity of 92%. Two of the 49 patients who entered the study had, however, no fluid retrieved with protected BAL.

V. THE ARGUMENT FOR BRONCHOSCOPY IN THE DIAGNOSIS OF VENTILATOR- AND NONVENTILATOR-ASSOCIATED NOSOCOMIAL PNEUMONIA

The use of invasive techniques, such as fiberoptic bronchoscopy, coupled with quantitative cultures of PSB or BAL specimens helps direct the initial antibiotic therapy in addition to confirming the actual diagnosis of nosocomial pneumonia. When cultures results are available, they allow for the precise identification of the offending organisms and their susceptibility patterns. Such data are invaluable for optimal antibiotic selection. They also increase the confidence and comfort level of health care workers in managing patients with suspected nosocomial pneumonia. Rello et al. found that 43% of patients required a change in their initial antibiotic regimen based on the results of bronchoscopic evaluation: 27% of patients were receiving ineffective antibiotic therapy, 9% of patients were receiving less than optimal antibiotic therapy, and 7% of patients were receiving unnecessary antibiotic therapy (91). Similar results were found by Alvarez et al. in a large series of 499 patients with proven ventilator-associated pneumonia (92). Therefore, antibiotic therapy that is directed by quantitative culture results may be more effective than empirical treatment. The inadequate initial management of VAP is associated with increased mortality rate, and there is evidence that the clinical recognition of treatment failure may be delayed. Recent studies have found that initial empirical antibiotic treatment often requires modification when quantitative culture results are available (33,91–93). What is less clear is whether such delayed modification of initial treatment impacts outcome (84,94). The results of gram-stained bronchoscopic specimens may provide an earlier guide to antibiotic management, but the impact of this information on physician practice and patient outcomes has not been studied.

The second most compelling argument for invasive bronchoscopic techniques is that they can reduce excessive antibiotic use. There is little disagreement that the clinical diagnosis of nosocomial pneumonia is overly sensitive and leads to the unnecessary use of broad-spectrum antibiotics. Because bronchoscopic techniques may be more specific, their use would reduce antibiotic pressure in the intensive care unit, thereby limiting the emergence of drug-resistant strains and the attendant increased risks of superinfection (95–97). Most epidemiological investigations have clearly demonstrated that the indiscriminate use of antimicrobial agents in ICU patients may have immediate as well as long-term consequences, which contribute to the emergence of multiresistant pathogens and increasing the risk of serious superinfections (95). This increased risk is not limited to one patient but may increase the risk of colonization or infection by multidrug-resistant bacterial strains in patients throughout the ICU and even the entire hospital. Virtually all reports emphasize that better antibiotic control programs to limit bacterial resistance are urgently needed in ICUs and that patients without true infection should not receive antimicrobial treatment (43).

The more targeted use of antibiotics also could reduce overall costs, despite the expense of bronchoscopy and quantitative cultures, and minimize antibiotic-related toxicity. This is particularly true in the case of patients who have late-onset ventilator-associated pneumonia, in whom expensive combination therapy is recommended by most authorities in the field. A conservative cost analysis performed in a trauma ICU suggested that the discontinuation of antibiotics upon the return of negative bronchoscopic quantitative culture results could lead to a savings of more than $1,700 per patient suspected of VAP (98).

Finally, probably the most important risk of not performing bronchoscopy for the patient is that another site of infection may be missed. The major benefit of a negative bronchoscopy may be to direct attention away from the lungs as the source of fever. Many hospitalized patients with negative bronchoscopic cultures have other potential sites of infection that can be identified via a simple diagnostic protocol. In a study of 50 patients with suspected ventilator-associated pneumonia who underwent a systematic diagnostic protocol designed to identify all potential causes of fever and pulmonary densities, Meduri et al. confirmed that lung infection was present in only 42% of cases and that the frequent occurrence of multiple infectious and noninfectious processes justifies a systematic search for the source of fever in this setting (35). Delay in the diagnosis of definitive treatment of the true site of infection may lead to prolonged antibiotic therapy, more antibiotic-associated complications, and induction of further organ dysfunction.

VI. THE ARGUMENT AGAINST BRONCHOSCOPY IN THE DIAGNOSIS OF VENTILATOR- AND NONVENTILATOR-ASSOCIATED NOSOCOMIAL PNEUMONIA

Reasons not to use invasive diagnostic techniques include the following: (1) the accuracy of bronchoscopic techniques is questionable in patients on prior antibiotics, especially when new antibiotics have been introduced after the onset of the symptoms suggestive of nosocomial pneumonia, before pulmonary secretions were collected; (2) bronchoscopy may transiently worsen patient's status, although several studies suggest that the incidence of such complications is quite low; (3) an invasive approach to diagnosing nosocomial pneumonia may increase costs of caring for critically ill patients, at least in some institutions in which fees for bronchoscopy are very high; and (4) although patient management may change based on results from invasive tests, data suggesting that these changes lead to an improvement in patient outcome are lacking.

The presence of prior antimicrobial treatment in patients clinically suspected of nosocomial pneumonia is frequently presented as a major limitation to accurate diagnosis, because it may lead to a high number of false-negative results. As demonstrated by Johanson et al. and other investigators, culture results of respiratory secretions are mostly not modified when pneumonia develops as a superinfection in patients who have been receiving systemic antibiotics for several days before the appearance of the new pulmonary infiltrates, the reason being that the bacteria responsible for the new infection are then resistant to the antibiotics given previously (58,84). In one study of 76 cases of proven ventilator-associated pneumonia, of the 33 pathogens that yielded $\geq 10^3$ cfu/mL from the initial PSB in the 22 patients who had received antibiotics for several days before the appearance of the new pulmonary infiltrates, 27 (82%) were resistant to these antibiotics, as were 10 of 12 microorganisms that yielded $< 10^3$ cfu/mL (84). To further evaluate the effects of antibiotic treatment received before the suspicion of pneumonia on the diagnostic yield of PSB, direct examination, and culture of lavage fluid, Timsit et al. studied two groups of ventilated patients with suspected nosocomial pneumonia: Sixty-five patients had received antibiotics for an earlier septic episode and 96 patients had not (99). Bronchoscopy was always performed before any treatment for suspected pneumonia was given. As in previous studies, all but two strains recovered from distal samples of patients with definite pneumonia were highly resistant to previous antibiotics. The sensitivity and specificity of each test did not differ between the two groups of patients, confirming that previous antibiotics used to treat an earlier septic episode unrelated to suspected pneumonia do not affect the diagnostic yield of PSB and BAL.

On the other hand, performing microbiological cultures of pulmonary secretions for diagnostic purposes after initiation of new antibiotic therapy in patients suspected of having nosocomial pneumonia can clearly lead to a high number of false-negative results, regardless of the way in which these secretions are obtained. In fact, all microbiological techniques are probably of little value in patients with a recent pulmonary infiltrate who have received new antibiotics for that reason, even for less than 24 hours. In this case, a negative finding could indicate either that pneumonia has been successfully treated and the bacteria eradicated, or that the patient had no lung infection to begin with. In one study in which follow-up cultures of protected bronchoscopic specimens were obtained in 43 cases of proven nosocomial pneumonia, 24 and 48 hours after the onset of antimicrobial treatment, nearly 40% of cultures were negative after only 24 hours of treatment and 65% after 48 hours (100). Similar results were obtained by Montravers et al. in a series of 76 consecutive patients with ventilator-associated pneumonia evaluated by fiberoptic bronchoscopy after 3 days of treatment (84). In this study, using follow-up PSB sample cultures to directly assess the infection site in the lung, 88% of patients had negative cultures after the onset of treatment. Using both PSB and BAL, Souweine et al. prospectively investigated 63 episodes of suspected ventilator-associated pneumonia (101). Based on prior antibiotic treatment, three groups were defined: no previous antibiotic treatments, n = 12; antibiotic treatment initiated >72 hours earlier, n = 31; and new antibiotic treatment class started within the last 24 hours, n = 20. Results were entirely consistent with the studies referenced earlier. If patients had been given antibiotics but did not have a recent change in antibiotic class, then the sensitivity of PSB and BAL culture (83 and 77%, respectively) were similar to the sensitivity of these methods when applied to patients not given antibiotics. In other words, prior therapy did not reduce the yield of diagnostic testing among those receiving current antibiotics given to treat a prior infection. On the other hand, if therapy was recent, the sensitivity of invasive diagnostic methods using traditional thresholds was only 38% with BAL and 40% with PSB (101).

These two clinical situations should be clearly distinguished before interpreting pulmonary secretion culture results, however they were obtained (Fig. 6). In the second situation, when the patient had received new antibiotics after the appearance of the signs suggesting the presence of pulmonary infection, no conclusion concerning the presence or absence of pneumonia can be drawn if culture results are negative. Pulmonary secretions therefore need to be obtained before new antibiotics are administered, as is the case for all types of microbiological samples.

Several investigators argue that the use of bronchoscopy in the evaluation of nosocomial pneumonia is limited by the lack of standardized, reproducible methods and diagnostic criteria (24). There is no doubt that the literature is replete with variations on this theme: what are the advantages of bronchoalveolar lavage (BAL) versus protected specimen brush (PSB); whether to collect secretions with the PSB under direct vision or wedge it distally; what

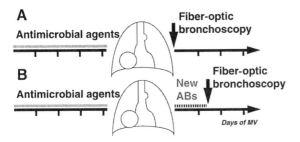

Figure 6   Patients already receiving antimicrobial therapy. (**A**) When pneumonia develops as a superinfection in a patient who has been receiving antimicrobial agents for several days before the appearance of new infiltrates and fiberoptic bronchoscopy is performed immediately without any modifications of the treatment, bacteria responsible for the new infection are then mostly resistant to the antibiotics given previously and culture results will not be modified. (**B**) In contrast, when fiberoptic bronchoscopy is done after the introduction of new antimicrobial agents, bacteria responsible for the infection are then frequently sensitive to the new antibiotics given and culture results are negative in a high number of cases.

volume of saline to use for BAL; which transport medium to use; whether to set up cultures using quantitative loops or serial dilutions; and whether to express the results in colony-forming units per milliliter (CFU/mL) or construct a bacterial index composed of the sum of the exponents from each quantitated isolate. Although a general consensus has emerged on the use of 1,000 CFU/mL as the cutoff for a PSB culture and 10,000 CFU/mL for BAL specimens, concern has been raised about reproducibility of results, particularly near the diagnosis thresholds (87,88). Whether the clinical suspicion of VAP should influence the interpretation of quantitative culture results also has not been entirely clarified (102). It is likely that no single method will emerge as superior to others. What is most important is that physicians using these techniques establish a protocol that is supported by the reported literature and within the capabilities of the local microbiology laboratory. Many microbiology laboratories may not be able to promptly and accurately process quantitative cultures, although the techniques used can be very similar to those applied routinely to urine cultures.

Some experts also question the willingness of physicians to stop antibiotic therapy in the face of a negative bronchoscopic culture. Indeed, there is evidence that physicians are reluctant to discontinue antibiotics for suspected nosocomial pneumonia solely because of a negative culture. The development of algorithms incorporating clinical suspicion into the interpretation of culture results may improve the acceptability of negative results. However, the value of bronchoscopy in the evaluation of suspected nosocomial pneumonia is limited if physicians only accept positive results.

Others have suggested that any potential value of bronchoscopy in the management of nosocomial pneumonia would be limited to late-onset infections, because infections that occur within 4 days of admission often are caused by community-acquired pathogens and are easier to diagnose and manage than is pneumonia occurring later in the hospital course. Although it is true that community-acquired pathogens often are identified in early onset pneumonia, hospital-acquired pathogens cannot be excluded in the early time frame (44). Furthermore, early onset pneumonia is a less common problem than late-onset infection, because risk of pneumonia (and risk of infection with hospital-acquired pathogens) increases with the duration of hospitalization.

VII. RECOMMENDATIONS

The diagnosis of bacterial pneumonia in the severely ill *mechanically ventilated patient* remains a difficult dilemma for the clinician. Our personal bias is that the use of bronchoscopic techniques to obtain PSB and BAL specimens from the affected area in the lung in ventilated patients with signs suggestive of pneumonia allows definition of a therapeutic strategy superior to that based exclusively on clinical evaluation. These bronchoscopic techniques, when they are performed before introduction of new antibiotics, enable physicians to identify most patients who need immediate treatment and help to select optimal therapy, in a manner that is safe and well tolerated by patients. On the other hand, these techniques prevent resorting to broad-spectrum drug coverage in all patients in whom there is a clinical suspicion of infection. Therefore, although the true impact of this decision tree on patient outcome has not yet been established, available data clearly suggest that being able to withhold antimicrobial treatment in some patients without infection may constitute a distinct advantage in the long term, by minimizing the emergence of resistant microorganisms in the ICU. In patients with clinical evidence of severe sepsis with rapid worsening organ dysfunction, hypoperfusion, or hypotension, the initiation of antibiotic therapy should not, however, be delayed while awaiting bronchoscopy and patients should be given immediate treatment with antibiotics. It is probably in this latter situation that simplified nonbronchoscopic diagnostic procedures could find their best justification, allowing distal pulmonary secretions to be obtained on a 24-hours basis, just before starting new antimicrobial therapy.

The best strategy to use in *nonventilated patients* who are clinically suspected of having pneumonia is probably more difficult to choose. However, as in ventilated patients, the most important problems in nonventilated patients are (1) to clinically identify patients with pneumonia, (2) to differentiate colonization from true distal lung infection, and (3) in case of infection, to select the most appropriate antimicrobial treatment.

A minimum requirement for the diagnosis of nosocomial pneumonia in a nonventilated patient is the presence of a new chest radiographic infiltrate. However, many noninfectious conditions commonly affect hospitalized patients and cause roentgenographic infiltrates. Thus, it is not difficult to appreciate that, in the presence of diseases such as ARDS, atelectasis, pulmonary embolism, congestive heart failure, community-acquired pneumonia, or lung contusion, which may be associated with lung infiltrates, nosocomial pneumonia can be overlooked. Elderly or immunosuppressed patients may have only a few clinical symptoms and signs suggestive of infection when pneumonia develops in the hospital. In these patients, the diagnosis of nosocomial pneumonia should be based on bacteriological confirmation by using "invasive" diagnostic methods, such as transtracheal aspiration, or bronchoscopic techniques, besides blood cultures and pleural fluid examination. Fiberoptic bronchoscopy is also the technique of choice in perplexing infections. Most investigators agree that the technique of BAL is of greatest value in establishing a bacterial or nonbacterial cause of infection, especially in the immunocompromised host or the patient with acquired immunodeficiency syndrome, in which it can also reliably diagnose *Pneumocystis carinii* pneumonia, cytomegalovirus infection, and drug-induced lung disease. In the same way, oropharyngeal and lower respiratory tract colonization is particularly common in postoperative patients who were recently extubated, in patients with suspected repeated microaspirations because of impaired consciousness or coma, and in patients with chronic colonization of the respiratory tract such as patients with chronic obstructive pulmonary disease. In these patients, sputum examination is unreliable for distinguishing between colonizing pathogens and infecting pathogens, and the use of bronchoscopic techniques to obtain PSB and BAL specimens from the affected area in the lung is probably justified in most cases.

However, conditions placing the patient at risk for fiberoptic complications are limitations for using "invasive" diagnostic techniques in nonventilated patients, because performance of bronchoscopy may paradoxically be more dangerous in this setting than in patients receiving mechanical ventilation. Our personal bias would be to use a policy based only on clinical evaluation and results of sputum analysis to select treatment in critically ill patients with impending respiratory failure who are not receiving ventilation. Rather than listing all the absolute contraindications, the place of fiberoptic bronchoscopy in this setting should probably be analyzed in terms of risk-benefit. The risk is probably very high in patients with severe hypoxemia ($Pao_2 < 60$ mmHg), active bronchospasm, recent acute myocardial infarction, unstable arrhythmias, agitation, coagulation disorders (platelet count <20,000/mL), and shock; in these cases, expected benefit must be at least equally high to justify the use of FOB.

ACKNOWLEDGMENTS

The authors wish to thank A. Failin for her invaluable help in the preparation of the manuscript.

REFERENCES

1. Pennington JE. Nosocomial respiratory infection. In: Mandell GL, Douglas RG Jr, Bennett JE, eds. Principles and Practice of Infectious Diseases. 3rd ed. Churchill Livingstone, 1990:2199–2205.
2. Haley RW, Hooton TM, Culter DH, et al. Nosocomial infections in US hospitals, 1975–1976: estimated frequency by selected characteristics of patients. Am J Med 1981; 70:947–959.
3. Horan TC, White JW, Jarvis WR, et al. Nosocomial infection surveillance. MMWR 1986; 35:175S–195S.
4. Craven DE, Driks MR. Nosocomial pneumonia in the intubated patient. Semin Respir Infect Dis 1987; 2:20–33.
5. Chastre J, Fagon JY. Pneumonia in the ventilator-dependent patient. In: Tobin MJ, ed. Principles and Practice of Mechanical Ventilation. New York: McGraw-Hill, 1994:857–890.
6. Vincent JL, Bihari DJ, Suter PM, et al. The prevalence of nosocomial infection in intensive care units in Europe. Results of the European Prevalence of Infection in Intensive Care (EPIC) study. JAMA 1995; 274:639–644.
7. Chevret S, Hemmer M, Carlet J, Langer M, the European Cooperative Group on Nosocomial Pneumonia. Incidence and risk factors of pneumonia acquired in intensive care units. Results from a multicenter prospective study on 996 patients. Intensive Care Med 1993; 19:256–264.
8. Cross AS, Roup B. Role of respiratory assistance devices in endemic nosocomial pneumonia. Am J Med 1981; 70:681–685.
9. Langer T, Mosconi P, Cigada M, Mandelli M, the Intensive Care Unit Group of Infection Control. Long-term respiratory support and the risk of pneumonia in critically ill patients. Am Rev Respir Dis 1987; 140:302–305.

10. Torres A, Aznar R, Gatell JM, et al. Incidence, risk and prognosis factors of nosocomial pneumonia in mechanically ventilated patients. Am Rev Respir Dis 1990; 142:523–528.

11. Craven DE, Kuncher LM, Lichtenberg DA, et al. Nosocomial infection and fatality in medical and surgical intensive care unit patients. Arch Intern Med 1988; 148:1161–1168.

12. Garibaldi RA, Britt MR, Coleman ML, et al. Risk factors for postoperative pneumonia. Am J Med 1987; 70:677–680.

13. Celis R, Torres A, Gatell JH, Almela M, Rodriguez-Roisin R, Augusti-Vidal A. Nosocomial pneumonia. A multivariate analysis of risk and prognosis. Chest 1988; 93:318–324.

14. Fagon JY, Chastre J, Domart Y, et al. Nosocomial pneumonia in patients receiving continuous mechanical ventilation. Prospective analysis of 52 episodes with use of a protected specimen brush and quantitative culture techniques. Am Rev Respir Dis 1989; 139:877–884.

15. Bell RC, Coalson JJ, Smith JD, et al. Multiple organ system failure and infection in adult respiratory distress syndrome. Ann Intern Med 1983; 99:293–298.

16. Sutherland KR, Steinberg KP, Maunder RJ, Milberg JA, Allen DL, Hudson LD. Pulmonary infection during the acute respiratory distress syndrome. Am J Respir Crit Care Med 1995; 152:550–556.

17. Craig CP, Connelly S. Effect of intensive care unit nosocomial pneumonia on duration of stay and mortality. Am J Infect Control 1984; 12:233–238.

18. Leu HS, Kaiser DL, Mori M, Woolson RF, Wenzel RP. Hospital-acquired pneumonia. Attributable mortality and morbidity. Am J Epidemiol 1989; 129:1258–1267.

19. Gross PA, Neu HC, Aswapokee P, et al. Deaths from nosocomial infections: experience in a university hospital and a community hospital. Am J Med 1980; 68:219–223.

20. Gross PA, Van Antwerpen C. Nosocomial infections and hospital deaths. A case control study. Am J Med 1983; 75:658–661.

21. Fagon JY, Chastre J, Hance AJ, Montravers P, Novara A, Gibert C. Nosocomial pneumonia in ventilated patients. A cohort study evaluating attributable mortality and hospital stay. Am J Med 1993; 94:281–288.

22. Kollef MH, Silver P, Murphy DM, Trouillion E. The effect of late-onset ventilator-associated pneumonia in determining patient mortality. Chest 1995; 108: 1655–1662.

23. Fagon JY, Chastre J, Vuagnat A, et al. Nosocomial pneumonia and mortality among patients in intensive care units. JAMA 1996; 275:866–869.

24. Niederman MS, Torres A, Summer W. Invasive diagnostic testing is not needed routinely to manage suspected ventilator-associated pneumonia. Am J Respir Crit Care Med 1994; 150:565–569.

25. Chastre J, Fagon JY. Invasive diagnostic testing should be routinely used to manage ventilated patients with suspected pneumonia. Am J Respir Crit Care Med 1994; 150:570–574.

26. Andrew C, Coalson J, Smith J, Johanson WG Jr. Diagnosis of nosocomial pneumonia in acute, diffuse lung injury. Chest 1981; 80:254–258.
27. Ayala A, Perrin MM, Meldrum DR, et al. Hemorrhage induces an increase in serum TNF which is not associated with increased levels of endotoxin. Cytokine 1990; 2:170–174.
28. Joshi M, Ciesla E, Caplan E. Diagnosis of pneumonia in critically ill patients. Chest 1988; 94:4S.
29. Mock CN, Burchard KW, Hassan F, Reed M. Surgical intensive care unit pneumonia. Surgery 1988; 104:494–499.
30. Wunderink RG, Woldenberg LS, Zeiss J, Day CM, Ciemins J, Lacher DA. The radiologic diagnosis of autopsy-proven ventilator-associated pneumonia. Chest 1992; 101:458–463.
31. Meduri GU, Belenchia JM, Estres RJ, et al. Fibroproliferative phase of ARDS: clinical findings and effects of corticosteroids. Chest 1991; 100:943–952.
32. Johanson WG Jr, Pierce AK, Sanford JP, et al. Nosocomial respiratory infections with gram-negative bacilli. The significance of colonization of the respiratory tract. Ann Intern Med 1972; 77:701–706.
33. Fagon JY, Chastre J, Hance AJ, Domart Y, Trouillet JL, Gibert C. Evaluation of clinical judgment in the identification and treatment of nosocomial pneumonia in ventilated patients. Chest 1993; 103:547–553.
34. Fagon JY, Chastre J, Hance AJ, et al. Detection of nosocomial lung infection in ventilated patients. Use of a protected specimen brush and quantitative culture techniques in 147 patients. Am Rev Respir Dis 1988; 138:110–116.
35. Meduri GU, Mauldin GL, Wunderink RG, Leeper KV, Jones CG, Tolley E, Mayhall G. Causes of fever and pulmonary densities in patients with clinical manifestations of ventilator-associated pneumonia. Chest 1994; 1006:221–235.
36. Pugin J, Auckenthaler R, Mili N, et al. Diagnosis of ventilator-associated pneumonia by bacteriologic analysis of bronchoscopic and nonbronchoscopic "blind" bronchoalveolar lavage fluid. Am Rev Respir Dis 1991; 143:1121–1129.
37. Bartlett JG, Finegold SM. Bacteriology of expectorated sputum with quantitative culture and wash technique compared to transtracheal aspirates. Am Rev Respir Dis 1978; 117:1019–1027.
38. Bryan CS, Reynolds KL. Bacteremic nosocomial pneumonia. Am Rev Respir Dis 1984; 129:668–671.
39. Pollock HM, Hawkins EL, Bonner JR, et al. Diagnosis of bacterial pulmonary infections with quantitative protected catheter cultures obtained during bronchoscopy. J Clin Microbiol 1983; 17:255–259.
40. Hill JD, Radliff JL, Parrott JCW, et al. Pulmonary pathology in acute respiratory insufficiency: lung biopsy as a diagnostic tool. J Thorac Cardiovasc Surg 1976; 71:64–71.
41. Salata RA, Lederman MM, Shlaes DM, et al. Diagnosis of nosocomial pneumonia in intubated, intensive care unit patients. Am Rev Respir Dis 1987; 135:426–432.
42. Jones RN, Kehrberg EN, Erwin ME, Anderson SC, the Fluoroquinolone Resis-

tance Surveillance Group. Prevalence of important pathogens and antimicrobial activity of parenteral drugs at numerous medical centers in the United States. Diagn Microbiol Infect Dis 1994; 19:203–215.

43. Neu HC. The crisis in antibiotic resistance. Science 1992; 257:1064–1073.

44. Trouillet JL, Chastre J, Vuagnat, et al. Ventilator-associated pneumonia caused by potentially drug-resistant bacteria. Am J Respir Crit Care Med 1998; 157: 531–539.

45. Kirtland SH, Corley DE, Winterbauer RH, et al. The diagnosis of ventilator-associated pneumonia; a comparison of histologic, microbiologic, and clinical criteria. Chest 1997; 112:445–457.

46. Wunderink RG, Russell GB, Mezger E, et al. The diagnostic utility of the anti-body-coated bacteria test in intubated patients. Chest 1991; 99:84–88.

47. Lambert RS, Vereen LE, George RB. Comparison of tracheal aspirates and protected brush catheter specimens for identifying pathogenic bacteria in mechanically ventilated patients. Am J Med Sci 1989; 297:377–382.

48. Marquette C, Georges H, Wallet F, et al. Diagnostic efficiency of endotracheal aspirates with quantitative bacterial cultures in intubated patients with suspected pneumonia. Am Rev Respir Dis 1993; 148:138–144.

49. El-Ebiary M, Torres A, Gonzales J, et al. Quantitative cultures of endotracheal aspirates for the diagnosing of ventilator associated pneumonia. Am Rev Respir Dis 1993; 148:1552–1557.

50. Torres A, Puig de la Bellacasa J, Rodriguez-Roisin R, Jimenez DE, Anta MT, Agusti-Vidal A. Diagnostic value of telescoping plugged catheters in mechanically ventilated patients with bacterial pneumonia using the Metras catheter. Am Rev Respir Dis 1988; 138:117–120.

51. Jourdain B, Novara A, Joly-Guillou, et al. Role of quantitative cultures of endo-tracheal aspirates for the diagnosis of nosocomial pneumonia. Am J Respir Crit Care Med 1995; 152:241–246.

52. Borderon E, Leprince A, Guevelier C, Borderon J. Valeurs des examens bactéri-ologiques des sécrétions trachéales. Rev Fr Mal Resp 1981; 9:229–239.

53. Kollef MH, Bock KR, Richards RD, Hearns ML. The safety and accuracy of minibronchoalveolar lavage in patients with suspected ventilator-associated pneumonia. Ann Intern Med 1995; 122:743–748.

54. Pham LH, Brun Buisson C, Legrand P, et al. Diagnosis of nosocomial pneumo-nia in mechanically ventilated patients. Comparison of a plugged telescoping catheter with the protected specimen brush. Am Rev Respir Dis 1991; 143: 1055–1061.

55. Marquette CH, Herengt F, Saulnier F, et al. Protected specimen brush in the assessment of ventilator-associated pneumonia: selection of a certain lung seg-ment for bronchoscopic sampling is unnecessary. Chest 1993; 103:243–247.

56. Jorda R, Parras F, Ibanez J, Reina J, Bergada J, Rawrich JM. Diagnosis of nosocomial pneumonia in mechanically ventilated patients by the blind pro-tected telescoping catheter. Intensive Care Med 1993; 19:377–382.

57. Rouby JJ, Martin de Lassale E, Poete P, et al. Nosocomial bronchopneumonia

in the critically ill. Histologic and bacteriologic aspects. Am Rev Respir Dis 1992; 148:1059–1066.

58. Johanson WG Jr, Seidenfeld JJ, Gomez P, De Los Santos R, Coalson JJ. Bacteriologic diagnosis of nosocomial pneumonia following prolonged mechanical ventilation. Am Rev Respir Dis 1988; 137:259–264.

59. Baughman RP, Thorpe JE, Staneck J, et al. Use of the protected specimen brush in patients with endotracheal or tracheostomy tubes. Chest 1987; 91:233–236.

60. Belenchia JM, Wunderink RG, Meduri GU, Leeper KV. Alternative causes of fever in ARDS patients suspected of having pneumonia (abstr). Am Rev Respir Dis 1991; 143:A683.

61. Bartlett JG, Alexander J, Mayhew J, Sollivan-Sigler N, Gorbach SL. Should fiberoptic bronchoscopy aspirates be cultured? Am Rev Respir Dis 1976; 114:73–78.

62. Meduri GU, Chastre J. The standardization of bronchoscopic techniques for ventilator-associated pneumonia. Chest 1982; 102 (suppl 1):557S–564S.

63. Kirkpatrick MB, Bass JB. Quantitative bacterial cultures of bronchoalveolar lavage fluids and protected brush catheter specimens from normal subjects. Am Rev Respir Dis 1989; 139:546–548.

64. Marquette CH, Copin MC, Wallet F, et al. Diagnostic tests for pneumonia in ventilated patients: prospective evaluation of diagnostic accuracy using histology as a diagnostic gold standard. Am J Respir Crit Care Med 1995; 151:1878–1888.

65. Trouillet JL, Guiguet M, Gibert C, et al. Fiberoptic bronchoscopy in ventilated patients: evaluation of cardiopulmonary risk under midazolam sedation. Chest 1990; 97:927–933.

66. Steinberg KP, Mitchell DR, Maunder RJ, Millberg JA, Whitcomb ME, Hudson LD. Safety of bronchoalveolar lavage in patients with adult respiratory distress syndrome. Am Rev Respir Dis 1993; 148:556–561.

67. Standiford TJ, Kunkel SL, Strieter RM. Elevated serum levels of tumor necrosis factor alpha after bronchoscopy and bronchoalveolar lavage. Chest 1991; 99: 1529–1530.

68. Wimberley N, Faling LJ, Bartlett JG. A fiberoptic bronchoscopy technique to obtain uncontaminated lower airway secretions for bacterial culture. Am Rev Respir Dis 1979; 119:337–343.

69. Linder J, Rennard SI. Development and application of bronchoalveolar lavage. In: Bronchoalveolar Lavage. Chicago: ASCP Press, 1988:1–16.

70. Baselski V, Wunderink RG. Bronchoscopic diagnosis of pneumonia. Clin Microbiol Rev 1994; 7:533–558.

71. Davis GS, Giancola MS, Costanza MC, Low RB. Analyses of sequential bronchoalveolar lavage samples from healthy human volunteers. Am Rev Respir Dis 1982; 126:611–616.

72. Monroe PW, Muchmore HG, Felton FG, Pirtle JK. Quantitation of microorganisms in sputum. Appl Microbiol 1969; 18:214–220.

73. Moser KM, Maurer J, Jassy L, et al. Sensitivity, specificity, and risk of diagnostic procedures in a canine model of *Streptococcus pneumoniae* pneumonia. Am Rev Respir Dis 1982; 125:436–442.

74. Higuchi JH, Coalson JJ, Johanson WG Jr. Bacteriologic diagnosis of nosocomial pneumonia in primates. Usefulness of the protected specimen brush. Am Rev Respir Dis 1982; 125:53–57.
75. Chastre J, Viau F, Brun P, et al. Prospective evaluation of the protected specimen brush for the diagnosis of pulmonary infections in ventilated patients. Am Rev Respir Dis 1984; 130:924–929.
76. Kahn FW, Jones JM. Diagnosing bacterial respiratory infection by bronchoalveolar lavage. J Infect Dis 1987; 155:862–869.
77. Chastre J, Fagon JY, Soler P, et al. Diagnosis of nosocomial bacterial pneumonia in intubated patients undergoing ventilation: comparison of the usefulness of bronchoalveolar lavage and the protected specimen brush. Am J Med 1988; 85:499–506.
78. Torres A, El-Ebiary M, Padro L, et al. Validation of different techniques for the diagnosis of ventilator-associated pneumonia. Am J Respir Crit Care Med 1994; 149:324–331.
79. Chastre J, Fagon JY, Bornet-Lecso M, et al. Evaluation of bronchoscopic techniques for the diagnosis of nosocomial pneumonia. Am J Respir Crit Care Med 1995; 152:231–240.
80. Torres A, Puig de la Bellacasa J, Rodriguez-Roisin R, Jimenez DE, Anta MT, Agusti-Vidal A. Diagnostic value of telescoping plugged catheters in mechanically ventilated patients with bacterial pneumonia using the Metras catheter. Am Rev Respir Dis 1988; 138:117–120.
81. Cook DJ, Fitzgerald JM, Guyatt GH, Walter S. Evaluation of the protected brush catheter and bronchoalveolar lavage in the diagnosis of pneumonia. J Intensive Care Med 1991; 6:196–205.
82. Middleton R, Broughton WA, Kirkpatrick MB. Comparison of four methods for assessing airway bacteriology in intubated, mechanically ventilated patients. Am J Med Sci 1992; 304:239–245.
83. Papazian L, Thomas P, Garbe L, et al. Bronchoscopic or blind sampling techniques for the diagnosis of ventilator-associated pneumonia. Am J Respir Crit Care Med 1995; 152:1982–1991.
84. Montravers P, Fagon JY, Chastre J, et al. Follow-up protected specimen brushes to assess treatment in nosocomial pneumonia. Am Rev Respir Dis 1993; 147:38–44.
85. Torres A, Martos J, Puig de la Bellacasa, et al. Specificity of endotracheal aspiration, protected specimen brush and bronchoalveolar lavage cultures in mechanically ventilated patients without pneumonia. Am Rev Respir Dis 1993; 147:952–957.
86. Dreyfuss D, Mier L, Le Bourdelles G, et al. Clinical significance of borderline quantitative protected brush specimen culture results. Am Rev Respir Dis 1993; 147:941–951.
87. Marquette CH, Herengt F, Mathieu D, Saulnier F, Courcol R, Ranon P. Diagnosis of pneumonia in mechanically ventilated patients. Repeatability of the protected specimen brush. Am Rev Respir Dis 1993; 147:211–214.

88. Timsit JF, Misset B, Francoual S, Goldstein W, Vaury P, Carlet J. Is protected specimen brush a reproducible method to diagnose ICU-acquired pneumonia. Chest 1993; 104:104–108.

89. Jourdain B, Joly-Guillou ML, Dombret MC, Calvat S, Trouillet JL, Gibert C, Chastre J. Usefulness of quantitative cultures of bronchoalveolar lavage fluid for diagnosing nosocomial pneumonia in ventilated patients. Chest 1997; 111: 411–418.

90. Meduri GU, Beals DH, Maijub AG, Baselski V. Protected bronchoalveolar lavage. A new bronchoscopic technique to retrieve uncontaminated specimens in ICU patients: A review. Crit Care Med 1994; 22:1683–1691.

91. Rello J, Gallego M, Mariscal D, Sonora R, Valles J. The value of routine microbial investigation in ventilator-associated pneumonia. Am J Respir Crit Care Med 1997; 156:196–200.

92. Alvarez-Lerma and The ICU-Acquired Pneumonia Group. Modification of empiric antibiotic treatment in patients with pneumonia acquired in the ICU. Intensive Care Med 1996; 22:387–394.

93. Bonten MJM, Bergmans DCJJ, Stobberingh EE, et al. Implementation of bronchoscopic techniques in the diagnosis of ventilator-associated pneumonia to reduce antibiotic use. Am J Respir Crit Care Med 1997; 156:1820–1824.

94. Luna CM, Vujacich P, Niederman MS, et al. Impact of BAL data on the therapy and outcome of ventilator-associated pneumonia. Chest 1997; 111:676–685.

95. McGowan JE Jr. Antimicrobial resistance in hospital organisms and its relation to antibiotic use. Rev Infect Dis 1983; 5:1033–1048.

96. Meyer KS, Urban C, Eagan JA, Berger BJ, Rahal JJ. Nosocomial outbreak of *Klebsiella* infection resistant to late-generation cephalosporins. Ann Intern Med 1993; 119:353–358.

97. Kollef MH. Ventilator-associated pneumonia. A multivariate analysis. JAMA 1993; 270:1965–1970.

98. Croce MA, Fabian TC, Shaw B, et al. Analysis of charges associated with diagnosis of nosocomial pneumonia: can routine bronchoscopy be justified? J Trauma 1994; 37:721–727.

99. Timsit JF, Misset B, Renaud B, Goldstein FW, Carlet J. Effect of previous antimicrobial therapy on the accuracy of the main procedures used to diagnose nosocomial pneumonia in patients who are using ventilation. Chest 1995; 108: 1036–1040.

100. Blavia R, Dorca J, Verdaguer R, Carratala J, Gudiol F, Manresa F. Bacteriological follow-up of nosocomial pneumonia by successive protected specimen brushes (abstr). Eur Respir J 1991; 4:A823.

101. Souweine B, Veber B, Bedos JP, et al. Diagnostic accuracy of protected specimen brush and bronchoalveolar lavage in nosocomial pneumonia: impact of previous antimicrobial treatments. Crit Care Med 1998; 26:236–244.

102. Baker AM, Bowton DL, Haponik EF. Decision making in nosocomial pneumonia: an analytic approach to the interpretation of quantitative bronchoscopic cultures. Chest 1995; 107:85–95.

2

Surveillance and Its Impact

OLIVIA KEITA-PERSE and ROBERT P. GAYNES

Centers for Disease Control and Prevention
Atlanta, Georgia

I. INTRODUCTION

Nosocomial pneumonia is the second most common nosocomial infection (1) and the most common nosocomial infection in intensive care units (ICUs). It affects more than 250,000 acute care patients annually in the United States (2). The Centers for Disease Control and Prevention (CDC) recently estimated that nosocomial pneumonia is a primary or contributing cause for more than 30,000 deaths annually in the United States (3). To decrease the incidence of nosocomial pneumonia, hospitals must focus their considerable prevention efforts. However, these efforts begin by appropriate monitoring of this costly complication of hospital care. This task is even more involved because nosocomial pneumonia is probably more than one syndrome with multiple pathogeneses.

II. METHODS FOR SURVEILLANCE FOR NOSOCOMIAL PNEUMONIA

Compared to most hospitalized patients, rates of nosocomial pneumonia are 10- to 20-fold higher in intensive care unit patients, and 7- to 21-fold higher in the intubated patients (4–6). Therefore, intubated patients in intensive care should be a major focus of surveillance for nosocomial pneumonia. Unit-targeted surveillance, the type that focuses on detecting nosocomial infection occurring among patients in one unit of the hospital, can help focus limited resources for surveillance around the areas where risk of nosocomial pneumonia is greatest, such as intensive care units. In this type of surveillance, patients usually are monitored for the presence of all types of infection, although some hospitals may choose to focus only on a particular infection (e.g., ventilator-associated pneumonia). However, for units or areas of the hospital with patients at lower risk, another approach might be to focus only on nosocomial pneumonia, varying the amount and type of surveillance according to the relative seriousness of the problem.

Three categories of data comprise the usual information collected on a patient with a nosocomial pneumonia: demographic, clinical, and laboratory. Information describing important risk factors for infection should also be collected, but only if it will be analyzed and used by the hospital personnel. Corresponding denominator data should also be collected so that infection rates can be calculated.

For the numerator of a nosocomial pneumonia rate, accurate and consistent case finding of nosocomial pneumonia in the population under study is needed. Consistent definitions for case finding are essential. Therefore, it is imperative that there be available a uniform set of criteria that define nosocomial pneumonia. The most widely used definitions currently in use are the definitions used by National Nosocomial Infection Surveillance (NNIS) system hospitals, the complete version of which was published in Hospital Epidemiology and Infection Control in 1996. The current definition for nosocomial pneumonia is shown on Table 1.

Nosocomial pneumonia is difficult to define. For consistency, physician diagnosis alone is *not* an acceptable criterion for nosocomial pneumonia. Many other pneumonic processes may mimic infectious pneumonia and be a precursor to or exacerbated by it. However, surveillance personnel should be able to distinguish pneumonia from other disease entities or changes in clinical status such as myocardial infarction, congestive heart failure, respiratory distress syndrome, pulmonary embolism, atelectasis, malignancy, or hyaline membrane disease in the neonates. The criteria for nosocomial pneumonia diagnosis are clinical and include fever, cough, and development of purulent sputum, in combination with radiological evidence of a new or progressive pulmonary infiltrate, a suggestive Gram's stain, and positive cultures of sputum, tracheal aspirate, pleural fluid, or blood. Although clinical criteria together with cultures of tracheal specimens may be sensitive for bacterial pathogens, they are not specific, especially in patients with mechanically assisted ventilation. Conversely, cultures of blood or pleural fluid have

Table 1 Pneumonia Must Meet One of the Following Criteria:

1. Rales or dullness to percussion on physical examination of chest and any of the following:
   a. New onset of purulent sputum or change in character of sputum
   b. Organism isolated from blood culture
   c. Isolation of pathogen from specimen obtained by transtracheal aspirate, bronchial brushing, or biopsy
2. Chest radiography examination shows new or progressive infiltrate, consolidation, cavitation, or pleural effusion and any of the following:
   a. New onset of purulent sputum or change in character of sputum
   b. Organism isolated from blood culture
   c. Isolation of pathogen from specimen obtained by transtracheal aspirate, bronchial brushing, or biopsy
   d. Isolation of virus or detection of viral antigen in respiratory secretions
   e. Diagnostic single antibody titer (IgM) or four-fold increase in paired serum samples (IgG) for pathogen
   f. Histopathological evidence of pneumonia
3. Patient younger than 12 months of age has two of the following: apnea, tachypnea, bradycardia, wheezing, rhonchi, or cough and any of the following:
   a. Increased production of respiratory secretions
   b. New onset of purulent sputum or change in character of sputum
   c. Organism isolated from blood culture
   d. Isolation of pathogen from specimen obtained by transtracheal aspirate, bronchial brushing, or biopsy
   e. Isolation of virus or detection of viral antigen in respiratory secretions
   f. Diagnostic single antibody titer (IgM) or four-fold increase in paired serum samples (IgG) for pathogen
   g. Histopathological evidence of pneumonia
4. Patient older than 12 months of age has chest radiological examination that shows new or progressive infiltrate, cavitation, consolidation, or pleural effusion and any of the following:
   a. Increased production of respiratory secretions
   b. New onset of purulent sputum or change in character of sputum
   c. Organism isolated from blood culture
   d. Isolation of pathogen from specimen obtained by transtracheal aspirate, bronchial brushing, or biopsy
   e. Isolation of virus or detection of viral antigen in respiratory secretions
   f. Diagnostic single antibody titer (IgM) or four-fold increase in paired serum samples (IgG) for pathogen
   g. Histopathological evidence of pneumonia

very low sensitivity but are generally quite specific for nosocomial pneumonia (7).

Because of these problems, a group of investigators recently formulated recommendations for standardization of methods used to diagnose ventilator-associated pneumonia. These methods involve bronchoscopic techniques (e.g., quantitative culture of protected-specimen brushings, bronchoalveolar lavage, and protected bronchoalveolar lavage). The reported sensitivities and specificities of these methods have ranged from 70% to 100% and 60% to 100%, respectively (7).

Although very useful in clinical research settings, the widespread use of bronchoscopic techniques for diagnosis of pneumonia has been hampered by several factors. Complications of bronchoscopic techniques include hypoxemia, bleeding, or arrhythmia. In addition, the sensitivity of the protected specimen brushings procedure may decrease for patients receiving antibiotic therapy. Nonbronchoscopic procedures, for example, protected bronchoalveolar lavage or protected specimen brushings, which use blind catheterization of the distal airways, and quantitative culture of endotracheal aspirate, have been developed recently (8,9). Of these, endotracheal aspirate culture may be the most practical. However, further studies are needed to determine each test applicability in daily clinical practice. The CDC is currently reviewing and revising the NNIS definitions, with a focus on the definition of pneumonia. When revising the criteria, signs, symptoms, and diagnostic and radiographical test results and their timing will be considered to more clearly define pneumonia. Also, the importance of reviewing a patient's record and radiographical reports serially will be emphasized, and items relying on subjective or difficult to interpret documentation will be clarified. More specific or relevant signs or symptoms will be considered for infants (10).

III. DEFINING AND CALCULATING NOSOCOMIAL PNEUMONIA RATES

A rate is an expression of the occurrence of an event. The time period must be specified and be identical for the numerator and denominator for the rate to be meaningful. Three kinds of rates are used in nosocomial infection surveillance: *incidence*, *prevalence*, and *incidence density*.

Incidence is the number of *new* cases of disease that occur in a defined population during a specified period. The incidence of nosocomial infection is simply the number of new nosocomial infections in a given period divided by the number of patients at risk during that period.

Prevalence is the total number of active (existing and new) cases of the disease in a defined population, either during a specified period (period prevalence) or at a specified point in time (point prevalence). The prevalence nosocomial infection rate is calculated simply by dividing the number of active nosocomial infections in patients surveyed by the number of patients surveyed. Because nosocomial pneumonias occur relatively infrequently, the period chosen for surveillance must be large enough for an adequate estimation of a hospital's prevalence rate and usually varies depending on the number of occupied beds in a hospital. In addition, these rates require risk adjustment, which is currently not available for interhospital comparison of prevalence rates.

Incidence density is the instantaneous rate at which disease is occurring, relative to the size of the disease-free population. Incidence density is measured in units of the number of cases of disease per person per unit of time. An example of an incidence density that is commonly used in hospitals is the number of nosocomial pneumonias per 1000 ventilator-days. Incidence density is useful when the infection rate varies in a linear fashion to the length of time a patient is exposed to a risk factor (i.e., the longer the patient is exposed, the greater the chance of acquiring infection). For example:

$$\frac{\text{\# ventilator associated pneumonia}}{\text{\# ventilator-days}} \times 1000$$

To compare a rate among patient groups within a hospital, over time, or across hospitals, infection control practitioners (ICPs) must adjust the rate for the variations in the major risk factors that lead to the infection. A patient's predisposition for becoming infected is strongly influenced by certain risk factors, such as personal characteristics and exposures. These risk factors are roughly divided into two categories: *intrinsic* and *extrinsic*.

Intrinsic risk factors are those that are inherent in the patient, such as underlying disease conditions and advanced age. Knowledge of intrinsic risk factors enables separate risk-specific rates to be calculated, which permits the comparison of rates among patients with similar risks in different hospitals or different time periods. There has been considerable discussion but limited progress on the difficult task of developing a practical risk index representing patients' intrinsic risks that can be used to adjust the overall nosocomial infection rate. In a review of the literature, Keita-Perse and Gaynes found that nosocomial pneumonia was the only site of nosocomial infection for which a significant number of studies attempted to correlate that single site with a score for severity of illness. Whereas most of the studies found a score for severity of illness that tended to predict nosocomial pneumonia, a scoring system that was developed for another outcome such as mortality for APACHE II, may include factors irrelevant to the outcome of interest. However, the preponderance of evidence suggests that some measure of severity of illness or underlying disease will correlate with nosocomial pneumonia but may not be widely available unless infection control practitioners calculate it themselves (11). Although no scoring system for risk adjusting nosocomial pneumonia rates exists, numerous risk factors have been described (26). Individual intrinsic risk factors for adjusting nosocomial pneumonia are shown in Table 2. Further studies are needed to develop better means of risk adjustment.

Extrinsic risk factors may be staff based (practices of an individual caregiver) or institution based (practices in an entire hospital). Although many extrinsic factors contribute to nosocomial infections, the factors that have been most frequently implicated and studied are certain high-risk medical interventions such as surgical operations or the use of invasive devices (12,13). Ventilators have been associated with a 3- to 21-fold increased risk for nosocomial pneumonia. Therefore, it is necessary to adjust nosocomial pneumonia risk for the use of a ventilator because it is a major risk factor for nosocomial pneumonia (14,15). The importance of this type of risk adjustment can be demonstrated in Figure 1, which shows the distribution of several rates for hospital ICUs. Examining the rates for Hospital Unit A and Hospital Unit B on each of the histograms shows that the comparison of infection rates between the two units change with risk adjustment. The rate for Unit A on the top histogram, which uses the number of patients in the denominator, was nearly four times higher than the median. However, the middle histogram shows that Hospital Unit A had the highest rate of ventilator utilization; that is, more than 70% patient-days were also ventilator-days. Using ventilator-days as the denominator of the rate helps to control for exposure to this major risk factor for nosocomial pneumonia, that is, high utilization of ventilators among the unit's patients. Hospital Unit A's ventilator-associated pneumonia rate (per 1000 ventilator days) was slightly lower than the median (bottom histogram). However, Hospital Unit A's high ventilator use may need to be reviewed for appropriateness. On the other hand, for Hospital Unit B, the ventilator-associated pneumonia rate (top histogram) was near the median, and its ventilator use (middle histogram) was low. When its rate was calculated controlling for ventilator-days in the denominator, it was quite high, suggesting the need to review ventilator maintenance and/or respiratory therapy practices.

Hospitals use surveillance data to assess their infection control program by comparing infection rates among similar patient populations within the

Table 2 Risk Factors for Nosocomial Pneumonia for Ventilated and Nonventilated Patients

Risk Factor	Ventilated (V), Nonventilated (NV), or both (B)
Duration of mechanical ventilation	V
Chronic lung disease	B
Severity of illness	B
Upper abdominal or thoracic surgery	B
Duration of surgery	NV
Age	B
Poor nutritional state or hypoalbuminemia	NV
Immunosuppressive therapy	NV
Depressed level of consciousness	NV
Impaired airway reflexes or difficulty handling secretions	NV
Duration of hospitalization	NV
Severe head trauma or intracranial pressure monitor	V
Large volume aspiration	NV
Nasoenteric tube	B
Neuromuscular disease	NV
Gender	NV
Barbiturate therapy after head trauma	V
Gastric acid inhibitor therapy or elevated gastric pH	V
Gross aspiration of gastric contents	V
Reintubation or self-extubation	V
Ventilator circuit changes at intervals of less than 48 hours	V
Prior antibiotic therapy	V
Bronchoscopy	V
Shock or intramucosal gastric acidosis	V
Emergent endotracheal intubation after trauma	V
Blunt trauma	V
Stress ulcer with macroscopic bleeding	V

Adapted from Ref. 25.

hospital (two separate ICUs) or among different hospitals. Testing for significance among infection rates is discussed elsewhere (16). However, the interpretation of statistical tests should be carefully considered. Many hospitals assume that any difference in the rates represents success or failure in the patient-care staff or institutional practices to prevent nosocomial pneumonia. However, other factors could account for the differences in the rates, including

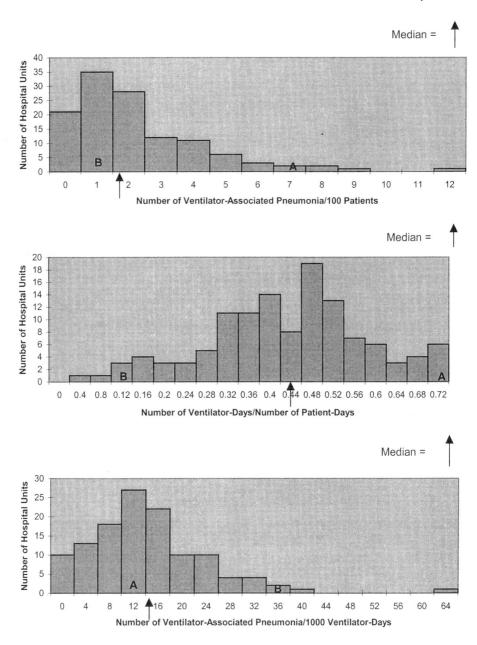

Figure 1 Comparison of the distributions of pneumonia rates (based on patients and on ventilator-days) and ventilator utilization in surgical intensive care units. A and B indicate the specific location of individual hospital unit rates. NNIS Data on Surgical Intensive Care Units, 1987–1995.

different surveillance definitions or techniques, inaccurate or insufficient information about clinical and laboratory evidence of infections in the patient's medical record, or not adjusting for patients' intrinsic risks for infection. Intrinsic risks are usually outside of the control of the hospital and vary among hospitals, but they are important factors in determining whether infections will develop.

It is also important to remember that surveillance of nosocomial infections measures the *endemic* rate of nosocomial infection. Less than 10% of all nosocomial infections occur in recognized outbreaks (17). This is important to remember when one attempts to devise a prevention and control strategy to reduce the infection rate. If an outbreak occurs in a hospital, it is often because of failure of one prevention strategy over a short period of time. Because surveillance is ongoing and measures the endemic rate, usually multiple problems must be addressed to lower a high rate of infection.

IV. VENTILATOR-ASSOCIATED AND NONVENTILATOR-ASSOCIATED NOSOCOMIAL PNEUMONIA RATES

Most of the published studies report the incidence rate of nosocomial pneumonia, that is, the number of cases of nosocomial pneumonia per 100 hospitalized patients. In six studies summarized in Table 3, the incidence of ventilator-associated pneumonia ranged from 9% to 24% (20). These rates fail to adjust for the duration of ventilation and are therefore difficult to interpret. Device-associated incidence density rates of nosocomial pneumonia, that is, the number of cases of ventilator-associated pneumonia per 1000 ventilator-days, are reported only for three studies and range from 10 to 30 per 1000 ventilator-days (14,21). In the NNIS, rates of ventilator-associated pneumonia per 1000 ventilator-days range from 9.4 in medical ICUs to 14.9 in surgical ICUs, 16.9 in trauma ICUs and 20.9 in burn ICUs.

Incidence density rates of ventilator-associated pneumonia and nonventilator-associated pneumonia (reported by the NNIS system) from 1990 to 1996 are shown in Figure 2. On average, ventilator-associated pneumonia rates are 9.3 times higher than nonventilator-associated pneumonia rates, ranging from 2.6 times higher in respiratory ICUs to 19 times higher in burn ICUs.

Experience with the NNIS has shown that targeted surveillance is better than hospital-wide surveillance for three main reasons. First, case-finding is

Table 3 Incidence and Mortality Rate of Ventilator-Associated Pneumonia

Reference	Study Years	# of patients	Incidence of VAP (%)	Diagnostic criteria	Mortality Rate (%)
23	1983 to 1984	233	21	Clinical	55
27	1983 to 1984	724	23	Clinical	44
21	1981 to 1985	567	9	PSB	71
28	1985 to 1987	130	18	Clinical	56
22	1987 to 1988	322	24	Clinical, PSB	33
29	1992 to 1993	277	15.5	Clinical	37

PSB, protected specimen brush; VAP, ventilator-associated pneumonia
Adapted from Ref. 22.

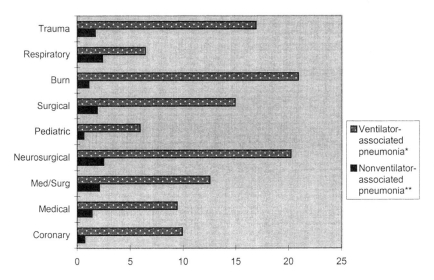

Figure 2 Ventilator and nonventilator associated pneumonia rates by type of ICU, NNIS 1990–1996.
*(Number of ventilator-associated pneumonia/number of ventilator-days) × 1000
**(Number of nonventilator associated pneumonia/number of nonventilator-days) × 1000

more accurate if targeted in a specific area. Second, in practical terms, targeting a specialized unit is more efficient for the infection control practitioner and for allocation of resources. And third, risk adjustment is feasible for targeted units; one cannot risk-adjust hospital-wide data. In the NNIS, ICU, High Risk Nursery (HRN), and surgical patients components increased dramatically after 1986, suggesting the feasibility of collection and interest in data that allow risk-adjustment and interhospital comparisons (18).

V. DISTRIBUTIONS OF PATHOGENS FOR NOSOCOMIAL PNEUMONIA

The distributions of the most commonly reported pathogens associated with nosocomial pneumonia differ between adult and pediatric ICUs, as shown in Figure 3. Although the significance of the common reporting of coagulase-negative *Staphylococci* is unknown for pediatric ICUs, group B streptococci and other streptococcal species are commonly reported as respiratory pathogens in children (19). The predominance of gram-negative pathogens such as *Pseudomonas aeruginosa* among adults is also well described and may relate, in part, to environmental contamination of ventilator circuits (23).

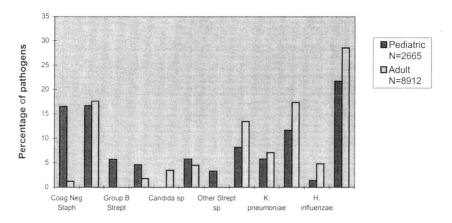

Figure 3 Pathogen distributions in adult and pediatric ICUs, NNIS 1986–1995.

VI. MORBIDITY AND MORTALITY ASSOCIATED WITH NOSOCOMIAL PNEUMONIA

Epidemiological studies evaluating adverse effects of nosocomial infections indicate that pneumonia is the leading cause of death from infections acquired during the hospital stay. Table 3 summarizes six studies that have reported crude mortality rates of ventilator-associated pneumonia ranging from 33% to 71% (20).

Several clinical factors have been associated with a greater risk of mortality, such as severity of underlying disease or age, but there is also a relationship between etiological agents and mortality from nosocomial pneumonia (14). The prognosis associated with aerobic gram-negative bacillary pneumonia is considerably worse than that associated with gram-positive pneumonia, with an 87% mortality rate for bacteriologically documented ventilator-associated pneumonias associated with *Pseudomonas* or *Acinetobacter* species, compared to 55% mortality rate for pneumonias caused by other organisms (21).

Besides the role of pathogens, worsening of respiratory failure caused by nosocomial pneumonia, presence of shock, and an inappropriate antibiotic treatment were associated with higher fatality rate (22). The attributable mortality rate of nosocomial pneumonia is still not known from most of these studies, because of the well-known relationship between severity of illness and pneumonia. In addition, it is difficult to establish whether such critically ill patients would have survived if nosocomial pneumonia had not occurred (9,23). However, more recent studies have further clarified the influence of nosocomial pneumonia on death. Fagon et al. reported that the mortality rate attributable to nosocomial pneumonia exceeded 25%, corresponding to a relative risk of death equal to 2.0, (respectively 40% and 2.5 in cases of pneumonia caused by *Pseudomonas* or *Acinetobacter* species) (24). Bueno-Cavanillas supported these results by reporting that the risk of mortality was almost three times higher in patients with pneumonia than in noninfected patients (relative risk 2.95; CI 95, 1.73–5.03) (25).

VII. COST

Nosocomial pneumonia is also associated with substantial morbidity, and the associated costs are remarkable. According to estimates made by the CDC, an average of 5.9 days of increased length of stay and $5683 in extra hospital charges (in 1992 dollars) result from each episode of nosocomial pneumonia

(9). Published estimates of excess duration of hospitalization attributed to nosocomial pneumonia have ranged from 4 to 13 days, with a median of 7.6 days (26).

REFERENCES

1. Horan TC, White JW, Jarvis WR, et al. Nosocomial infection surveillance, 1984. CDC Surveillance Summaries. MMWR 1986; 35(1SS):17–29.
2. Wenzel RP. Hospital acquired pneumonia: overview of the current state of the art of prevention and control. Eur J Clin Microbiol Infect Dis 1989; 8:56–60.
3. Public health focus: surveillance, prevention, and control of nosocomial infections. MMWR 1992; 41:783–787.
4. Celis R, Torres A, Gatell JM, Almela M, Rodriguez-Roisin R, Augusti-Vidal A. Nosocomial pneumonia: a multivariate analysis of risk and prognosis. Chest 1988; 93:318–324.
5. Cross AS, Roupe B. Role of respiratory assistance devices in endemic nosocomial pneumonia. Am J Med 1981; 70:681–685.
6. Craven DE, Kunches LM, Lichtenberg DA, et al. Nosocomial infection and fatality in medical and surgical intensive care unit patients. Arch Intern Med 1988; 148:1161–1168.
7. Tablan OC, Anderson LJ, Arden NH, et al. Guideline for prevention of nosocomial infection. Respir Care 1994; 39,12:1191–1236.
8. El-ebiary M, Torres A, Gonzalez J, et al. Quantitative cultures of endotracheal aspirates for the diagnosis of ventilator-associated pneumonia. Am Rev Respir Dis 1993; 148:1552–1557.
9. Marquette CH, Georges H, Wallet F, et al. Diagnostic efficiency of endotracheal aspirates with quantitative bacterial cultures in intubated patients with suspected pneumonia. Am Rev Respir Dis 1993; 148:138–144.
10. Horan TC, Emori TG. Definitions of nosocomial infections. In: Abrutyn E, ed. Infection Control Reference Service. Philadelphia: WB Saunders, 1996.
11. Keita-Perse O, Gaynes RP. Severity of illness scoring systems to adjust nosocomial infection rates: a review and commentary. Am J Infect Control 1996; 24:429–434.
12. Kunin CM, McCormick RD. Prevention of catheter-induced urinary-tract infections by sterile closed drainage. N Engl J Med 1996; 274:1155–1161.
13. Maki DG, Goldmann DA, Rhame FS. Infection control in intravenous therapy. Ann Intern Med 1973; 79:867–887.
14. George DL. Epidemiology of nosocomial ventilator-associated pneumonia. Infect Control Hosp Epidemiol 1993; 14:163–169.
15. Gaynes RP, Culver DH, Banerjee S, Edwards JR, Henderson TS. Meaningful

interhospital comparisons of infection rates in intensive care units. Am J Infect Control 1993; 21(1):43–44.

16. Martin SM, Plikaytis BD, Bean NH. Statistical considerations for analysis of nosocomial infection data. In: Bennett JV, Brachman PS, eds. Hospital Infections. Boston: Little, Brown, 1992:135–159.

17. Stamm WE, Weinstein RA, Dixon RE. Comparison of endemic and epidemic nosocomial infections. Am J Med 1981; 70:393–397.

18. Sartor C, Edwards JR, Gaynes RP, Culver DH. Evolution of hospital participation in the National Nosocomial Infections Surveillance System, 1986 to 1993. Am J Infect Control 1995; 23,6:364–368.

19. Levy J. The pediatric patient. In: Wenzel RP, ed. Prevention and Control of Nosocomial Infections. Baltimore: William & Wilkins, 1997:1039–1058.

20. Fagon J-Y, Novara A, Stephan F, Girou E, Safar M. Mortality attributable to nosocomial infections in the ICU. Infect Control Hosp Epidemiol 1994; 15:428–434.

21. Fagon J-Y, Chastre J, Domart Y, et al. Nosocomial pneumonia in patients receiving continuous mechanical ventilation: prospective analysis of 52 episodes with use of a protected specimen brush and quantitative culture techniques. Am Rev Respir Dis 1989; 139:877–884.

22. Torres A, Aznar R, Gatel JM, et al. Incidence, risk, and prognosis factors of nosocomial pneumonia in mechanically ventilated patients. Am Rev Respir Dis 1990; 142:523–528.

23. Craven DE, Kunches LM, Kilinsky V, et al. Risk factors for pneumonia and fatality in patients receiving continuous mechanical ventilation. Am Rev Respir Dis 1986; 133:792–796.

24. Fagon J-Y, Chastre J, Hance AJ, Montravers P, Novara A, Gibert C. Nosocomial pneumonia in ventilated patients: a cohort study evaluating attributable mortality and hospital stay. Am J Med 1993; 94:281–288.

25. Bueno-Cavanillas A, Delgado-Rodriguez M, Lopez-Luque A, et al. Influence of nosocomial infection on mortality rate in an intensive care unit. Crit Care Med 1994; 22:55–60.

26. George DL. Nosocomial pneumonia. In: Mayhall GC, ed. Hospital Epidemiology and Infection Control. Baltimore: Williams & Wilkins, 1996:175–195.

27. Langer M, Mosconi P, Cigada M, Mandelli M. Long-term respiratory support and risk of pneumonia in initially ill patients. Intensive Care Unit Group of Infection Control. Am Rev Respir Dis 1989; 140:302–305.

28. Driks MR, Craven DE, Celli BR, Manning M, Burke RA, et al. Nosocomial pneumonia in intubated patients given sucralfate as compared with antacids or histamine 2 blockers. The role of gastric colonization. N Engl J Med 1987; 317: 1376–1382.

29. Kollef MH. Ventilator-associated pneumonia. A multivariate analysis. JAMA 1993; 270:1965–1970.

3

Host- and Device-Associated Risk Factors for Nosocomial Pneumonia
Cost-Effective Strategies for Prevention

CATHERINE A. FLEMING, KATHLEEN A. STEGER, and DONALD E. CRAVEN

Boston Medical Center
Boston, Massachusetts

I. INTRODUCTION

Nosocomial pneumonia (NP) is defined as an infection of lung parenchyma that was neither present nor incubating at the time of hospital admission. As the second most frequent hospital-acquired infection in the United States, NP accounts for approximately 15% of all hospital-associated infections (1,2). Despite improvements in diagnosis and treatment, the associated mortality and morbidity rates remain high and related costs have been estimated to be about $1.2 billion per year (3).

Nosocomial pneumonia is usually caused by one or more species of bacteria, and less commonly by pathogens such as *Legionella pneumophila*, respiratory viruses, and *Aspergillus fumigatus* (1,2,4). Accurate diagnosis of NP is difficult to make clinically but is essential for differentiating between lower respiratory tract colonization and infection, for interpreting the results of clinical trials, and for formulating appropriate prevention strategies. Meth-

53

ods such as bronchoscopy, blind bronchoalveolar lavage (BAL), protected specimen brush (PSB), and quantitative endotracheal aspiration have dramatically improved the specificity for diagnosing ventilator-associated pneumonia (VAP), although their widespread use may be limited by cost and availability (5–7). Evaluation of these quantitative techniques in terms of their impact on morbidity, mortality, and cost compared to clinical diagnosis and broad-spectrum antibiotic treatment will require further assessment and outcome-based research (8,9).

Epidemiolgical studies have identified specific groups of hospitalized patients who are at particular risk of acquiring NP (6,10–19). This increased susceptibility may reflect endogenous host factors such as age, coexisting illness, and use of medications, or it may result from external factors such as procedures, cross infection, and use of diagnostic or therapeutic devices. Effective prevention involves the recognition of these potential risk factors and the implementation of appropriate preventive strategies (1,2,20). Efficacy of prevention strategies is often difficult to assess because crude mortality rates for NP range from 20% to 50%, and often reflect the severity and acuity of the patient's underlying disease, as well as the difference in prognosis associated with specific pathogens (10,15,17–19,21–25). The mortality rate attributable to pneumonia or "attributable mortality" has been estimated at approximately 30% and may represent a more useful parameter in the evaluation of prevention policies. However, this mortality rate may vary according to the diagnostic methods used and the appropriateness of the initial antibiotic therapy (15,21,26).

Radical changes in current health care practices, leading to decreased length of stay and increased outpatient management, may result in a decreased incidence of nosocomial infections. However, earlier discharge from hospital may also result in the blurring of distinctions between community-acquired and hospital-acquired infections, while changing the rates and the natural history of hospital-acquired pneumonia. Accurate evaluation of the merits and cost effectiveness of preventive strategies may require a revision of the definition of nosocomial infections to "health care facility"—acquired infections, which would include nursing homes and other long-term care facilities.

This chapter reviews the risk factors for NP, classifying them as host or device related, and correlates each group with appropriate preventive strategies. Interventions should be feasible, cost effective, and based on good scientific data. In view of the higher incidence and mortality rates of NP in mechanically ventilated patients, this subset of patients is given special attention. Particular emphasis is directed at bacterial pathogens and a brief overview is

Table 1 Host-Associated Risk Factors and Preventive Measures for Nosocomial Pneumonia Caused by Bacteria

Risk factor	Preventive measure	CDC/ HICPAC[a]	Kollef category (VAP)*
Age >60	Primary prevention; health care maintenance	NS	NS
Smoking	Smoking cessation	NS	NS
Underlying disease	Treat COPD; incentive spirometry	II	NS
	Influenza, pneumococcal vaccination	IA	D
Immunosuppression	Taper steroids	NS	NS
	Minimize duration of neutropenia ± G-CSF	NS	D
	Reduce exposure to nosocomial pathogens	NS	NS
HIV/AIDS	See text	NS	NS
Immobility	Lateral rotational bed	NR	B
Depressed consciousness	Cautious use of CNS depressants	NS	NS
	Position patient upright at 30°–45°	1B/1A**	B/A
Medications:			
Antibiotics	Antibiotic prophylaxis for NP not recommended	IA	B
	Judicious administration of antibiotics	NS	C
Sedatives	Judicious administration	NS	NS
Neuromuscular blockers	Judicious administration	NS	NS
Stress bleeding prophylaxis	Use of nonalkylinating cytoprotective agents	II	NS
	Use only when specifically indicated	NS	B
Abdominal/thoracic surgery	Adequate analgesia	IB	NS
	Encourage coughing and deep breathing	IB	NS
Ororpharyngeal/gastric colonization	Avoid selective decontamination of digestive tract	NR	B

[a] Centers for Disease Control and Prevention/Hospital Infection Control Practices Advisory Committee (CDC/ HICPAC) guidelines: Category IA is ''strongly recommended for all hospitals and strongly supported by well-designed experimental or epidemiologic studies.'' Category IB is ''strongly recommended for all hospitals and viewed as effective by experts in the field and a consensus of HICPAC based on strong rationale and suggestive evidence, even though definitive scientific studies may not have been done.'' Category II is ''suggested for implementation in many hospitals. Recommendations may be supported by suggestive clinical or epidemiologic studies, a strong theoretical rationale, or definitive studies applicable to some but not all hospitals.'' No recommendation (NR); unresolved issue is defined as practices for which insufficient evidence or consensus regarding efficacy exists.''
NS = not specified in HICPAC or Kollef guideline; COPD = chronic obstructive pulmonary disease; G-CSF = granulocyte–colony-stimulating factor; CNS = central nervous system; NP = nosocomial pneumonia.
* See Appendix on p. 80 for Kollef grading scheme.
** Recommendation upgraded by new data since original recommendation.

provided for more unusual pathogens such as *Legionella*, viruses, and fungi. The discussion of prevention focuses primarily on those measures discussed in the Centers for Disease Control and Prevention (CDC) and the Hospital Infection Control Practices Advisory Committee (HICPAC) ''1994 Guideline for the Prevention of Hospital-Acquired Pneumonia'' (2). This guideline was reviewed and approved by experts from a number of important infection control, pulmonary, and infectious disease organizations, and is the most comprehensive prevention document currently available. CDC/HICPAC classification categories IA, 1B, II, and NR are defined in Table 1 and are based on the merit of the relevant data available in the medical literature as of 1994. The category ''not specified'' (NS) has been added to denote recommendations that merit consideration but are not specified in the CDC/HICPAC guideline or other areas of prevention. In addition we have included Kollef's recommendations for the prevention of ventilator associated pneumonia (VAP) where appropriate (183; Appendix).

II. TARGETS FOR INTERVENTION

Although NP may result from bacteremia or inhalation of bacteria-containing aerosols, aspiration of bacteria colonizing the oropharynx or stomach is the most frequent route of infection and therefore an equally important target for prevention (Fig. 1) (24,27–33). Time of onset of hospital acquired pneumonia (HAP), prior hospitalization, and previous antibiotic therapy should also be considered in targeting prevention strategies. Early onset HAP, usually occurring during the first 4 days of the hospital stay, is more likely to be caused by *Streptococcus pneumoniae*, *Moraxella catarrhalis*, *Haemophilus influenzae*, or *anaerobes* (12,29,34–36). Conversely, late-onset bacterial pneumonia is more commonly caused by *Staphylococcus aureus* and gram-negative bacilli such as *Klebsiella*, *Acinetobacter* spp., or *Pseudomonas aeruginosa* (Table 2) (34,35,37).

Factors that predispose a patient to aspiration include host factors such as impaired consciousness or recent thoracoabdominal surgery and external factors such as respiratory or gastrointestinal tract instrumentation and mechanical ventilation (27,29–31,38–40). Host factors, medications, devices, and breeches in infection control all have an impact on bacterial colonization of the pharynx and trachea. In some mechanically ventilated patients, the stomach and gastrointestinal tract may affect oropharyngeal and tracheal colonization with gram-negative bacilli (24,31,39,41–48).

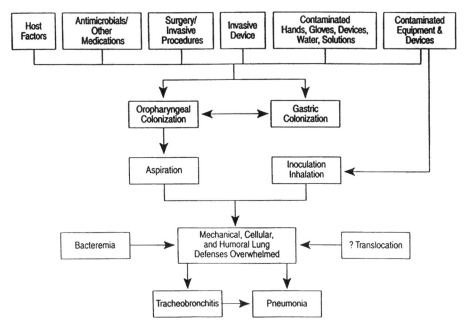

Figure 1 Summary of risk factors contributing to colonization and infection of the lower respiratory tract. Important risk factors include the inoculum and virulence of the infecting agents, response of the pulmonary host defenses in the lung. (From Ref. 181, with permission.)

Most identified risk factors for bacterial NP affect colonization, aspiration, or both. The likelihood that NP will develop depends on the presence of predisposing risk factors and the individual's pulmonary host defenses (e.g., mechanical removal, humoral factors, cytokines, and cellular defenses) (49–53).

III. HOST FACTORS

A. Medical Patients

Risk factors for bacterial nosocomial pneumonia have been identified by several large studies (10,11,14–17,22,36,39,54–56) (see Table 1). The presence of advanced age, underlying diseases, immune suppression, and malnutrition

Table 2 Selected Pathogens Commonly Associated with Bacterial Nosocomial
Pneumonia Classified by Time of Onset

Pathogens	Rate[a]	Comments
Early-onset		
Streptococcus pneumoniae (*Pneumococcus*)	5%–15%	Person–person spread documented; penicillin resistant and MDR strains problematic; subtyping and antibiograms helpful to document transmission
Haemophilis influenzae (type b and nontypeable)	<5%	Nosocomial outbreaks reported in pediatric and elderly patients
Anaerobes	0%–35%	Rare cause of VAP
Late-onset		
Aerobic gram-negative bacilli: (*Pseudomonas aeruginosa, Escherichia coli, Enterobacter* spp., *Acinetobacter* spp., *Klebsiella pneumoniae, Serratia marcescens*)	40%–60%	Endogenous colonization and nosocomial transmission; present in food, water, and enteral feedings; on hands of hospital personnel, equipment, and devices; MDR strains are of concern; molecular typing helpful in understanding epidemiology
Staphylococcus aureus	20%–40%	Sources include patients, hospital personnel, fomites; molecular typing useful; MRSA frequently seen
Legionella pneumophilia	0%–10%	Sources include potable water, showers, faucets, cooling towers

[a] Crude rates of pneumonia taken in part from CDC's data and may vary in part by hospital, patient population, and method of diagnosis.
Abbreviations: MDR = multidrug resistant; VAP = ventilator-associated pneumonia; MRSA = methicillin-resistant *S. aureus*
Source: Adapted from Ref. 76.

are associated with an increased risk of development of NP. Colonization with gram-negative bacteria is significantly increased in patients with hypotension, acidosis, azotemia, alcoholism, diabetes mellitus, leukopenia, or pulmonary disease (27,38,40,57,58). Conditions such as advanced age, being a smoker, malnutrition, severe illness, or postoperative state may increase the adherence of bacteria to oropharyngeal and respiratory tract epithelial cells (59–64).

Gastric colonization may result from increased gastric pH, which may facilitate bacterial multiplication (24,32,43,44,46,48,65–71). This is seen in elderly patients, in those with achlorhydria, ileus, and upper gastrointestinal disease, or in patients receiving antacids or enteral feeding. Aspiration is more likely to occur in immobilized patients and in those who have had recent surgery or who have decreased consciousness (42,67,72,73). Finally, these patients may be less able to mount a specific host response. This combination of risk factors, while difficult to modify, should alert the clinician to the potential for NP and the need to minimize exposure to additional risk factors.

Selected simple, cost-effective measures, the implementation of which should decrease the incidence of NP in susceptible persons, are summarized in Table 1 (1,2,74,75). It is recommended that pneumococcal and influenza vaccinations be offered to all persons 65 years of age or older or those with chronic underlying disease. Optimizing health care maintenance strategies may decrease the need for hospital admission. Smoking cessation should be encouraged in all patients and particularly in those in whom elective surgery is planned. Patients with chronic obstructive pulmonary disease may benefit from incentive spirometry, positive end-expiratory pressure, or continuous positive airway pressure by face mask (1,2,74,75).

B. Surgical Patients

Postoperative patients, notably those who have undergone thoracic or abdominal surgery, or who have underlying chronic obstructive airways disease, are at particularly high risk of NP (1,2,74,75). Bacterial pathogens may enter the airway during intubation or after aspiration. Sedation, an anesthetized airway after extubation, vomiting, recumbent position, and head and neck, abdominal, and thoracic surgery are all significant risk factors for aspiration (184). Postoperative atelectasis, retained secretions, and pain may all increase the risk of NP by impairing the host's ability to clear bacteria and secretions effectively.

Preventive measures to reduce the risk of NP include maintaining semiupright patient position to reduce aspiration, frequent coughing, chest physiotherapy, and early ambulation to prevent atelectasis and retained secretions. Deep breathing exercises, incentive spirometry, and intermittent positive pressure breathing (IPPB) may benefit patients with underlying pulmonary dysfunction. Effective pain control also facilitates coughing and the expectoration of aspirated secretions (2).

Immobilized trauma patients are at high risk of development of hospital-acquired infections, including pneumonia. Kinetic or lateral rotational beds are hypothesized to increase tidal volume and improve the drainage of secretions in the lungs by intermittent or continuous rotation on the longitudinal axis (76–79). Studies looking at the benefit of kinetic beds in preventing pneumonia have yielded variable results, and this issue was classified as unresolved (NR) in the CDC/HICPAC guidelines.

C. Acquired Immunodeficiency Syndrome

Acquired immunodeficiency syndrome (AIDS) patients may be at greater risk of development of NP because they may have underlying medical diseases, prior antibiotic therapy, invasive devices, surgery, or mechanical ventilation, as well as concurrent intravenous drug use and neutropenia (80–84). The use of trimethoprim-sulfamethoxazole for *Pneumocystis carinii* pneumonia (PCP) prophylaxis may decrease bacterial colonization and infection rates but may predispose to infection with multi-drug resistant (MDR) organisms (85–87). Gram-negative bacilli and *S. aureus* are common in patients who have been hospitalized previously or have received broad-spectrum antibiotics, and community-acquired respiratory pathogens such as pneumococcus and *H. influenzae* may be acquired and transmitted among immunosuppressed hospitalized patients (1,88,89). Much attention has recently been focused on the high incidence, relapse rate, and mortality rate of pseudomonal infections in AIDS patients (90–92). Risk factors for pseudomonal infection among patients infected with human immunodeficiency virus (HIV) include advanced HIV disease, presence of central venous catheter, urinary catheter, and steroid therapy (93,94).

Nosocomial outbreaks of *Mycobacterium tuberculosis* infection (MTB) involving HIV-infected persons have been characterized by high attack and mortality rates, rapid progression to active disease, and significant spread to both patients and health care workers (95,96). Factors that contributed to these outbreaks include an increasing number of HIV-infected patients exposed to MTB and delays in proper isolation, diagnosis, and treatment (97,98). Prevention guidelines published by the Centers for Disease Control (CDC) stress early identification of active disease, prompt isolation, and expeditious initiation of effective therapy (97). In addition, routine skin testing for MTB exposure among health care workers is recommended as is contact investigation and appropriate preventive therapy following an exposure (99).

Clusters or hospital outbreaks of PCP in the United States were initially reported in immunosuppressed children and more recently in patients with AIDS. Several studies have suggested possible nosocomial transmission between AIDS patients and other immuncompromised patients sharing the same waiting rooms in outpatient clinics (100,101). Although these data are inconclusive, there is circumstantial evidence to support implementation of precautions designed to prevent the nosocomial spread of *P. carinii* among immunosuppressed patients.

Immunosuppressed patients are at increased risk of acquiring unusual nosocomial infections including aspergillosis, legionellosis, and viral infections, which are discussed later. To avoid infectious complications in all immunosuppressed patients, the intensity and duration of immunosuppression and neutropenia should be minimized whenever possible and exposure to potential nosocomial pathogens should be avoided. Although the use of granulocyte colony-stimulating factors is controversial, it may be indicated in prolonged neutropenia.

IV. MEDICATIONS

A. Antibiotics

The use of antibiotics to prevent NP in susceptible patients is controversial. Clearly, some antibiotics have had a role in reducing colonization with early onset pathogens such as *S. pneumoniae* and *H. influenzae* (14,22,34,102). Thus, although broad-spectrum antibiotics, such as cephalosporins, may decrease the risk of early onset HAP, they may, in turn, increase the prevalence of colonization and infection resulting from nosocomial, MDR pathogens (10,22,34,102).

Given the risk of superinfection, antibiotics should be used judiciously, particularly in intensive care unit (ICU) patients who are at high risk for development of pneumonia (103). Controlling antibiotic use in sites such as the ICU is frequently associated with a decrease in patient colonization and incidence of infections with MDR pathogens (104–106). In accordance with the CDC/HICPAC guideline, we also discourage the use of prophylactic antibiotics for HAP. We advocate treatment of NP as outlined in the American Thoracic Society guidelines (8). However, with the increasing prevalence of MDR nosocomial infections, more stringent and widespread control of antibiotic use may become necessary (107).

Combinations of local and systemic antibiotics for selective decontamination of the digestive tract (SDD) have been advocated to reduce or prevent HAP and other nosocomial infections (108–114). The SDD often uses combinations of nonabsorbable antibiotics, such as aminoglycoside, polymyxin B, and amphotericin B in a paste, which is applied to the oropharynx, and a liquid, which is given orally, with and without systemic cefotaxime, trimethoprim, or a quinolone. Several studies and review articles of SDD report dramatically reduced rates of respiratory tract colonization and infection, but these studies are difficult to compare because of differences in study design and study population, and inconsistent definitions of respiratory tract infection that could include tracheobronchitis (108–110). The potential effect of SDD to facilitate the emergence of MDR strains of bacteria raises further concerns about its risk-benefit ratio (110–115). In accordance with the CDC/HICPAC recommendation for SDD, we do not advocate its routine use.

B. Sedatives

Sedatives may increase the risk of aspiration and decrease cough and clearance of secretions from the lower respiratory tract. This effect is profound in elderly patients or those with impaired swallowing. Prevention strategies should include judicious use of sedation and proper positioning of patients in a semirecumbant position to minimize the risk of aspiration. In mechanically ventilated patients, the use of sedatives may influence clinical outcome. Barrientos-Vega et al. recently reported that propofol decreased weaning time and was economically more favorable than midazolam (116). Although more studies are required, it appears that careful use of sedatives may decrease the incidence of NP in both ventilated and nonventilated patients.

C. Neuromuscular Blockers

Limited data are available on neuromuscular blockers as a risk factor for VAP. In a retrospective review of severely head-injured patients, the occurrence of pneumonia was significantly higher (29% versus 15%) in those patients pharmacologically paralyzed on admission compared to the nonparalyzed group. The implications of this study, however, are limited by its design and the absence of uniform diagnostic criteria for pneumonia. Prekates and co-workers recently studied risk factors for VAP (diagnosed by bronchoscopy with PSB and BAL) in 92 postoperative trauma patients (117). Ventilator-associated pneumonia occurred in 23% of these patients. Independent predictors of VAP, after stepwise logistic regression, were flail chest ($p < 0.001$) and the use of neuromuscular blockers ($p < 0.001$). In the absence of additional data, it is difficult to make specific recommendations regarding the use of neuromuscular blocking agents. Although prospective randomized studies are needed to further evaluate this issue, we suggest these drugs should be used cautiously after sedation and analgesia has been maximized in accordance with the practice guidelines recently published by the Society of Critical Care Medicine (118).

D. Stress Bleeding Prophylaxis

Antacids and histamine type 2 (H_2) blockers are frequently administered for prevention of stress bleeding in critically ill patients. The possibility that these agents predispose patients to NP is controversial. The benefits of prescribing stress bleeding prophylaxis in ICU patients is an unresolved issue, and the specific indications need to be determined (119). Several studies have reported significantly lower rates of clinically diagnosed VAP in patients given prophylaxis with sucralfate, a nonalkylinating cytoprotective agent that may have bactericidal activity (24,35,120–125). In the largest study to date, sucralfate had the greatest effect on reducing late-onset VAP; no difference was noted for early onset VAP (35). The differences in outcomes among groups given sucralfate, antacids, and H_2 blockers may be related to gastric pH, reflux, level of bacterial overgrowth, or the bactericidal activity of sucralfate (24,35,47,48,70,121,126,127). Other investigators have observed no difference in rates of VAP in patients given either antacids and/or H_2 blockers or sucralfate (28,32,46,47). Bonten and coworkers, in a double-blind study using bronchoscopy and quantitative cultures for diagnosis, reported no difference in rates of VAP between patients given prophylaxis with sucralfate versus antacids, and concluded that the stomach was not an important contributor to the pathogenesis of VAP (46,47). However, the dose of antacids was lower than in other studies and patients were not stratified by time of onset of VAP. The CDC/HICPAC guideline suggests that, if stress bleeding prophylaxis is indicated, nonalkylinating agents should be used (category II) (2).

V. DEVICE-ASSOCIATED RISK FACTORS

Devices that circumvent host defenses and facilitate the transmission of bacteria into the lung have been identified as risk factors for NP (17,22,24,29–31,35,41,55,59,74,128) (Tables 3 and 4). This includes devices in contact with the respiratory tract for diagnostic purposes (e.g., bronchoscopes) or therapeutic purposes (e.g., endotracheal tubes, nebulizers). Devices are readily colonized by nosocomial bacteria with transmission frequently occurring by way of contaminated hands of health care workers from other patients, devices, or other body sites of the same patient. Certain devices also predispose the patient

Table 3 Device-Associated Risk Factors and Preventive Measures for Nosocomial
Pneumonia Caused by Bacteria

Risk factor	Preventive measure	CDC/ HICPAC[a]	Kollef category (VAP)*
Enteral feeding	Verify tube placement	IB	NS
	Use sterile water	NS	NS
	Use orogastric tube if possible	NS	D
	Position patient at 30°–45°	IB	B
	Remove residual	IB	NS
Oxygen delivery system	Change tubing between patients	IB	NS
Invasive devices	Appropriate cleaning and sterilization	IA	NS
	Expeditious removal	IB	C
Spirometer	Clean; sterilize/disinfect between patients	IB	NS
Temperature/O₂ sensor	Clean; sterilize/disinfect between patients	IB	NS
Resuscitation bag	Clean; sterilize/disinfect between patients	IA	NS
Bronchoscopy	Judicious use	NS	NS
Endotracheal intubation	See Table 4		
Tracheostomy care	Aseptic technique when changing tube	IB	NS
Cross infection	Educate and train personnel	IA	NS
	Surveillance with feedback to staff	IA	NS
	Handwashing, use of gloves and gowns	IA	B

[a] CDC/HICPAC guideline criteria as defined in Table 1.
* Kollef guidelines as defined in Appendix, p. 80.

to aspiration and gastric reflux (Fig. 2). Bacteria may also directly enter the
lower respiratory tract as aerosols generated by contaminated respiratory therapy equipment.

Mechanically ventilated patients are exposed to multiple devices and
are at particular risk of development of ventilator-associated pneumonia
(VAP), the risk of which is proportional to the duration of assisted ventilation
(see Table 4). The rates of nosocomial infections may be influenced by the
type of intensive care unit in which the patient undergoes treatment, with
higher rates observed in surgical intensive care than in medical ICU patients
(22,129,130). We examine specific devices that have been associated with NP

Table 4 Ventilator-Associated Risk Factors and Preventive Measures for Nosocomial Pneumonia

Risk factor	Preventive measure	CDC/ HICPAC[a]	Kollef category (VAP)*
Endotracheal intubation	Keep cuff pressure optimal; aspirate sub-glottic secretions before deflating cuff	IB	C
	CASS	NR[b]	A
	Oral intubation	NR[b]	D
	Semirecumbent patient positioning	IB	B/A**
Ventilator circuit	Do not change more often than every 48 hours	IA	A
	Drain/discard condensate away from patients	IB	C
	Use heat-moisture exchanger	NR	A
In-line medication/ nebulizer	Disinfect between treatments; sterilize between patients	IB	NS
Tracheal suction catheter	Aseptic technique	IA	NS
	Sterile single-use catheter for open system	11	NS
	Closed-circuit tracheal suction catheter	NR	NS

[a] CDC/HICPAC guideline criteria as defined in Table 1.
[b] We suggest that CASS and oral intubation should be implemented whenever possible.
Abbreviation: CASS = continuous aspiration of subglottic secretions.
* Kollef guidelines defined in Appendix, p. 80.
** Recommendation upgraded by new data since original recommendation.

and recommend strategies to minimize those risks. Appropriate cleaning and sterilization or disinfection of reusable equipment is mandatory. We also consider the issue of cross infection by health care workers because this greatly influences the incidence and bacteriology of device-related pneumonia.

A. Nasogastric and Orogastric Tubes and Enteral Feeding

Many critically ill patients have a nasogastric tube in place to manage secretions, prevent gastric distention, or provide nutritional support. Placement of a nasogastric tube may increase nasopharyngeal colonization, cause reflux of gastric contents, and act as a conduit for bacteria to migrate to the oropharynx (see Table 3) (16,128,131,132).

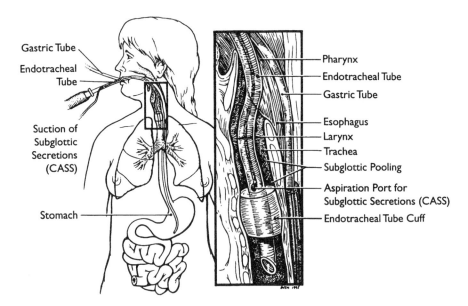

Figure 2   Example of an intubated patient with continuous aspiration of subglottic secretions as reported by Valles and coworkers (29). Removal of subglottic secretions decreases colonization of the trachea and the risk of ventilator-associated pneumonia. This system has recently become available in the United States. Ideally, an endotracheal tube is preferred to a nasotracheal tube and placing the gastric tube through the mouth rather than the nose may reduce the risk of nosocomial sinusitis and pneumonia. (From Ref. 20, with permission.)

The administration of enteral feedings may also predispose the patient to NP (72,133–135). Feedings may become contaminated during preparation, as illustrated by a recent case report describing a cluster of ventilator-associated. *P. aeruginosa* respiratory infections, the investigation of which implicated contaminated food coloring dye (45). Enteral feeding may also elevate gastric pH, leading to colonization and gastric distention, and thus increasing the risk of reflux and aspiration (2,134,135). Gastric reflux and aspiration are common in hospitalized patients (1,31,43,72,73,136–138). In one study, oropharyngeal reflux was described in approximately 70% of patients receiving tube feedings, 40% of whom had evidence of pulmonary aspiration (137). However, enteral feeding, when compared with parenteral nutrition, appears to reduce the risk of nosocomial pneumonia, and early initiation of enteral feeding may help maintain the gastrointestinal epithelium and prevent bacterial translocation (138–140).

To minimize the risk of NP associated with enteral feeds, we recommend the routine use of sterile water for the preparation of both feeds and nasogastric tube flushes, because tap water may be a potential source of nosocomial gram-negative bacilli, *Legionella*, and mycobacterium avium–intracellular complex (MAC) (45,133). Measures that may decrease the risk of regurgitation include monitoring residual volume in the stomach and removal of gastric residual if the volume is large or bowel sounds are not auscultated (2,22,31,137,141). Maintaining the patient in a semiupright position may reduce reflux, aspiration, and NP (22,31,138,184). Enteral feeding remains a controversial treatment with many unresolved issues such as the use of continuous versus intermittent enteral feeding, the need to acidify enteral feedings, and the optimal site and position of the feeding tube (2,135,141). Placement of an orogastric tube may be preferable to nasogastric intubation to reduce sinusitis and possibly pneumonia as discussed later.

B. Endotracheal Tube

The risk of development of NP is increased 4- to 21-fold for intubated patients and increases with the duration of mechanical ventilation (2,16,25,55). The incidence has been estimated to be 6 to 52 cases per 100 patients, depending on the population studied, and results in a 2- to 10-fold increase in mortality rate and a two- to three-fold increase in hospital stay (142,143). Identification and implementation of preventive measures could greatly affect ICU mortality and morbidity rates but also have a favorable cost-benefit ratio. However, as reintubation has also been shown to be a risk factor for VAP, early extubation to minimize duration of ventilation must be weighed against the risk of reintubation (144).

An endotracheal tube facilitates the entry of bacteria into the trachea, decreases clearance of bacteria and secretions from the lower airway, and acts as a surface on which bacteria may collect and form a protective biofilm (1,16,25,29,30,128,136,145,146). Leakage around the endotracheal tube cuff enables pooled secretions and bacteria to enter the trachea, increasing tracheal colonization and leading to VAP (see Fig. 2). Maintaining appropriate cuff pressures may also decrease leakage of pooled subglottic secretions into the trachea and prevent VAP (102). In a recent study by Rello and coworkers, there was a significantly higher rate of VAP noted in patients who failed the continuous aspiration of subglottic secretions (CASS) technique during the first 8 days of mechanical ventilation, and there was a trend toward a higher risk of VAP for patients with cuff pressures <20 cm H_2O (102). These data underscore the importance of maintaining adequate cuff pressure to reduce aspiration around the endotracheal tube cuff.

Attention has been focused on the possible benefit of manual intermittent or continuous aspiration of subglottic secretions to decrease colonization and the risk of VAP. Mahul et al. reported that the occurrence of VAP was both decreased and delayed using manual intermittent aspiration of subglottic secretions (30). An endotracheal tube that incorporates a dorsal separate lumen ending in the subglottic area and that opens above the cuff allowing continuous aspiration of secretions is available in the United States. Valles et al. reported that CASS significantly reduced the incidence of VAP from 39.6 episodes per 1000 days in control subjects to 19.6 episodes per 1000 ventilator-days in the CASS group with infections in the CASS group occurring on average 6 days later (29). Efficacy was most pronounced during the first 2 weeks after intubation. In 85% of infections, the causative organism was previously isolated in cultures of subglottic secretions, indicating their importance in the pathogenesis of VAP. Although CASS was classified as an unresolved issue in the CDC/HICPAC recommendations, we suggest that it be adopted based on the excellent risk and cost-benefit ratio.

Colonization of the surface of the endotracheal tube may be an important risk factor for VAP (145,146). Many endotracheal tubes become rapidly colonized with nosocomial pathogens encased in a biofilm that protects bacteria from both antibiotics and host defense (145,146). These aggregates of bacteria may become dislodged from the endotracheal tube by ventilation flow, tracheal suctioning, or bronchoscopy, then embolize to the lower respiratory tract. More than 95% of the endotracheal tubes examined by scanning electron microscopy in one study had partial bacterial colonization and 84% were completely covered by bacteria encased in a biofilm or glucocalyx (145). Research is in progress to alter the composition of the endotracheal tube to be more resistant to colonization and biofilm formation. However, more simple measures such as gentle tracheal suctioning and the use of aseptic technique to reduce cross contamination may also reduce the incidence of VAP.

C. Nasal Intubation and Sinusitis

Nasotracheal intubation and placement of a nasogastric tube are underappreciated risk factors for nosocomial sinusitis and VAP (128,147). The association between the development of sinusitis and VAP is difficult to demonstrate. However, the presence of sinusitis has been shown to be associated with a substantial increase in the number of nosocomial pathogens that are identified in patients with VAP. In a study by Rouby and coworkers, maxillary sinusitis, diagnosed by baseline and serial computer axial tomographic scan and needle aspiration, was linked to the placement and duration of nasotracheal and nasogastric intubation (128). Ventilator-associated pneumonia occurred significantly more frequently in the patients with maxillary sinusitis. In addition, the most common organisms isolated from maxillary sinus aspirates were *P. aeruginosa*, *Acinetobacter* spp., *S. aureus*, and *Candida albicans*, correlating well with organisms causing VAP. Finally, placement of orotracheal and orogastric tubes significantly decreased the incidence of bacterial maxillary sinusitis. Although demonstrating a causal link between the presence of sinusitis and VAP is difficult, we believe the association makes intuitive sense and that orotracheal and orogastric intubation should be preferentially performed whenever possible.

D. Ventilator Tubing Condensate and Heat–Moisture Exchangers

Mechanical ventilators that have heated bubble humidifiers generate condensate as a result of the difference in temperatures of the inspired gas and the ambient air (148). The tubing and condensate are rapidly colonized with the patient's oropharyngeal flora, resulting in bacterial concentrations of 10^3 to 10^6 organisms/mL. The contaminated condensate can enter the respiratory tract when the tubing is manipulated, resulting in VAP. To minimize this risk, reflux of condensate should be avoided by educating health care workers to drain condensate away from the patient and to routinely wash their hands after handling the condensate. Other tools that decrease the incidence of VAP include heated ventilator tubing, which significantly reduces condensate formation, and heat–moisture exchangers (HMEs), which eliminate tubing condensate (2,20,74) (Fig. 3).

Heat–moisture exchangers recycle exhaled moisture and heat, eliminating the need for a humidifier and avoiding formation of circuit condensate (2,149). Heat–moisture exchangers are well tolerated by most patients, easy to use, and particularly useful in postoperative or lower risk patients who require less humidity (150). Recently, Kirton et al. conducted a prospective randomized trial comparing HME with heated wire humidifiers in mechanically ventilated trauma patients. The incidence of nosocomial VAP in the HME group was 6% compared to 16% for the conventional humidifier ($p <$ 0.05); the total number of ICU days was also significantly reduced in the HME group and disposable ventilator circuit costs were reduced (151). In addition, the incidence of partial endotracheal tube occlusion was not significantly different between the groups. Heat–moisture exchangers may, therefore, be a

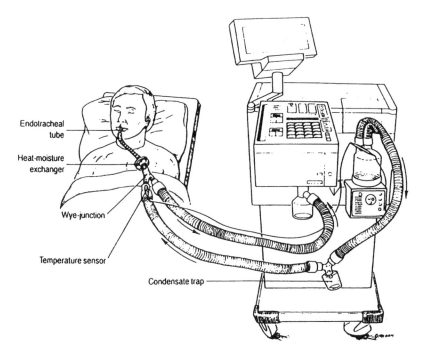

Figure 3 Mechanically ventilated patient in the upright position. The ventilator hu-
midifies the air which is carried through the inspiratory tubing to the wye junction into
the endotracheal tube and the patient's lower respiratory tract. The humidified air is
expired out the expiratory phase tube to a "trap." If a heat–moisture exchanger (HME)
is inserted between the swivel adapter and wye junction, the humidifier can be turned
off and there is no condensate in the circuit. (From Ref. 181, with permission.)

cost-effective way to decrease the incidence of VAP in specific groups of
patients.

   The effect of changing ventilator tubing in the prevention of VAP has
been explored. There appears to be no advantage in changing ventilator circuits more frequently than every 48 hours. Furthermore, we support the current
data suggesting that they may not need to be changed at all (2,152–154).

E. Bronchoscopy

Bronchoscopy is frequently performed in mechanically ventilated patients for
diagnostic purposes, or to remove mucous plugs or excessive secretions. Three

studies have addressed the possibility that bronchoscopy may predispose to NP in mechanically ventilated patients. In the first study, bronchoscopy, performed for therapeutic lavage, was identified as a risk factor for HAP (56). More recently, Pujol et al. reported that bronchoscopy was an independent risk factor in the development of methicillin-resistant *S. aureus* (MRSA) VAP, although it is possible that this may be biased because the indication for the bronchoscopy was not cited (155). Finally, Sanchez-Nieto et al. recently conducted a pilot study in which 51 patients suspected of having VAP were randomized to receive either quantitative endotracheal aspirate (QEA) with bronchoscopy and bronchoalveolar lavage (group A) or QEA alone (group B). The observed crude mortality rate was 46% in group A and 26% in group B, and the adjusted mortality rate was 29% and 10%, respectively. Although these differences are not statistically significant, possibly reflecting the small sample size, they suggest a trend toward increased mortality rate in ventilated patients undergoing bronchoscopy (9).

Several factors could explain the possible association between bronchoscopy and VAP, including the use of large volumes of BAL that impede the clearance of bacteria from the lower respiratory tract and the introduction of nosocomial pathogens into the lower airway by dislodging bacterial aggregates from the endotracheal tube surface. As discussed previously, when bacteria encased in biofilm embolize to different areas of the lung, they may be particularly difficult for host defenses to clear effectively (145,146). These pathogenic mechanisms are theoretical, and prospective clinical studies are required to evaluate the actual risk of bronchoscopy in ventilated patients.

F. Nebulizers and Miscellaneous Respiratory Therapy Equipment

Small volume "in-line" medication nebulizers, which are inserted into the mechanical ventilator circuit, are readily colonized from contaminated condensate and allow bacterial aerosols direct access to the lower airway, bypassing the normal host defenses (1,156,157). Both hand-held and "in-line" should be sterilized between patients and their use limited to clear indications.

Appropriate cleaning and sterilization or disinfection of all reusable respiratory therapy equipment is essential to reduce transmission of infectious agents. Resuscitation bags, spirometers, temperature sensors, and oxygen analyzers, if not properly sterilized or if transferred between patients, are also potential sources of cross infection (1,2,158,159). In summary, respiratory therapy devices should not be transferred between patients and proper cleaning and sterilization is strongly recommended.

Tracheal suction catheters may inoculate bacteria directly into the respiratory tract and aseptic technique, including wearing gloves, is recommended during suctioning. A closed multiuse suction system may be more convenient than a single-use catheter and it may cause less hypoxia for the patient, but it has not been shown to decrease the risk of VAP (2,160).

VI. CROSS INFECTION FROM PATIENTS AND STAFF

Gram-negative bacilli and *S. aureus*, the organisms most commonly responsible for NP, are ubiquitous in hospitals but concentrate in intensive care units (129,161–163). These organisms may colonize in persons with impaired host defenses, or devices may become contaminated. Pathogens are transmitted on the hands or gloves of hospital personnel, with procedures such as suctioning and manipulation of devices increasing the risk of cross contamination (1). Organisms may also be spread from device to patient, from patient to patient, or from one body site to the respiratory tract of the same patient by way of device or hand. Cross colonization or cross infection is a key mechanism in the pathogenesis of nosocomial infection and the spread of highly resistant pathogens. Handwashing before and after patient contact is an effective means of removing transient bacteria, but, because of poor compliance with handwashing among hospital personnel, some investigators have advocated the use of barrier precautions (gloves and gowns) for contact with all patients. This practice has been associated with significantly decreased rates of nosocomial infections in pediatric intensive care units (164). Care must be taken to change gloves between patients because they may become colonized, and handwashing is still required because even gloved hands may be contaminated by way of leaks (1).

Previous studies have indicated that hospitals with effective surveillance and infection control programs have rates of pneumonia 20% lower than hospitals without such programs (2). Effective targeted surveillance for high-risk patients, coupled with staff education, use of proper isolation techniques, and effective infection control practices, is the cornerstone for the prevention of nosocomial pneumonia (1,162,165).

Sherertz et al. reported a nosocomial outbreak of MRSA in which epidemiological investigation identified a colonized physician who shed MRSA in association with a viral upper respiratory infection (URI), illustrating the role of surveillance and epidemiological investigation in halting an outbreak (166). Because of the changes in the health care system and the increasing impact of managed care programs, infection control staff have been decreased. We recommend that targeted surveillance of high-risk areas, such as the intensive care units, remain a priority and that ICU staff should be involved in collection and analysis of surveillance data, with prompt feedback of results. Monitoring of MDR pathogens and device-related infections should be carried out throughout the hospital (1).

VII. SPECIAL PATHOGENS

A. *Legionella pneumophila*

L. pneumophila is an important cause of nosocomial pneumonia, although the incidence is underestimated because sputum culture, serology, and/or urinary antigen test for *Legionella* are not routinely performed (2,133,167–172). Underlying disease, particularly end-stage renal disease, hematological malignancies, cytoxic chemotherapy, and advanced age, are all associated with an increased risk of acquiring *Legionella* pneumonia (Table 5). Because *Legionella* is not spread person to person, the occurrence of cases in an institution indicates an environmental source, which, if not identified and addressed, may result in more cases. The organism is ubiquitous in water and may be increased during active construction around the hospital. Nosocomial legionellosis has been traced to airborne spread of organisms from contaminated cooling towers (2,133,168,173). Inhalation of aerosols from showers, faucets, and respiratory therapy equipment, and aspiration of contaminated potable water have all been proposed as methods of transmission (2).

To prevent nosocomial legionellosis, a high index of suspicion must be directed at all cases of nosocomial pneumonia with appropriate testing and access to a specialized laboratory being required. The CDC/HICPAC has recently published guidelines for prevention of legionellosis (2). Although some investigators have suggested routine environmental sampling of hospital water supply, CDC/HICPAC recommends culturing potable water if nosocomial cases are observed (173). Periodic cleaning and hyperchlorination of cooling towers are also recommended with careful evaluation of the location of hospital air intake vents in relation to the effluent from cooling towers.

Methods that may be used to disinfect water distribution systems known to be contaminated with *Legionella* include superheating and hyperchlorination (2). The use of hyperchlorination is limited by the fact that *Legionella* is relatively chlorine tolerant and the concentrations required to kill *Legionella* result in significant corrosion of the plumbing system. Superheating and flush-

Table 5 Risk Factors and Preventive Measures for Nosocomial *Legionella* and Viral Pneumonia

Pathogen	Issues/risk factors	Preventive measures	CDC/HICPAC[a]
Legionella			
Primary prevention	Chronic disease/immune suppression	Increased awareness of risk factors and high index of suspicion	IA
	Colonization of hospital water supplies	No recommendation for routine environmental culturing, water treatments or maintaining certain temperature of potable water {1899}	NR
	Nebulization/other semi critical devices	Proper cleaning/disinfection, use sterile H_2O for nebulization	IA
		Avoid large-volume room-air humidifiers unless sterilized	IA
	Cooling towers	Position so that drift is away from hospital's air intake system, use an effective biocide, & follow recommended maintenance.	IB
Secondary prevention	Single laboratory confirmed case or >2 possible cases within 6 months	Conduct epidemiologic/environmental investigation to determine source	IB
		If source identified, decontaminate† and continue surveillance	IB
		If source not found, continue surveillance for at least two months	II

Influenza			
Primary Prevention	Elderly, immunosuppressed	Yearly vaccination of those at risk as well as health care workers	IA
Secondary Prevention	Person-person spread via droplet	Private rooms suspected/diagnosed cases; use masks for entering room	IB
	Nosocomial outbreak	Vaccinate susceptible patients/staff	IB
		Administer oseltamivir/zanamivir to susceptible patients/staff	IA[‡]
Respiratory Syncytial Virus (RSV)			
	Common in infants/young children	Educate personnel; handwashing, gloves for handling secretions	IA
	Seasonal outbreaks	Gown before anticipated soiling by respiratory secretions	IB
	Abundant in respiratory secretions	Restrict staff with URI symptoms from caring for patients at risk	IB
	Person-person spread	Private room/cohorting during outbreak; defer elective admission	II

* CDC/HICPAC guideline criteria as defined in Table 1.
[†] Refer to MMWR 1997; 46:54–57 for detailed description
Abbreviation: URI = upper respiratory illness
[‡] Recommendation upgraded by new data since original recommendation.

ing, in which the temperature of water in the tank is heated to greater than 70°C, followed by the running of all shower heads and faucets to kill *Legionella*, has emerged as the most widely used method for disinfection of water heating systems. Consultation with state, local, and federal health officials and with hospitals which have had experience dealing with environmental legionellosis is strongly recommended.

B. Influenza

Influenza usually begins in the community and, like respiratory syncytial virus, spreads to the hospital from infected patients, staff, or visitors (2,174). Influenza is spread person to person by large droplet nuclei introduced into the respiratory tract of close contacts, but direct contact transmission may also occur. Closed units such as nursing homes, chronic disease facilities, intensive care units, and pediatric wards predispose to increased risk. Influenza is usually diagnosed clinically and confirmatory cultures, if done, are performed on the first cases.

The control of influenza relies on prevention by immunization and chemoprophylaxis (see Table 5) (2,175). Influenza vaccine should be given annually to long-term care residents, persons who are 65 years of age or older, and all high-risk patients, including those with cardiac, pulmonary, renal, or metabolic disease. Because influenza can be introduced by hospital personnel, it is recommended that health care workers be immunized to decrease risk to hospitalized patients. Influenza vaccine is effective in preventing severe influenza-related complications, and adverse reactions are infrequent and minor. Chemoprophylaxis with oseltamivir or zanamavir is recommended for high-risk unvaccinated populations during an outbreak with the concurrent administration of vaccine. These agents are effective against influenza A and B (176,177,185,186).

C. Respiratory Syncytial Virus

Respiratory syncytial virus (RSV) is a highly contagious virus that causes lower respiratory tract infection in young children and infants each winter or spring and is a common cause of nosocomial infection on pediatric units (2,178). In recent years, adults who are immunocompromised, elderly, or with chronic obstructive pulmonary disease have also been shown to be at risk for severe RSV infection.

Respiratory syncytial virus is present in high concentrations in respiratory secretions and can be transmitted directly by large respiratory droplets during close contact with infected persons or indirectly by contaminated hands or fomites (2,174). The conjunctiva and nasal mucosa are the most important portals of entry. Culture of RSV remains the gold standard for diagnosis, but antigen detection systems are widely used because they have high sensitivity and specificity, and results may be available more rapidly. Following the identification of a laboratory-confirmed case in a hospitalized patient, subsequent cases may be diagnosed presumptively.

Prevention efforts, as outlined in the CDC/HICPAC guideline, should be directed at containing the reservoir of virus in infected patients (see Table 5) (2). This requires surveillance for infection (category 1B) and staff education (category 1B). Staff are advised to wash hands (category 1A), wear gloves (category 1A), and wear gowns (category 1B) (178). Gloves must be changed between seeing patients and precautions taken to avoid inoculation of eyes or nose. Special efforts, such as assigning private rooms or cohorting infected patients and staff (category II), may be needed to prevent infection of high-risk patients.

D. *Aspergillus*

Aspergillus spores are found universally in unfiltered air and, when inhaled, they penetrate to the lower respiratory tract (179,180). Once introduced into an environment, these spores persist for long periods of time. High concentrations in the hospital have been found in false ceiling dust, polysyrene linings of fireproofed doors, and fireproofing material, spore concentrations are increased during hospital construction and renovation (180). Immunocompromised patients, particularly those with prolonged neutropenia from chemotherapy, organ transplantation, or AIDS, are at highest risk for aspergillosis.

Although *Aspergillus* pneumonia is uncommon, it has a high mortality rate resulting from the necrotizing nature of the infection and its poor response to antifungal therapy. A single case of nosocomial *Aspergillus* pneumonia should prompt a search for other cases. Prevention of nosocomial aspergillosis requires the evaluation of hospital airflow systems as summarized in the CDC/HICPAC guideline (2). In addition, proper staff education (category 1A) and surveillance (category 1B) are recommended. Prevention efforts should be aimed at minimizing fungal spore counts by using high-efficiency air filtration (category 1B), minimizing the time that high-risk patients spend outside their rooms for diagnostic procedures and other activities (category 1B), and taking optimal precautions for patients during periods of hospital construction or renovation (category 1B) (2).

VIII. BARRIERS TO PREVENTION

Advances in the understanding of the pathogenesis and risk factors for NP have not resulted in a dramatic change in the incidence of infections in susceptible populations. There are many barriers impeding the effective implementation of prevention strategies as shown in Figure 4. Prevention is undervalued in the US health care system and by health care providers who are trained in and focused on the challenges of diagnosis and treatment. When caring for acutely ill patients, it may be difficult for providers to appreciate the importance of preventive measures. Progress can only be made when prevention is deemed equally important and sustained efforts to change attitudes and practices are introduced. This could be facilitated by the introduction of, and adher-

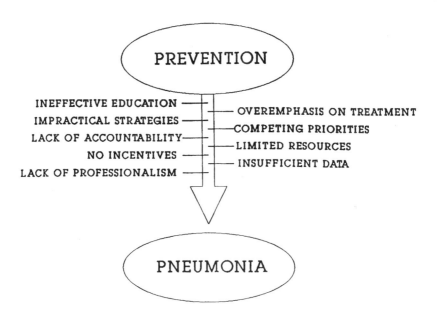

Figure 4   Summary of notable barriers to the prevention of nosocomial pneumonia. (From Ref. 182, with permission.)

ence to, patient management protocols designed to standardize implementation of the various prevention strategies discussed in this chapter.

The current health care environment may make it more difficult to prevent hospital-acquired infections. Hospital downsizing and understaffing may result in an increase in nosocomial infections in high-risk patients. Adherence to infection control procedures is likely to be compromised as staff numbers shrink and continuing education of health care workers becomes a lower priority. The effect of earlier discharge on infection rates is unclear. Increased surveillance of recently discharged patients and changes in the current definition of NP may be required to accurately evaluate this effect.

Use of devices is the most important risk factor for NP; however, the development of improved devices has been slow. Future possibilities include antibiotic impregnated devices that may retard colonization and endotracheal tubes that resist the accumulation of biofilm. Increased acceptance of techniques such as CASS, the routine use of HME, and maintainance of adequate cuff pressures may also minimize device-associated risks for NP. The successful implementation of these devices requires the acceptance and cooperation of physicians, respiratory technicians, and nurses.

IX. SUMMARY

Nosocomial pneumonia persists as the second most frequent hospital-acquired infection, with many preventive strategies remaining controversial. In the 1980s, significant strides were made in the understanding of the pathogenesis of nosocomial pneumonia, although many of these advances have not been translated into more effective prevention. Host- and device-associated risk factors for pneumonia are increasingly prevalent as the population ages, those with chronic illness survive longer, and the art of medicine becomes more invasive. The emergence and spread of multidrug-resistant (MDR) organisms in hospitalized patients reinforces the need for heightened awareness and prevention. However, with the changing health care system, resources may be diverted away from surveillance, education, and prevention.

Clinical research designed to further identify both host- and device-associated risk factors and to assess the benefit of specific preventive measures is required. Unfortunately, funding and institutional support for research may receive a lower priority under managed care and capitation policies. There is a need for increased recognition of host-associated risk factors, necessitating involvement of primary care physicians, and for increased emphasis on preventive strategies such as smoking cessation, vaccination, and postoperative care. Device-associated risk factors should also be minimized, with particular attention being given to patients receiving mechanical ventilation because they are at highest risk from use of multiple devices. The effect of earlier discharge and more intensive outpatient therapy on the development of pneumonia needs to be assessed, with a possible reevaluation of the classifications of community-acquired and nosocomial.

The implementation of many of the prevention guidelines outlined in this chapter should reduce morbidity and mortality rates associated with NP. Intervention strategies should be adjusted to each institution and integrated into a continuing comprehensive education program. Although data are limited, we believe these recommendations to be both cost effective and acceptable to patients and health care workers.

APPENDIX: KOLLEF GRADING SCHEME

A, supported by at least two randomized, controlled investigations; B, supported by at least one randomized, controlled investigation; C, supported by nonrandomized, concurrent-cohort investigations, historical-cohort investigations or case-series; D, supported by randomized, controlled investigations of other nosocomial infections; U, undetermined or not yet studied in clinical investigations.

REFERENCES

1. Craven DE, Steger KA. Epidemiology of nosocomial pneumonia: new concepts on an old disease. Chest 1995; 108:1S–16S.
2. Tablan OC, Anderson LJ, Arden NH, Breiman RF, Butler JC, McNeil MM, et al. Guideline for prevention of nosocomial pneumonia: Part I. Issues on prevention of nosocomial pneumonia, 1994. Infect Control Hosp Epidemiol 1994; 15: 588–625.
3. Martone WJ, Jarvis WR, Culver DH, Haley RW. Incidence and nature of endemic and epidemic nosocomial infections. In: Bennett JV, Brachman PS, eds. Hospital Infections. 3rd ed. Boston: Little, Brown, 1993:577–596.
4. Horan T, Culver D, Jarvis W, Emori TG, Banergee S, Martone W, et al. Pathogens causing nosocomial infections. CDC: The Antimicrobic Newsletter 1988; 5:65–67.
5. Niederman MS, Torres A, Summer W. Invasive diagnostic testing is not needed routinely to manage suspect ventilator-associated pneumonia. Am J Respir Crit Care Med 1994; 150:565–569.
6. Chastre J, Fagon JY. Invasive diagnostic testing should be routinely used to

manage ventilated patients with suspected pneumonia. Am J Respir Crit Care Med 1994; 150:570–574.

7. Kollef MH, Bock KR, Richards RD, Hearns ML. The safety and diagnostic accuracy of minibronchoalveolar lavage in patients with suspected ventilator-associated pneumonia. Ann Intern Med 1995; 122:743–748.

8. The American Thoracic Society (was adopted by the ATS Board of Directors). Hospital-acquired pneumonia in adults: diagnosis, assessment of severity, initial antimicrobial therapy, and preventative strategies: a consensus statement. Am J Respir Crit Care Med 1996; 153:1711–1725.

9. Sanchez-Nieto JM, Torres A, Garcia-Cordoba F, El-ebiary M, Carrillo A, Ruiz J, et al. Impact of invasive and noninvasive quantitative culture sampling on outcome of ventilator-associated pneumonia: a pilot study. Am J Respir Crit Care Med 1997; 156:1–6.

10. Torres A, Aznar R, Gatell JM, Jimenez P, Gonzalez J, Ferrer A, et al. Incidence, risk, and prognostic factors of nosocomial pneumonia in mechanically ventilated patients. Am Rev Respir Dis 1990; 142:523–528.

11. Rello J, Quintana E, Ausina V, Castella J, Luquin M, Net A, et al. Incidence, etiology, and outcome of nosocomial pneumonia in mechanically ventilated patients. Chest 1991; 100:439–444.

12. Rello J, Quintana E, Ausina V, Puzo C, Net A, Prats G. Risk factors for *Staphylococcus aureus* pneumonia in critically ill patients. Am Rev Respir Dis 1990; 142:1320–1324.

13. Jimenez P, Torres A, Rodriguez-Roisin R, De La Bellacasa JP, Aznar R, Gatell JM, et al. Incidence and etiology of pneumonia acquired during mechanical ventilation. Crit Care Med 1989; 17:882–885.

14. Torres A, Aznar R, Gatell JM, Jimenez P, Gonzalez J, Ferrer A, et al. Incidence, risk, and prognosis factors of nosocomial pneumonia in mechanically ventilated patients. Am Rev Respir Dis 1990; 142:523–528.

15. Fagon JY, Chastre J, Hance AJ, Montravers P, Nowara A, Gilbert C. Nosocomial pneumonia in ventilated patients: a cohort study evaluating attributable mortality and hospital stay. Am J Med 1993; 94:281–288.

16. Celis R, Torres A, Gatell JM, Almela M, Rodriguez-Roisin R, Augusti-Vidal A. Nosocomial pneumonia: a multivariate analysis of risk and prognosis. Chest 1988; 93:318–324.

17. Craven DE, Kunches LM, Kilinsky V, Lichtenberg DA, Make BJ, McCabe WR. Risk factors for pneumonia and fatality in patients receiving continuous mechanical ventilation. Am Rev Respir Dis 1986; 133:792–796.

18. Graybill JR, Marshall LW, Charache P, et al. Nosocomial pneumonia: a continuing major problem. Am Rev Respir Dis 1973; 108:1130–1140.

19. Stevens RM, Teres D, Skillman JJ, et al. Pneumonia in an intensive care unit: a thirty-month experience. Arch Intern Med 1974; 134:106–111.

20. Craven DE, Steger KA. Nosocomial pneumonia in mechanically ventilated adult patients: Epidemiology and prevention in 1996. Semin Respir Infect 1996; 11:32–53.

21. Leu HS, Kaiser DL, Mori M, Woolson RF, Wenzel RP. Hospital-acquired pneumonia: attributable mortality and morbidity. Am J Epidemiol 1989; 129:1258–1267.

22. Kollef MH. Ventilator-associated pneumonia. JAMA 1993; 270:1965–1970.

23. Fagon J, Chastre J, Domart Y, Trouillet J, Gibert C. Mortality due to ventilator-associated pneumonia or colonization with *Pseudomonas* or *Acinetobacter* species: assessment by quantitative culture of samples obtained by a protected specimen brush. Clin Infect Dis 1996; 23:538–542.

24. Driks MR, Craven DE, Celli BR, Manning M, Burke RA, Garvin GG, et al. Nosocomial pneumonia in intubated patients given sucralfate as compared with antacids or histamine type 2 blockers: the role of gastric colonization. N Engl J Med 1987; 317:1376–1382.

25. Haley RW, Hooton TM, Culver DH, et al. Nosocomial infections in US hospitals, 1975–1976: estimated frequency by selected characteristics of patients. Am J Med 1981; 70:947–959.

26. Gouin F, Bregeon F, Thirion X, Saux P, Denis JP, Papazian L. Ventilator-associated pneumonia and mortality (abstr). 35th Interscience Conference on Antimicrobial Agents and Chemotherapy, San Francisco 1995; J119:278.

27. Johanson WGJ, Pierce AK, Sanford J, Thomas GD. Nosocomial respiratory infections with gram-negative bacilli: the significance of colonization of the respiratory tract. Ann Intern Med 1972; 77:701–706.

28. Reusser P, Zimmerli W, Scheidegger D, Marbet GA, Buser M, Gyr K. Role of gastric colonization in nosocomial infections and endotoxemia: a prospective study in neurosurgical patients on mechanical ventilation. J Infect Dis 1989; 160:414–421.

29. Valles J, Artigas A, Rello J, Bonsoms N, Fontanals D, Blanch LI, et al. Continuous aspiration of subglottic secretions in the prevention of ventilator-associated pneumonia. Ann Intern Med 1995; 122:179–186.

30. Mahul PH, Auboyer C, Jospe R, Ros A, Guerin C, El Khouri Z, et al. Prevention of nosocomial pneumonia in intubated patients: respective role of mechanical subglottic secretions drainage and stress ulcer prophylaxis. Inten Care Med 1992; 18:20–25.

31. Torres A, Serra-Battles J, Ros E, Piera C, Puig de la Bellacasa J, Cobos A, et al. Pulmonary aspiration of gastric contents in patients receiving mechanical ventilation: the effect of body position. Ann Intern Med 1992; 116:540–542.

32. Bonten MJM, Gaillard CA, de Leeuw PW, Stobberingh EE. The role of colonization of the upper intestinal tract in the pathogenesis of ventilator-associated pneumonia. Clin Infect Dis 1997; 24:309–319.

33. Cameron J, Zuidema G. Aspiration pneumonia: magnitude and frequency of the problem. JAMA 1972; 219:1194–1198.

34. Pugin J, Auckenthaler R, Mili N, Janssens JP, Lew PD, Suter PM. Diagnosis of ventilator-associated pneumonia by bacteriologic analysis of bronchoalveolar lavage fluid. Am Rev Respir Dis 1991; 143:1121–1129.

35. Prod'hom G, Leuenberger PH, Koerfer J, et al. Nosocomial pneumonia in me-

chanically ventilated patients receiving antacid, ranitidine, or sucralfate as prophylaxis for stress ulcer. Ann Intern Med 1994; 120:653–662.

36. Schleupner CJ, Cobb DK. A study of the etiologies and treatment of nosocomial
pneumonia in a community-based teaching hospital. Infect Control Hosp Epidemiol 1992; 13:515–525.

37. Rello J, Torres A, Ricart M, Valles J, Gonzalez J, Artigas A, et al. Ventilator-
associated pneumonia by *Staphylococcus aureus*: comparison of methicillin-
resistant and methicillin-sensitive episodes. Am J Respir Crit Care Med 1994;
150:1545–1549.

38. Johanson WG, Pierce AK, Sanford JP. Changing pharyngeal bacterial flora of
hospitalized patients: emergence of gram-negative bacilli. N Engl J Med 1969;
281:1137–1140.

39. Torres A, El-ebiary M, Gonzalez J, Ferrer M, Puig de la Bellacasa J, Gene A,
et al. Gastric and pharyngeal flora in nosocomial pneumonia acquired during
mechanical ventilation. Am Rev Respir Dis 1993; 148:352–357.

40. Mackowiak PA, Martin RM, Jones SR, et al. Pharyngeal colonization by gram-
negative bacilli in aspiration-prone persons. Arch Intern Med 1978; 138:1224–
1227.

41. Niederman MS. Gram-negative colonization of the respiratory tract: pathogenesis and clinical consequences. Semin Respir Infect 1990; 5:173–184.

42. Atherton ST, White DJ. Stomach as a source of bacteria colonizing respiratory
tract during artificial ventilation. Lancet 1978; 2:968–969.

43. du Moulin GC, Paterson DG, Hedley-Whyte J, Lisbon A. Aspiration of gastric
bacteria in antacid-treated patients: a frequent cause of postoperative colonization of the airway. Lancet 1982; 1:242–245.

44. Tryba M. The gastropulmonary route of infection—fact or fiction? Am J Med
1991; 91(suppl 2A):135S–146S.

45. File TJ, Tan J, Thomson RJ, Stephens C, Thompson P. An outbreak of *Pseudomonas aeruginosa* ventilator-associated respiratory infections due to contaminated food coloring dye—further evidence of the significance of gastric colonization preceding nosocomial pneumonia. Infect Control Hosp Epidemiol 1995;
16:417–418.

46. Bonten MJM, Gaillard CA, van Tiel FH, Smeets HGW, van der Geest S, Stobberingh EE. The stomach as a source for colonization of the upper respiratory
tract and pneumonia in ICU patients. Chest 1994; 105:878–884.

47. Bonten MJM, Bergmans DCJJ, Ambergen AW, de Leeuw PW, van der Geest
S, Stobberingh EE, et al. Risk factors for pneumonia, and colonization of respi-
ratory tract and stomach in mechanically ventilated ICU patients. Am J Respir
Crit Care Med 1996; 154:1339–1346.

48. Niederman MS, Craven DE. Devising strategies for nosocomial pneumonia
prevention: should we ignore the stomach? Clin Infect Dis 1997; 24:320–323.

49. Toews GB. Role of the polymorphonuclear leukocyte: interaction with nosocomial pathogens. Eur J Clin Microbiol Infect Dis 1989; 8:21–24.

50. Rose RM. Pulmonary macrophages in nosocomial pneumonia: defense function

and dysfunction, and prospects for activation. Eur J Clin Microbiol Infect Dis 1989; 8:25–28.

51. Fick RB. Lung humoral response to *Pseudomonas* species. Eur J Clin Microbiol Infect Dis 1989; 8:29–34.

52. Reynolds HY. Normal and defective respiratory host defenses. In: Pennington JE, ed. Respiratory Infections: Diagnosis & Management. 2nd ed. New York: Raven Press, 1989:1–33.

53. Kunkel SL, Strieter RM. Cytokine networking in lung inflammation. Hosp Pract 1990; 25:63–76.

54. George DL. Epidemiology of nosocomial ventilator-associated pneumonia. Infect Control Hosp Epidemiol 1993; 14:163–169.

55. Cross AS, Roupe B. Role of respiratory assistance devices in endemic nosocomial pneumonia. Am J Med 1981; 70:681–685.

56. Joshi N, Localio AR, Hamory BH. A predictive risk index for nosocomial pneumonia in the intensive care unit. Am J Med 1992; 93:135–142.

57. Louria DB, Kaminski T. The effects of four antimicrobial drug regimens on sputum superinfection in hospitalized patients. Am Rev Respir Dis 1962; 85: 649–665.

58. Valenti WM, Trudell RG, Bentley DW. Factors predisposing to oropharyngeal colonization with gram-negative bacilli in the aged. N Engl J Med 1978; 298: 1108–1111.

59. Niederman MS, Mantovani R, Schoch P, et al. Patterns and routes of tracheobronchial colonization in mechanically ventilated patients: the role of nutritional status in colonization of the lower airway by *Pseudomonas* species. Chest 1989; 95:155–161.

60. Niederman MS, Merrill WW, Ferranti RD, Pagano KM, Palmer LB, Reynolds HY. Nutritional status and bacterial binding in the lower respiratory tract in patients with chronic tracheostomy. Ann Intern Med 1984; 100:795–800.

61. Abraham SN, Beachey EH, Simpson WA. Adherence of *Streptococcus pyogenes, Escherichia coli*, and *Pseudomonas aeruginosa* to fibronectin-coated and uncoated epithelial cells. Infect Immun 1983; 41:1261–1268.

62. Woods DE, Straus DC, Johanson WG Jr, et al. Role of pili in adherence of *Pseudomonas aeruginosa* to mammalian buccal epithelial cells. Infect Immun 1980; 29:1146–1151.

63. Woods DE, Straus DC, Johanson WG Jr, et al. Role of fibronectin in the prevention of adherence of *Pseudomonas aeruginosa* to buccal cells. J Infect Dis 1981; 143:784–790.

64. Reynolds HY. Bacterial adherence to respiratory tract mucosa: a dynamic interaction leading to colonization. Semin Respir Infect 1987; 2:8–19.

65. Giannella RA, Broitman SA, Zamcheck N. Influence of gastric acidity on bacterial and parasitic enteric infections: a perspective. Ann Intern Med 1973; 78: 271–276.

66. Arnold I. The bacterial flora within the stomach and small intestine: the effect of experimental alterations of acid-base balance and the age of the subject. Am J Med Sci 1993; 186:471–481.

67. Bishop RF, Anderson CM. The bacterial flora of the stomach and small intestine in children with obstruction. Arch Dis Child 1960; 35:487–491.

68. Seley GP, Colp R. The bacteriology of peptic ulcers and gastric malignancies: possible bearing on complications following gastric surgery. Surgery 1941; 10: 369–380.

69. Gracey M, Suhurjano S, Stone DE. Microbial contamination of the gut: another feature of malnutrition. Am J Clin Nutr 1973; 26:1170–1174.

70. Daschner F, Kappstein I, Engels I, Reuschenbach K, Pfisterer J, Krieg N, et al. Stress ulcer prophylaxis and ventilation pneumonia: prevention by antibacterial cytoprotective agents. Infect Control 1988; 9:59–65.

71. Donowitz LG, Page MC, Mileur GL, Guenthner SH. Alteration of normal gastric flora in critical care patients receiving antacid and cimetidine therapy. Infect Control 1986; 7:23–26.

72. Olivares L, Segovia A, Revuelta R. Tube feeding and lethal aspiration in neurological patients: a review of 720 autopsy cases. Stroke 1974; 5:654–656.

73. Huxley EJ, Viroslav J, Gray WR, et al. Pharyngeal aspiration in normal adults and patients with depressed consciousness. Am J Med 1978; 64:564–568.

74. Craven DE, Steger KA, Fleming CA. Preventing hospital-acquired pneumonia: current concepts and strategies. Semin Respir Crit Care Med 1997; 18:185–200.

75. Craven DE, Steger KA, LaForce FM. Nosocomial pneumonia. In: Anonymous Hospital Infections. 4th ed. Boston: Little, Brown, 1997.

76. Kelley RE, Vibulsresth S, Bell L, Duncan RC. Evaluation of kinetic therapy in the prevention of complications of prolonged bed rest secondary to stroke. Stroke 1987; 18:638–642.

77. Gentilello L, Thompson DA, Tonnesen AS, et al. Effect of a rotating bed on the incidence of pulmonary complications in critically ill patients. Crit Care Med 1988; 16:783–786.

78. Summer WR, Curry P, Haponik EF, Nelson S, Elston R. Continuous mechanical turning of intensive care unit patients shortens length of stay in some diagnostic-related groups. J Crit Care 1989; 4:45–53.

79. Fink MP, Helsmoortel CM, Stein KL, Lee PC, Cohn SM. The efficacy of an oscillating bed in the prevention of lower respiratory tract infection in critically ill victims of blunt trauma: a prospective study. Chest 1990; 97:132–137.

80. Weber DJ, Becherer PR, Rutala WA, Samsa GP, Wilson MB, White II GC. Nosocomial infection rate as a function of human immunodeficiency virus type 1 status in hemophiliacs. Am J Med 1991; 91(suppl 3B):206–211.

81. Craven DE, Steger KA, Hirschhorn LR. Nosocomial colonization and infection in persons infected with human immunodeficiency virus. Infect Control Hosp Epidemiol 1996; 17:304–318.

82. Nichols L, Balogh K, Silverman M. Bacterial infections in the acquired immune deficiency syndrome: clinicopathologic correlations in a series of autopsy cases. Am J Clin Pathol 1989; 92:787–790.

83. Gaynes R, Martone W, Bisno A, Rimland D, Srivastara P, Culver D. Nosocomial infections among HIV-positive patients (abstr): Second Annual Meeting of SHEA, April 12–14, 1992, Baltimore, MD.

84. Stroud L, Srivastava P, Culver D, Bisno A, Rimland D, Simberkoff M, et al. Nosocomial infections in HIV-infected patients: preliminary results from a multicenter surveillance system (1989–1995). Infect Control Hosp Epidemiol 1997; 18:479–485.

85. Hirschtick RE, Glassroth J, Jordan MC, Wilcosky TC, Wallace JM, Kvale PA, et al. Bacterial pneumonia in persons infected with the human immunodeficiency virus. N Engl J Med 1995; 333:845–851.

86. Weinke T, Schiller R, Fehrenback FJ, Pohle HD. Association between *Staphylococcus aureus* nasopharyngeal colonization and septicemia in patients infected with the human immunodeficiency virus. Eur J Clin Microbiol Infect Dis 1992; 11:985–989.

87. Craven DE, Fagan M, Steger KA, Gunn J, Rolitsky C. Risk factors for nasopharyngeal (NP) colonization with *Staphylococcus aureus* in HIV-infected outpatients (abstr). Third Annual Meeting of SHEA Chicago, IL 1993:S51.

88. Blumberg HM, Rimland D. Nosocomial infection with penicillin-resistant pneumococci in patients with AIDS. J Infect Dis 1989; 160:725–726.

89. Goetz MB, O'Brien H, Musser JM, Ward JI. Nosocomial transmission of disease caused by nontypeable strains of *Haemophilus influenzae*. Am J Med 1994; 96:342–347.

90. Kielhofner M, Atmar RL, Hamill RJ, Musher DM. Life-threatening *Pseudomonas aeruginosa* infections in patients with human immunodeficiency virus infection. Clin Infect Dis 1992; 14:403–411.

91. Mendelson MH, Curtman A, Szabo S, Neibart E, Meyers BR, Policar M, et al. *Pseudomonas aeruginosa* bacteremia in patients with AIDS. Clin Infect Dis 1994; 18:886–895.

92. Baron AD, Hollander H. *Pseudomonas aeruginosa* bronchopulmonary infection in late human immunodeficiency virus disease. Am Rev Respir Dis 1993; 148:992–996.

93. Dropulic LK, Leslie JM, Eldred LJ, Zenilman J, Sears CL. Clinical manifestations and risk factors of *Pseudomonas aeruginosa* infection in patients with AIDS. J Infect Dis 1995; 171:930–937.

94. Fichtenbaum CJ, Woeltje KF, Powderly WG. Serious *Pseudomonas aeruginosa* infections in patients infected with human immunodeficiency virus: a case-control study. Clin Infect Dis 1994; 19:417–422.

95. Fischl MA, Daikos GL, Uttamchandani RB, Poblete RB, Moreno JN, Reyes RR, et al. Clinical presentation and outcome of patients with HIV infection and tuberculosis caused by multiple-drug-resistant bacilli. Ann Intern Med 1992; 117:184–190.

96. Daley CL, Small PM, Schecter GF, Schoolnik GK, McAdam RA, Jacobs WR, Jr et al. An outbreak of tuberculosis with accelerated progression among persons infected with the human immunodeficiency virus: an analysis using restriction fragment length polymorphisms. N Engl J Med 1992; 326:231–235.

97. Centers for Disease Control. Guidelines for preventing the transmission of tuberculous infection in health-care settings, with special focus on HIV-related issues. MMWR 1994; 43(No. RR-13):1–33.

98. Markowitz N, Hansen NI, Hopewell PC, Glassroth J, Kvale PA, Mangura BT, et al. Incidence of tuberculosis in the United States among HIV-infected persons. Ann Intern Med 1997; 126:123–132.

99. Blumberg HM, Watkins D, Berschling J, Antle A, Moore P, White N, et al. Preventing the nosocomial transmission of tuberculosis. Ann Intern Med 1995; 122:658–663.

100. Chave J, David S, Wauters J, Van Melle G, Francioli P. Transmission of *Pneumocystis carinii* from AIDS patients to other immunosuppressed patients: a cluster of *Pneumocystis carinii* pneumonia in renal transplant recipients. AIDS 1991; 5:927–932.

101. Haron E, Bodey GP, Luna MA, Dekmezian R, Elting L. Has the incidence of *Pneumocystis carinii* pneumonia in cancer patients increased with the AIDS epidemic? Lancet 1988; 15:904–905.

102. Rello J, Sonora R, Jubert P, Artigas A, Rue M, Valles J. Pneumonia in intubated patients: role of respiratory airway care. Am J Respir Crit Care Med 1996; 154: 111–115.

103. Tillotson JR, Finland M. Bacterial colonization and clinical superinfection of the respiratory tract complicating antibiotic treatment of pneumonia. J Infect Dis 1969; 119:597–624.

104. Oliphant CM, Postelnick M, Noskin GA, Peterson LR. The impact of use reduction on the antipseudomonal activity of fluoroquinolones (abstr). 35th Interscience Conference on Antimicrobial Agents and Chemotherapy, San Francisco, 1995; C52:48.

105. White AC Jr, Atmar RL, Cate TR, Okpara A, Wilson J, Stager C, et al. Impact of faculty-enforced antibiotic restrictions on antibiotic costs and sensitivities (abstr). 35th Interscience Conference on Antimicrobial Agents and Chemotherapy, San Francisco, 1995; N17:348.

106. Bertino JS Jr, Foltzer MA, Kozak AJ, Reese RE, Vamvakias A. Cost & resistance (R) implications of a multidisciplinary antibiotic use program (MDAUP) (abstr). 36th ICAAC, New Orleans 1996; N3:293.

107. Hospital Infection Control Practices Advisory Committee (HICPAC). Recommendations for preventing the spread of vancomycin resistance. Infect Control Hosp Epidemiol 1995; 16:105–113.

108. Selective Decontamination of the Digestive Tract Trialists' Collaborative Group. Meta-analysis of randomised controlled trials of selective decontamination of the digestive tract. BMJ 1993; 307:525–532.

109. van Saene HKF, Stoutenbeek CP, Stoller JK. Selective decontamination of the digestive tract in the intensive care unit: current status and future prospects. Crit Care Med 1992; 20:691–703.

110. The European Society of Intensive Care Medicine, The Societe Reanimation de Langue Francaise. The first European Consensus Conference in intensive care medicine: selective decontamination of the digestive tract in intensive care unit patients. Infect Control Hosp Epidemiol 1992; 13:609–611.

111. Stoutenbeek CP, van Saene HKF, Miranda DR, Zandstra DF. The effect of

selective decontamination of the digestive tract on colonization and infection rate in multiple trauma patients. Intensive Care Med 1984; 10:185–192.

112. Ferrer M, Torres A, Gonzalez J, Puig de la Bellacasa J, Gatell JM, Roca M, et al. Utility of selective digestive decontamination in a general population of mechanically ventilated patients. Am Rev Respir Dis 1992; 4:A112.

113. Cockerill FR, Muller SM, Anhalt JP, Marsh HM, Farnell MB, Mucha P, et al. Prevention of infection in critically ill patients by selective decontamination of the digestive tract. Ann Intern Med 1992; 117:545–553.

114. Gastinne H, Wolff M, Delatour F, Faurisson F, Chevret S. A controlled trial in intensive care units of selective decontamination of the digestive tract with nonabsorbable antibiotics. N Engl J Med 1992; 326:594–599.

115. Duncan RA, Steger KA, Craven DE. Selective decontamination of the digestive tract: risks outweigh benefits for intensive care unit patients. Semin Respir Infect 1993; 8:308–324.

116. Barrientos-Vega R, Sanchez-Soria MM, Morales-Garcia C, Robas-Gomez A, Cuena-Boy R, Ayensa-Rincon A. Prolonged sedation of critically ill patients with midazolam or propofol: impact on weaning and costs. Crit Care Med 1997; 25:33–40.

117. Prekates A, Nanas S, Floros J, Zakinthynos S, Argyropoulou A, Routchi C, et al. Predisposing factors for ventilator-associated pneumonia in general ICU. Am J Respir Crit Care Med 1996; 153:A562.

118. Shapiro BA, Warren J, Egol AB, Greenbaum DM, Jacobi J, Nasraway SA, et al. Practice parameters for sustained neuromuscular blockade in the adult critically ill patient: an executive summary. Crit Care Med 1995; 23:1601–1605.

119. Ben-Menachem T, Fogel R, Patel RV, Touchette M, Zarowitz BJ, Hadzijahic N, et al. Prophylaxis for stressed-related gastric hemorrhage in the medical intensive care unit. A randomized, controlled, single-blind study. Ann Intern Med 1994; 121:568–575.

120. Kappstein I, Friedrich T, Hellinger P, Benzing A, Geiger K, Schulgen G, et al. Incidence of pneumonia in mechanically ventilated patients treated with sucralfate or cimetidine as prophylaxis for stress bleeding: bacterial colonization of the stomach. Am J Med 1991; 91(suppl 2A):125–131.

121. Tryba M. Risk of acute stress bleeding and nosocomial pneumonia in ventilated intensive care unit patients: sucralfate versus antacids. Am J Med 1987; 83(suppl):117–124.

122. Gaynes R, Bizek B, Mowry-Hanley J, Kirsch M. Risk factors for nosocomial pneumonia after coronary artery bypass graft operations. Ann Thorac Surg 1991; 51:215–218.

123. Cook DJ, Reeve BK, Scholes LC. Histamine-2-receptor antagonists and antacids in the critically ill population: stress ulceration versus nosocomial pneumonia. Infect Control Hosp Epidemiol 1994; 15:437–442.

124. Tryba M. Sucralfate versus antacids or H_2-antagonists for stress ulcer prophylaxis: a meta-analysis on efficacy and pneumonia rate. Crit Care Med 1991; 19:942–949.

125. Hillman KM, Riordan T, O'Farrell SM, Tabaqchali S. Colonization of the gastric contents in critically ill patients. Crit Care Med 1982; 10:444–447.

126. Mantey-Stiers F, Tryba M. Antibacterial activity of sucralfate in human gastric juice. Am J Med 1987; 87:125–128.

127. West AP, Abdul S, Sherratt M, Inglis TJ. Antibacterial activity of sucralfate against *Escherichia coli*, *Staphylococcus aureus*, and *Pseudomonas aeruginosa* in batch and continuous culture. Eur J Clin Microbiol Infect Dis 1993; 12:869–871.

128. Rouby J, Laurent P, Gosnach M, Cambau E, Lamas G, Zouaoui A, et al. Risk factors and clinical relevance of nosocomial maxillary sinusitis in the critically ill. Am J Respir Crit Care Med 1994; 150:776–783.

129. Craven DE, Kunches LM, Lichtenberg DA, Kollisch NR, Barry MA, Heeren TC, et al. Nosocomial infection and fatality in medical and surgical intensive care unit patients. Arch Intern Med 1988; 148:1161–1168.

130. Kollef MH. The Identification of ICU-specific outcome predictors: a comparison of medical, surgical, and cardiothoracic ICU's from a single institution. Heart Lung 1995; 24:60–66.

131. Craven DE, Driks MR. Pneumonia in the intubated patient. Semin Respir Infect 1987; 2:20–33.

132. Cheadle WG, Vitale GC, Mackie CR, Cuschieri A. Prophylactic postoperative nasogastric decompression: a prospective study of its requirement and the influence of cimetidine in 200 patients. Ann Surg 1985; 202:361–366.

133. Venezia RA, Agresta MD, Hanley EM, Urquhart K, Schoonmaker D. Nosocomial legionellosis associated with aspiration of nasogastric feedings diluted in tap water. Infect Control Hosp Epidemiol 1994; 15:529–533.

134. Pingleton SK, Hinthorn DR, Liu C. Enteral nutrition in patients receiving mechanical ventilation: multiple sources of tracheal colonization include the stomach. Am J Med 1986; 80:827–832.

135. Anderson KR, Norris DJ, Godfrey LB, et al. Bacterial contamination of the tube-feeding formulas. J Parenter Enter Nutr 1984; 8:673–678.

136. Cameron JL, Reynolds J, Zuidema GD. Aspiration in patients with tracheostomies. Surg Gynecol Obstet 1973; 136:68–70.

137. Ibanez J, Penafiel A, Raurich J, et al. Gastroesophageal reflux and aspiration of gastric contents during nasogastric feeding; the effect of posture (abstr) Intensive Care Med 1988; 14 (suppl 2):296.

138. Border J, Hassett J, LaDuca J, et al. The gut origin septic states in blunt multiple trauma (ISS + 40) in the ICU. Ann Surg 1987; 206:427–448.

139. Deitch EA, Berg R. Bacterial translocation from the gut: a mechanism of infection. J Burn Care Rehab 1987; 8:475.

140. Fiddian-Green RG, Baaker S. Nosocomial pneumonia in the critically ill: product of aspiration or translocation? Crit Care Med 1991; 19:763–769.

141. Montecalvo MA, Korsberg TZ, Farber HW, Smith BF, Dennis RC, Fitzpatrick GF, et al. Nosocomial pneumonia and nutritional status of critical care patients randomized to gastric versus jejunal tube feedings. Crit Care Med 1992; 20: 1377–1387.

142. Freeman J, Rosner BA, McGowan JE. Adverse effects of nosocomial infection. J Infect Dis 1979; 140:732–740.
143. Craig CP, Connelly S. Effect of intensive care unit nosocomial pneumonia on duration of stay and mortality. Am J Infect Control 1984; 12:233–238.
144. Torres A, Gatell JM, Aznar E, El-ebiary M, Puig de la Bellacasa J, Gonzalez J, et al. Re-intubation increases the risk of nosocomial pneumonia in patients needing mechanical ventilation. Am J Respir Crit Care Med 1995; 152:137–141.
145. Sottile FD, Marrie TJ, Prough DS, et al. Nosocomial pulmonary infection: possible etiologic significance of bacterial adhesion to endotracheal tubes. Crit Care Med 1986; 14:265–270.
146. Inglis TJJ, Millar MR, Jones JG, Robinson DA. Tracheal tube biofilm as a source of bacterial colonization of the lung. J Clin Microbiol 1989; 27:2014–2018.
147. Holzapfel L, Chevret S, Madinier G, Ohen F, Demingeon G, Coupry A, et al. Influence of long-term oro- or nasotracheal intubation on nosocomial maxillary sinusitis and pneumonia: results of a prospective, randomized, clinical trial. Crit Care Med 1993; 21:1132–1138.
148. Craven DE, Goularte TA, Make BJ. Contaminated condensate in mechanical ventilator circuits: a risk factor for nosocomial pneumonia. Am Rev Respir Dis 1984; 129:625–628.
149. Branson RD, Campbell RS, Davis KJ, Johnson DJ, Porombka D. Humidification in the intensive care unit: prospective study of a new protocol utilizing heated humidification and a hygroscopic condenser humidifier. Chest 1993; 104:1800–1805.
150. Hurni J, Feihl F, Lazor R, Leuenberger P, Perret C. Safety of combined heat and moisture exchanger filters in long-term mechanical ventilation. Chest 1997; 111:686–691.
151. Kirton OC, DeHaven B, Morgan J, Morejon O, Civetta J. A prospective, randomized comparison of an in-line heat moisture exchange filter and heated wire humidifiers: Rates of ventilator associated early-onset (community-acquired) or late-onset (hospital-acquired) pneumonia and incidence of endotracheal tube occlusion. Chest. In Press.
152. Craven DE, Connolly MGJ, Lichtenberg DA, Primeau PJ, McCabe WR. Contamination of mechanical ventilators with tubing changes every 24 or 48 hours. N Engl J Med 1982; 306:1505–1509.
153. Dreyfuss D, Djedaini K, Weber P, Brun P, Lanore JJ, Rahmani J, et al. Prospective study of nosocomial pneumonia and of patient and circuit colonization during mechanical ventilation with circuit changes every 48 hours versus no change. Am Rev Respir Dis 1991; 143:738–743.
154. Kollef M, Shapiro S, Fraser V, Silver P, Murphy D, Trovillion E, et al. Mechanical ventilation with or without 7-day circuit changes: a randomized controlled trial. Ann Intern Med 1995; 123:168–174.
155. Pujol M, Pallares R, Pena C, Corbella X, Dorca J, Verdaguer R, et al. Risk factors for methicillin-resistant *Staphylococcus aureus* (MRSA) pneumonia in intubated patients (abstr). 34th ICAAC, Orlando, FL, 1994; J72:95.

156. Dhand R, Tobin MJ. Inhaled bronchodilator therapy in mechanically ventilated patients. Am J Respir Crit Care Med 1997; 156:3–10.

157. Craven DE, Lichtenberg DA, Goularte TA, Make BJ, McCabe WR. Contaminated medication nebulizers in mechanical ventilator circuits: a source of bacterial aerosols. Am J Med 1984; 77:834–838.

158. Korn C, Burke R, O'Donnell C, Small E. An outbreak of stenotrophomas (xanthomonas) maltophilia associated with reusable in-line ventilator temperature probes (abstr). 23rd Annual Education & International Conference, APIC, 1996.

159. Weems JJ Jr. Nosocomial outbreak of *Pseudomonas cepacia* associated with contamination of reusable electronic ventilator temperature probes. Infect Control Hosp Epidemiol 1993; 14:583–586.

160. Deppe SA, Kelly JW, Thoi LL, Chudy JH, Longfield RN, Ducey JP, et al. Incidence of colonization, nosocomial pneumonia, and mortality in critically ill patients using a Trach Care^R closed-suction system versus an open-suction system: a prospective, randomized study. Crit Care Med 1990; 18:1389–1394.

161. Maki DG, McCormick RD, Zilz MA, Stolz SM, Alvarado CJ. An MRSA outbreak in a SICU during universal precautions: new epidemiology for nosocomial MRSA. In: Anonymous. Program and abstracts of the 30th Interscience Conference on Antimicrobial Agents and Chemotherapy, Atlanta, October 21–24, 1991. Washington, DC: American Society for Microbiology, 1990:165.

162. Weinstein RA. Epidemiology and control of nosocomial infections in adult intensive care units. Am J Med 1991; 91:179S–184S.

163. Weinstein RA. Failure of infection control in intensive care units: can sucralfate improve the situation? Am J Med 1991; 91(suppl 2A):132S–134S.

164. Klein BS, Perloff WH, Maki DG, et al. Reduction of nosocomial infection during pediatric intensive care by protective isolation. N Engl J Med 1989; 320:1714–1721.

165. Albert RK, Condie F. Handwashing patterns in medical intensive care units. N Engl J Med 1981; 304:1465–1466.

166. Sherertz RJ, Reagan DR, Hampton KD, Robertson KL, Streed SA, Hoen HM, et al. A cloud adult: the *Staphylococcus aureus*-virus interaction revisited. Ann Intern Med 1996; 124:539–547.

167. Kirby BD, Synder KM, Meyer RD, et al. Legionnaires disease: report of sixty-five nosocomially acquired cases and review of the literature. Medicine 1980; 59:188–205.

168. Marrie TJ, MacDonald S, Clarke K, Haldane D. Nosocomial Legionnaires' disease: lessons from a four-year prospective study. Am J Infect Control 1991; 19:79–85.

169. Haley CE, Cohen ML, Halter J, Meyer RD. Nosocomial Legionnaires' disease: a continuing common-source epidemic at Wadsworth Medical Center. Medicine 1979; 90:583–586.

170. Breiman RF, Fields BS, Sanden G, Volmer L, Meier A, Spika J. An outbreak of Legionnaires' disease associated with shower use: possible role of amoebae. JAMA 1990; 263:2924–2926.

171. Brady MT. Nosocomial Legionnaires' disease in a children's hospital. J Pediatr 1989; 115:46–50.

172. Blatt SP, Parkinson MD, Pace E, Hoffman P, Dolan D, Lauderdale P, et al. Nosocomial Legionnaires' disease: aspiration as a primary mode of disease acquisition. Am J Med 1993; 95:16–22.

173. Yu VL, Beam TR Jr, Lumis RM, Vickers RM, Fleming J, McDermott C, et al. Routine culturing for *Legionella* in the hospital environment may be a good idea: a three-hospital prospective study. Am J Med Sci 1987; 294:97–99.

174. Hall CB, Douglas G, Geiman JM, et al. Nosocomial respiratory syncytial virus infections. N Engl J Med 1975; 293:1343–1346.

175. Centers for Disease Control. Prevention and control of influenza. Advisory Committee Immunization Practices 1995; 44:April 21:1–38.

176. Dolin R, Reichman RC, Madore HP, Maynard R, Linton PN, Webber-Jones J. A controlled trial of amantadine and rimantadine in the prophylaxis of influenza A infection. N Engl J Med 1990; 322:443–450.

177. Tominack RL, Hayden FG. Rimantadine hydrochloride and amantadine hydrochloride use in influenza A virus infections. Infect Dis Clin North Am 1987; 1:459–478.

178. Valenti WM, Betts RF, Hall CB, Hruska JF, Douglas RGJ. Nosocomial viral infections: II. Guidelines for prevention and control of respiratory viruses, herpes viruses, and hepatitis viruses. Infect Control 1981; 1:165–178.

179. Rhame FS. Prevention of nosocomial aspergillosis. J Hosp Infect 1991; 18: 466–472.

180. Arnow PM, Anderson RL, Mainous PD, et al. Pulmonary aspergillus during hospital renovation. Am Rev Respir Dis 1978; 118:49–53.

181. Craven DE, Steger KA. Hospital-acquired pneumonia: perspective for the epidemiologist. Infect Control Hosp Epidemiol 1997; 18:783–795.

182. Craven DE, Steger KA, Sullivan MM. Preventing nosocomial pneumonia: a dynamic strategy. In: Torres A, Woodhead M, eds. Eur Respir Mon 1997; 2: Chapter 7:118–156.

183. Kollef MH. The prevention of ventilator-associated pneumonia. N Engl J Med 1999; 340:627–634.

184. Drakulovic MB, Torres A, Bauer TT, Nicolas JM, Nogue S, Ferrer M. Supine body position as a risk factor for nosocomial pneumonia in mechanically ventilated patients: A randomised trial. Lancet 1999; 354:1851–1858.

185. Hayden FG, Atmar RL, Schilling M, Johnson C, Poretz D, Paar D, et al. Use of the selective oral neuraminidase inhibitor oseltamivir to prevent influenza. N Engl J Med 1999; 341:1336–1343.

186. The MIST (Management of Influenza in the Southern Hemisphere Trialists) Study Group. Randomised trial of efficacy and safety of inhaled zanamivir in treatment of influenza A and B virus infections. Lancet 1998; 352:1877–1881.

4

Antimicrobial Therapy of Nosocomial Pneumonia

RAYMOND CHINN

Sharp Memorial Hospital
San Diego, California

I. INTRODUCTION

Once the diagnosis of nosocomial pneumonia has been established, several important factors must be considered before a rational empirical antimicrobial regimen can be chosen. These include severity of illness and comorbid conditions of the patient, prior antibiotic use, early versus late onset of infection, results of the sputum Gram's stain, and the resident flora profile of the institution, particularly in the intensive care unit (Table 1). Empirical antimicrobial therapy for nosocomial pneumonia in a ventilated patient with renal failure in whom multiple intra-abdominal abscesses develop following colon resection is very different from the patient who aspirates following an otherwise uncomplicated cholecystectomy.

In addition to host and environmental factors, an understanding of the various properties of antibiotic classes and recognition of the more common mechanisms of resistance will provide added insight into the complex interplay between the host and microbe. Integration of pharmacokinetic and pharmacodynamic properties into microbiological data may improve antibiotic choice and, thereby, enhance the patient's prospects for recovery.

This chapter (1) presents examples of the more common antimicrobial resistance mechanisms, (2) highlights general concepts of antimicrobial therapy, (3) discusses emerging strategies to optimize antibiotic use, and (4) re-

Table 1   Factors that Influence Initial Choice of
Antimicrobial Therapy

Early versus late infection
Aspiration risk
Prior antibiotic pressure
Chronic illness (diabetes, renal failure, malnutrition)
Chronic obstructive pulmonary disease
Immunosuppressive therapy
Neutropenia
Advanced age
Residence in an intensive care unit
Mechanical ventilation
Results of initial Gram's stain
Recent nosocomial pathogens of the institution

views the treatment of early and late nosocomial pneumonia with a focus on problematic pathogens.

II. ANTIBIOTICS AND RESISTANCE

The resilience with which bacteria respond to continued pharmacological insults is a testament to their adaptive ability and survival advantage. In general, antimicrobial resistance may occur through two mechanisms (1): by the acquisition of exogenous genetic material, an example being vancomycin intermediate *Staphylococcus aureus* (VISA), or by the development of mutational resistance, an example being the producers of extended-spectrum β-lactamases (ESBLs).

Vancomycin intermediate *S. aureus*, first isolated in Japan in May 1996, then subsequently in the eastern United States (2,3), may be an example of transfer of exogenous genetic material. Transfer of vancomycin resistance from vancomycin-resistant enterococci (VRE) to *S. aureus* has been demonstrated in the laboratory (4,5). Because *S. aureus* is a leading cause of nosocomial pneumonia, 37.5% of which have become methicillin resistant (6), the threat of an increasing prevalence of VISA and the eventual appearance of vancomycin-resistant *S. aureus* (VRSA) have sobering implications. Detection of VISA will ensure proper isolation to prevent nosocomial spread and initiate appropriate, albeit less than optimal, therapy.

Of more clinical significance are the producers of ESBLs, which result in resistance of *Escherichia coli*, *Klebsiella pneumoniae*, and *Proteus* spp. to the extended-spectrum β-lactams (1,7–10). The production of the common plasma-mediated β-lactamases (*TEM-1* and *SHV-1*) by these organisms is associated with the typical pattern of resistance (i.e., to ampicillin, the first generation cephalosporins, and the extended-spectrum penicillins), leaving unaffected the cephamycins, oxyimino-β-lactams (extended-spectrum cephalosporins, monobactams, carbopenems), and β-lactam/β-lactamase inhibitors. It was believed that the oxyimino-β-lactams were resistant to hydrolysis by the β-lactamases. In contrast, the expected resistance of *Enterobacter cloacae*, *Citrobacter freundii*, and *Serratia marcescens* to these agents resulted from an increased production of *AmpC* chromosomal β-lactamase.

As the oxyimino-β-lactams became a cornerstone of antimicrobial therapy, resistance to these agents were detected in strains of *E. coli* and *K. pneumoniae*. Interestingly, it has been shown that derivatives of the existing plasmid-mediated β-lactamases, *TEM-1* and *SHV-1*, in these bacteria were responsible for the dramatic change in resistance traits rather than introduction of new β-lactamases. Transfer of ESBLs to other bacteria through multiresistance plasmids has occurred. Producers of ESBLs may also become resistant to the cephamycins (cefotetan, cefoxitin) by incorporation of an *AmpC* gene into plasmids, thereby increasing the pattern of resistance further.

The ability to detect ESBLs has clinical relevance because it will have an impact on antibiotic therapy. Producers of ESBLs are suspected when susceptibility testing indicates resistance to ceftazidime (but may be paradoxically susceptible to ceftriaxone and cefotaxime by the minimal inhibitory concentration [MIC] or disc diffusion) and susceptible to the cephamycins (11). More recently, a breakpoint of ≥2 μg/mL to cefpodoxime has been suggested as a standard. Another method of detection is the use of the E-test strip with a gradient of ceftazidime on one side and ceftazidime in combination with clavulanate on the other. The ESBLs are thought to be present when enhancement of inhibition is demonstrated. Table 2 highlights some of the more common resistance mechanisms for antimicrobial agents used commonly in the treatment of nosocomial pneumonia.

III. GENERAL CONCEPTS ON ANTIMICROBIAL THERAPY

Pharmacokinetic and pharmacodynamic properties should be incorporated into the selection of antibiotics for the treatment of nosocomial pneumonia (12).

Table 2   Selected Antimicrobial Mechanisms of Resistance

Antimicrobial class	Mechanism of resistance
Aminoglycosides	Aminoglycoside modifying enzymes
β-lactamase inhibitors	Overproduction of β-lactamase; new β-lactamases; chromosomal cephalosporinases
Carbopenems	Zinc metalloenzymes; other β-lactamases
Cephalosporins	Extended spectrum β-lactamases; chromosomal β-lactamases (*AmpC*); plasmid β-lactamases (*TEM-1, SHV-1*)
Quinolones	Alterations in DNA topoisomerase, efflux mechanisms, permeability changes
Vancomycin	Modified cell wall precursors with decreased affinity for vancomycin.

Source: Modified from Ref. 1.

Pharmacokinetics refer to the rate and degree of antibiotic delivery into the blood and extracellular systems as well as drug clearance. The efficacy of antimicrobial therapy is dependent on the drug concentration in the lung; however, estimation of such concentration has been a frustrating exercise because of the lack of standardization of varied methods used. Nevertheless, samples to determine antibiotic concentration have been obtained from multiple sites, including lung tissue, sputum and bronchial secretions, bronchial mucosa, epithelial lining fluid, and alveolar macrophages. Because assays of lung tissue consist of a homogenate of tissue, blood, intracellular fluid, and extracellular fluid, they are not reliable in assessing the antibiotic concentration in the target areas. In evaluating the impact of antibiotic concentration on the treatment of pneumonia, the concentration of drug in the epithelial lining fluid (obtained by bronchoalveolar lavage) or alveolar macrophages (important for intracellular pathogens such as *Legionella*) is considered more relevant. The determination of concentration in sputum and bronchial secretions is more appropriately applied to the therapy of acute bacterial exacerbations of chronic bronchitis and patients with cystic fibrosis.

The epithelial lining fluid of the lung is separated by the nonfenestrated capillary endothelium on one side and alveolar membrane on the other; both are permeable to lipid-soluble antibiotics such as macrolides, quinolones, clindamycin, and trimethoprim-sulfamethoxazole, but relatively impermeable to water-soluble agents such as the aminoglycosides and β-lactams. However, the contribution of antibiotic transport of the water-soluble agents by polymorphonuclear neutrophils, that is, the effects of inflammation into the critical sites, has yet to be characterized.

Epithelial lining fluid concentrations of β-lactams antibiotics are about 10% to 35% of serum levels; therefore, the achievable concentration of this group of drugs in the target area can be estimated if serum levels are known and, when the MIC is considered, it would then be theoretically possible to design an appropriate therapeutic regimen. Aminoglycosides, because of their lower protein binding when compared to the β-lactams and their lower molecular weight, achieve higher concentrations, ranging 25% to 50% of serum levels.

Antibiotic concentration, however, may not be the sole determinant of antibiotic efficacy because the host may augment antimicrobial activity by the bactericidal actions of macrophages and neutrophils. These strategies can be impaired by the certain characteristics exhibited by the chosen antibiotic. For example, an acid environment and anaerobic condition may lessen the effect of aminoglycosides.

Pharmacodynamics, which relate to the association between antibiotic concentration and response, resulting in either therapeutic efficacy or drug-associated toxicity, is the other important pharmacological element that should be considered in a review on the therapy of pneumonia. Antibiotics exhibit either concentration-dependent (dose-dependent) or concentration-independent (time-dependent) killing. Aminoglycosides and quinolones are examples of concentration-dependent killing, which achieve optimal bactericidal efficacy when the peak is ≥10 times the minimal inhibitory concentration (MIC) of the bacteria (13); this prevents subtherapeutic dosing, which can result in the development of resistance, a trait known as adaptive resistance when bacteria downregulates the incorporation of the drug into the cell wall (14). Another phenomenon associated with dose-dependent killing is the postantibiotic effect (PAE), during which bacterial growth continues to be suppressed even when the antibiotic concentration goes below the MIC. This property has been described for the aminoglycosides, quinolones, carbopenems, macrolides, and tetracyclines. An added advantage when aminoglycosides are used is that the duration of the PAE is related to the peak serum concentration (15). In contrast, the β-lactams and vancomycin exhibit concentration-independent killing, requiring antibiotic concentrations consistently four times higher than the MIC for continued bactericidal activity. To optimize the use of antibiotics based on these various traits, strategies proposed include combination therapy, single daily dosing of aminoglycosides, aerosolization and instillation of aminoglycosides, and, for those organisms with higher MICs susceptible to β-lactams, there may be a theoretical advantage for the use of continuous infusions of β-lactams or more frequent dosing intervals.

IV. MONOTHERAPY VERSUS COMBINATION THERAPY

Much discussion has been generated on the topic of monotherapy versus combination therapy in the treatment of nosocomial pneumonia (16–22). The stated theoretical advantages for the use of combination therapy include (1) the prevention of the emergence of resistant organisms and (2) the possible synergistic or additive effects of the drugs. On the other hand, cost and toxicity may narrow the cost-benefit ratio. In general, pathogens such as *Pseudomonas aeruginosa* and multiresistant *Acinetobacter*, *Enterobacter*, and *Serratia* may require combination therapy in seriously ill patients (see later text). Combination therapy could include (1) an aminoglycoside with a β-lactam, (2) an aminoglycoside with a quinolone, (3) a quinolone with a β-lactam, or (4) double β-lactams. The use of the latter regimen is not synergistic and may lead to antagonism. If one drug induces β-lactamase production, then both antibiotics may be inactivated as a result. In combination therapy, neither synergy nor additive effect is consistently observed. When imipenem alone was compared to a combination of imipenem and netilmicin, nephrotoxicity complicated the clinical picture without the benefits of an improved outcome, except in infections caused by *P. aeruginosa* (23).

V. SINGLE DAILY DOSE OF AMINOGLYCOSIDES

There is renewed interest in the use of aminoglycosides given the progressive resistant patterns of organisms such as *P. aeruginosa*, *Acinetobacter*, and *Enterobacter*; in addition to the advantages cited earlier, this class of antibiotics is little influenced by the inoculum effect and the emergence of resistance during therapy is rare. The disadvantages of aminoglycosides include (1) inactivation of the drug in acid environment, which is produced as part of the acute inflammatory response, (2) difficulty in achieving therapeutic tissue levels when conventional dosing guidelines are used, and (3) threat of nephrotoxicity in patients who have already been subjected to variety of pharmacological or vascular insults.

Acknowledging that nephrotoxicity of aminoglycosides is a sequela of the accumulation of the drug rather than the height of the peak serum concentration, the administration of a single daily dose (SDD) of aminoglycosides, which would also overcome the problem of inadequate drug levels, has been proposed. There have been a number of meta-analyses (15,24–29) of SDD in the therapy of various infections. Barza and colleagues (29) found that, when the relative percentages of *P. aeruginosa* isolates in the trials were larger, clinical success occurred more frequently with the SDD. Others reported that (1) clinical effectiveness was greater, nephrotoxicity was lower, and ototoxicity was not increased (15), (2) there was a small but statistically significant difference in outcome favoring the use of SDD without increased risks of nephrotoxicity, ototoxicity, and vestibular toxicity (24), and (3) there were equivalent outcomes in terms of bacteriological cure and a trend toward reduced mortality rates and toxicity (27). However, Ali and Goetz (24) in their meta-analysis remarked that, in those studies when combination antimicrobial therapy was excluded, there was no difference in microbiological or clinical response.

Unfortunately, there is a paucity of comparative data examining the outcome of patients, that is, clinical and microbiological cure, with lower respiratory infections treated with SDD versus conventional dosing of aminoglycosides. Nor has the impact of aminoglycosides in combination therapy been subjected to critical evaluation. In a study by Nicolau and colleagues (28), SDD was administered to 2184 adult patients, 58 of their first 500 patients were followed up clinically for evidence of clinical and microbiological cure. For these 58 patients, there were 70 documented or suspected sites of infection, 20 of which underwent treatment for lower respiratory infection. Interestingly, clinical and microbiological cure were noted in all patients with extrapulmonary infections whereas clinical failures were apparent in four patients (14%) who were ventilated and whose putative pathogens were *P. aeruginosa* (2), *Citrobacter* sp. (1), and *Acinetobacter* (1). Some animal studies indicated that SDD combined with β-lactam therapy show enhanced synergistic activity against *P. aeruginosa* (30). Questions remain as to whether the administration of SDD alone or in combination is associated with a more favorable clinical outcome in the treatment of nosocomial pneumonia when compared with standard aminoglycoside dosing regimens.

Monitoring of SDD is still in its infancy and quite different from conventional models in that peaks in excess of 20 μg/mL for gentamicin and tobramycin are anticipated. Dosages used varied from 3 to 7 mg/kg/day for gentamicin, tobramycin, and netilmicin and from 14 to 20 mg/kg/day for amikacin. Modification is recommended for increasing dosing interval to every 36 hours for creatinine clearance between 40 and 59 mL/min and to 48 hours for creatinine clearances between 20 and 39 mL/min (26). A proposed target to avoid toxicity is to ensure a level of <1 µg/mL at 18 hours for the every 24-hour dosing for gentamicin and tobramycin.

Reportedly, SDD of aminoglycosides results in less accumulation in renal cells because the reabsorption of aminoglycoside is saturation dependent (30,31). Animal studies have shown that SDD allows a longer period when there is no additional drug exposure; with reduced aminoglycoside burden for "cellular processing" (26), there is theoretically less inherent toxicity.

Most authorities agree that SDD of aminoglycosides should not be used in pediatrics, pregnancy, dialysis patients, burn patients involving >20% of the body surface area, patients with ascites, patients receiving nephrotoxic drugs, those exposed to contrast material, persons older than 60 years, quadriplegic or amputee patients, and those with neurological syndromes such as myasthenia gravis. Some data suggest that there may be increased nephrotoxicity in the elderly when aminoglycosides are administered as a SDD compared with the conventional dosing methods (32).

In summary, the theoretical advantages of SDD are attractive and meta-analyses have shown some improved clinical and microbiological outcomes without increasing (and perhaps even decreasing the risks of nephrotoxicity); however, there is little available comparative information on the treatment of pneumonia either as monotherapy or combination therapy. Clinical studies may not be forthcoming as Bertino and Rotschafer (33) point out in their editorial, because aminoglycosides are generic. In cases of multidrug-resistant nosocomial pneumonia in which the organism is sensitive to an aminoglycoside, the use of SDD may be warranted unless there are contraindications.

VI. AEROSOLIZED AND INSTILLED AMINOGLYCOSIDES

Several approaches have been tried to increase the therapeutic efficacy of the aminoglycosides in the treatment of nosocomial pneumonia. These include direct instillation of the aminoglycoside into the respiratory tract through the endotracheal tube or tracheostomy and the use of aerosolized delivery systems. The postulated advantage is that these methods would deliver high concentrations of the aminoglycoside directly into the lung at least in bronchial secretions; whether such concentrations are achievable in epithelial lining fluid awaits clarification (34). Instillation usually results in higher levels in bronchial secretions when compared with the aerosolized method of delivery.

Used successfully in the adjuvant treatment of exacerbation of chronic bronchitis and bronchiectasis in patients with cystic fibrosis, aerosolized tobramycin has been administered in dosages varying from 20 to 600 mg every 8 hours (35). High concentrations in lung tissue have been documented following nebulization of tobramycin as determined by lung scintigraphy after a 300-mg dose (36). Baran and colleagues (37) found a mean tobramycin concentration of 2 ± 2.26 µg/mL in epithelial lining fluid as obtained from bronchoalveolar lavage after jet nebulization of an 80-mg dose.

Lack of systemic absorption with gentamicin or tobramycin administered by endotracheal instillation was demonstrated by Crosby et al. (38) in 10 patients with creatinine clearance greater than 40 mL/min; however, Odio and colleagues (39) found that significant serum levels were achieved in patients with azotemia when gentamicin 40 mg was instilled every 6 hours.

There are two published studies assessing the impact of aminoglycoside instillation as adjunctive therapy for gram-negative bacillary pneumonia. Klastersky et al. (40) found that more patients given instillation of sisomicin in addition to systemic antibiotics improved when compared to patients receiving systemic therapy alone. Although the study by Brown et al. (41) did not demonstrate any difference in clinical outcome when comparing systemic plus endotracheal instillation of tobramycin to systemic therapy alone, there was a statistically significant microbiological cure in the instillation group (56% versus 25% in the control group). This study has been criticized for failure to follow an intention-to-treat analysis and the interpretation is therefore hampered by the fact that less than half of the patients completed the protocol.

In contrast to the prophylaxis study by Feeley and colleagues (42) using aerosolized polymyxin at doses 4–20 mg, six to eight times per day, in which the emergence of resistant organism during aerosolized treatment was encountered, these two studies showed that there was no increase in the emergence of resistant pathogens when compared to the placebo group. In the experimental guinea pig model, Makhoul et al. (43) found that, by adding aerosolized tobramycin to systemic therapy, there was more effective eradication of *P. aeruginosa* and inflammatory changes in the lung were significantly reduced.

Bronchospasm frequently complicates aerosolized polymyxin therapy as a result of mast cell degranulation and histamine release; as such, a bronchial challenge is recommended before initiating therapy. Tobramycin may offer an advantage over gentamicin when used in aerosolized therapy because tobramycin is suspended in neutral pH (a condition similar to the respiratory lining

Table 3 Continuous Infusion of
Antimicrobials and Steady-State
Serum Concentrations

Antibiotic and dose (g/24 hr)	Concentration (µg/mL)
Aztreonam 2 g	15–18
Cefotaxime 2 g	10–14
Cefuroxime 2 g	12–15
Cefotetan 1 g	15–18
Ceftazidime 2 g	12–14
Pieperacillin 6 g	16–20

Source: Modified from Ref. 44.

fluid) and has no preservatives, thereby minimizing the bronchospastic potential. In the absence of clinical studies demonstrating a therapeutic advantage, the precise role of aerosolized and instillation therapy remains to be determined.

VII. CONTINUOUS INFUSION OF β-LACTAMS

To exploit the time-dependent or concentration-independent killing property of the β-lactams, which exert their bactericidal effect when drug concentrations are constantly above four times the minimal inhibitory concentration (MIC), continuous infusion has been studied (44,45). Knowledge of the achievable tissue concentration may permit a dose prediction for continuous administration (46). Nicolau et al. (44) have calculated steady-state concentrations of β-lactams administered by continuous infusion in patients with normal renal function (Table 3). Assuming that the epithelial lining fluid attains 10% to 35% of serum levels, modifying the steady-state level to achieve tissue levels four times the MIC may offer a therapeutic advantage in severe nosocomial pneumonia requiring therapy with a β-lactam; however, comparative studies have not been done.

VIII. EARLY NOSOCOMIAL PNEUMONIA

Guidelines have provided a systematic approach to the diagnosis and therapy of nosocomial pneumonia (16,46,47). It is often helpful to categorize nosocomial pneumonia as (1) early, occurring within 5 days of admission, or (2) late, ≥ 5 days after admission. Early infections in mild to moderately ill patients without significant risk factors are more likely due to methicillin-sensitive *S. aureus* (MSSA), *Streptococcus pneumoniae*, *Haemophilus influenza*, and less commonly, enteric gram-negative rods (16,46,48,49). With this microbiological profile, initial therapy with a second generation (e.g., cefuroxime) or a third generation non-pseudomonal cephalosporin (e.g., ceftriaxone and cefotaxime), β-lactam/β-lactamase inhibitor (ampicillin/sulbactam) would be reasonable. Alternatives to the β-lactams include (1) the quinolones (e.g., ciprofloxacin) for suspected gram-negative bacillary infections, (2) clindamycin for suspected infections resulting from MSSA or *S. pneumoniae* for the penicillin- and cephalosporin-allergic individual, or (3) combination of clindamycin and aztreonam/quinolone for polymicrobial infections in individuals who have allergies to penicillin or the cephalosporins. Whether an antecedent viral illness predisposed to these pathogens of early nosocomial pneumonia or whether nosocomial pneumonia resulted from aspiration remains speculative.

When early nosocomial pneumonia develops in a patient on antibiotics or with a history of recent exposure to antimicrobials, an extension of the antimicrobial spectrum is often necessary. Contrast the empirical therapy of nosocomial pneumonia in a patient receiving cefazolin prophylaxis with that of a ventilated patient receiving clindamycin and gentamicin for peritonitis. In the former case, aerobic gram-negative pathogens sensitive to the extended-spectrum β-lactams +/− anaerobes are likely pathogens, whereas a variety of multidrug-resistant pathogens may be recovered in the latter case.

IX. ANAEROBES

A well-acknowledged mechanism for the development of early nosocomial pneumonia is aspiration of contents from the oropharynx or stomach. This is frequently observed in nonventilated patients with witnessed aspiration, or in heavily sedated, ventilated patients who aspirate around the tracheostomy tube despite an inflated cuff. The predisposition for anaerobic infection may be influenced by the extent of gingivitis and periodontal disease. Indeed, Baker et al. (50) found that, in ventilated trauma patients, the majority of the pneumonias occurring soon after intubation was due to oral flora. Many of the organisms recovered from the oropharynx are anaerobes, but the importance of this group of organisms in the pathogenesis of nosocomial pneumonia remains a topic of controversy. In a review of the literature addressing this issue, Mayhall (48) found that, in 14 published studies between 1984 and 1995, only nine anaerobic isolates (3.1%) from 293 cases of nosocomial pneumonia in five studies were recovered, suggesting a minimal role, if any, for anaerobes in nosocomial pneumonia.

In contrast, Bartlett (52), when using transtracheal aspiration in nonventilator-associated pneumonia patients before the institution of antibiotic therapy, was able to identify 35% of anaerobes of 159 episodes of nosocomial pneumonia; however, 93% were polymicrobial, which included isolation of aerobic organisms. The most commonly isolated anaerobes were *Peptostreptococcus*, *Peptococcus*, *Fusobacterium*, *Prevotella melaninogenica*, and *Bacteroides fragilis*.

A more recent study (53), which focused on the potential role of anaerobes in ventilator-associated pneumonia (VAP) by applying strict diagnostic criteria (i.e., the recovery of $>10^3$ CFU/mL from protected specimen brushes) and by incorporating optimal culture methods for the isolation of anaerobes, found that, of 130 patients, 100 of them (77%) had aerobic organisms isolated alone whereas anaerobes were identified in 30 (23%) cases. Of the latter 30 patients, 26 (87%) of the cases were associated with aerobic bacteria; anaerobes alone were recovered from the remaining four (13%) patients.

Perhaps as a result of prompt antimicrobial intervention, none of this latter group of patients had necrotizing pneumonia, the hallmark of severe anaerobic pneumonia caused by aspiration in a community setting. Of the 30 patients who had anaerobic organisms isolated, 16 patients were on some form of antibiotics with some activity against anaerobic bacteria 48 hours before the culture. The most frequently isolated anaerobes in this series were *Provotella melaninogenica* (36%), *Fusobacterium nucleatum* (17%), and *Veillonella parvula* (12%). Therefore, the extent to which anaerobes are recovered may be dependent on antibiotic therapy in that these organisms are often sensitive to the various recommended antimicrobial regimens for nosocomial pneumonia; this may account for the higher numbers of anaerobes isolated in the study by Bartlett (52) in that cultures were obtained before antibiotic therapy.

Univariate analysis associated the isolation of anaerobes to (1) the development of pneumonia within the first 5 days of admission to the intensive care units, (2) orotracheally intubated compared with nasotracheal intubation, (3) younger age, and (4) higher acuity. Multivariate analysis found that altered level of consciousness, higher acuity, and admission to the MICU (in contrast to thoracic surgery, orthopedic surgery, and abdominal surgery units) predisposed the patient to the development of nosocomial pneumonia in which anaerobes were identified.

Table 4 Antibiotic Regimens for Nosocomial Pneumonia with Anaerobic Coverage

Antibiotic regimen	Comments
Clindamycin[a] with •Aminoglycoside •Quinolone (e.g., ciprofloxacin) •Aztreonam •Ceftazidime	Covers aerobic gram-negative coverage including *Pseudomonas aeruginosa.*
Aminoglycoside with an extended spectrum penicillin: •Piperacillin[b]	Covers aerobic gram-negative rods including *Pseudomonas aeruginosa.*
β-lactam with β-lactamase inhibitor[a]: •Ampicillin/sulbactam •Ticarcillin/clavulinic acid •Piperacillin/tazobactam	May be used as monotherapy if aerobic gram-negative pathogens susceptible; combination gram-negative therapy may be necessary.
Metronidazole[a] with β-lactam: •Except aztreonam and ceftazidime	Metronidazole has poor activity against the aerobic and microaerophilic streptococci; aztreonam and ceftazidime have no and poor activity against aerobic gram-positive oropharyngeal flora respectively.
Cephamycins[b] (cefoxitin, cefotetan)	May be used as monotherapy.
Trovofloxacin[a]	May be used as monotherapy.
Carbopenems[a] (imipenem, meropenem)	Reserved for multidrug-resistant aerobic gram-negative rods.

[a] Usually active against all anaerobes.
[b] Nearly always active against all anaerobes.

If anaerobes are thought to be significant in a given clinical circumstance, a variety of therapeutic options are available as initial empirical therapy of nosocomial pneumonia and, depending on the patient risk and prior antibiotic usage, coverage of aerobic gram-negative rods (Table 4) may be desirable.

X. LATE-ONSET NOSOCOMIAL PNEUMONIA

Data from the National Nosocomial Infection Surveillance System (NNIS), Centers for Disease Control and Prevention (CDC) from January 1986 through April 1997 report that *S. aureus* and *P. aeruginosa* each accounted for about

17.4% of pathogens isolated; taken together, aerobic gram-negative rods (excluding *Haemophilus*) led the list with 42% of agents causing nosocomial pneumonia in intensive care units (Table 5). In contrast to early nosocomial pneumonia in mild to moderately ill individuals, gram-negative bacteria predominate the list of pathogens in pneumonia in seriously ill patients and patients with late-onset nosocomial pneumonia.

The prevalence of *P. aeruginosa* isolated from NNIS hospitals is in keeping with the recommendation of the American Thoracic Society (16), which advocates coverage for this pathogen, *Acinetobacter*, and other resistant flora unique to an institution, regardless of the onset, in severely ill patients (defined by the American Thoracic Society as requiring ≥35% oxygen to maintain an arterial oxygen saturation >90%, mechanical ventilation, rapid radiographic progression, or multilobar involvement, or cavitation, evidence of sepsis [hypotension <90 mmHg, pressor requirement >4 hours, urine output <20 mL/hr] and acute renal failure necessitating dialysis). The devastation of gram-negative bacillary pneumonia is in part due to the remarkable trophism of these organisms for the respiratory epithelium, resulting in severe necrosis and hemorrhage in the host.

Ventilator-associated nosocomial pneumonia presents a particularly difficult therapeutic challenge because of the heavy bacterial burden, exemplified by a patient with closed head trauma and increased intracranial hypertension who is unable to clear secretions because of therapeutic paralysis or heavy

Table 5 Pathogens in Ventilator-Associated Pneumonia from NNIS Hospitals, January 1996–April 1997

Pathogen	No.	%
Staphylococcus aureus	8,292	17.4
Pseudomonas aeruginosa	8,307	17.4
Enterobacter spp.	5,446	11.4
Klebsiella pneumoniae	3,195	6.7
Haemophilus influenzae	2,346	4.9
Acinetobacter	2,198	4.6
Stenotrophomonas	1,337	2.8
Others	16,660	34.8[a]
Total	47,781	100

[a] The organisms represented in this group comprised <2.8% each of the total.
Source: Ref. 6.

sedation. Consequently, the absence or a diminished cough reflex to effectively remove inspissated secretions results in the loss of an integral part of the defense system. Such high-density infections create an environment favoring proliferation of the pathogen and destruction of the lung parenchyma caused by the cascade of the inflammatory reaction.

Once cultures and sensitivity testing results become available, the antibiotic regimen is then modified to improve cost-benefits, enhance outcome, reduce toxicity from unnecessary drug exposure, and discourage the emergence of multidrug-resistant bacteria within a hospital environment.

XI. THERAPY OF SELECTED PATHOGENS IN NOSOCOMIAL PNEUMONIA

A. *Staphylococcus aureus*

In nosocomial pneumonias caused by *S. aureus*, methicillin-sensitive strains account for most of the early infections whereas methicillin-resistant *S. aureus* (MRSA) is responsible for late-onset infection. Rello and colleagues (54) found that MRSA was associated with a higher incidence of bacteremia and worse outcome, which may be in part because of the bacteriostatic nature of vancomycin. Rifampin, which is rapidly bactericidal for susceptible strains, has been used with vancomycin to treat refractory infections such as endocarditis (55,56), but there are no published studies on the treatment of severe MRSA pneumonia with combination therapy. When rifampin is used as a single agent, resistance quickly develops. Patients with non–life-threatening allergies to vancomycin may tolerate teicoplanin (a glycoprotein not commercially available in the United States). When severe allergies to the glycoproteins prevent their use, alternatives include, when the organism is susceptible, clindamycin, trimethoprim–sulfamethoxazole and quinolones such as ciprofloxacin. In one study, trimethoprim–sulfamethoxazole was comparable to vancomycin (57). As with rifampin, resistance frequently develops when quinolones are used for therapy; therefore, combination therapy with rifampin seems justified when the use of a quinolone is indicated.

B. Bacteria with Extended-Spectrum β-Lactamases

Typically, ESBL-producing isolates of *E. coli* and *K. pneumoniae* are resistant to ceftazidime and aztreonam; however, susceptibility testing may indicate that the organism is susceptible to other extended-spectrum β-lactams (cefotaxime, ceftriaxone). These agents should not be used in this situation because treatment failure is likely, except in urinary tract infections because of the high urinary concentrations.

It is unclear whether recent insights into treatment modalities for bacteremia caused by ESBL producers are applicable to nosocomial pneumonia, and further studies are needed before definitive guidelines can be issued. It appears that treatment of bacteremia caused by ESBL-producing *E. coli* is amenable to noncephalosporin monotherapy whereas the outcome for *Klebsiella* is improved when two susceptible agents are used (58). The carbopenems have shown consistent activity against ESBLs; other antibiotics that could be used (assuming in vitro susceptibility) include the quinolones, β-lactam/β-lactamase inhibitors (by descending order of inhibitory activity: piperacillin/tazobactam, ticarcillin/calvulinic acid, ampicillin/sulbactam), and possibly the cephamycins (cefoxitin, cefotetan). However, treatment of ESBL-producing *K. pneumoniae* (59) infections with the cephamycins have not been successful in that the same organisms were subsequently isolated, showing resistance to this group of agents.

C. *Pseudomonas Aeruginosa*

Nosocomial pneumonia caused by *P. aeruginosa* has a high attributable mortality rate among ventilated patients, especially when associated with bacteremia, despite the institution of appropriate antimicrobial therapy (60–62). Rello and colleagues (63) reported 26 intubated patients with pneumonia caused by infection with *P. aeruginosa* and found a mortality rate of 42.3% versus 28.1% in matched control subjects without pneumonia. Combination therapy is desirable because synergy has been demonstrated and its use may potentially avoid resistance during therapy (17,64). In a study of 405 patients, it was found that monotherapy with either ciprofloxacin or imipenem was equivalent in terms of efficacy for the therapy of gram-negative bacillary nosocomial pneumonia, except for *P. aeruginosa*, which had a negative impact on treatment success (17).

The ability to develop resistance when monotherapy (less often with aminoglycosides) is used to treat infections caused by *P. aeruginosa* is well described (17). Therefore, traditional therapy has consisted of a combination of an antipseudomonal β-lactam (or β-lactam/β-lactamase inhibitor, carbopenem, monobactam) with an aminoglycoside because of in vitro demonstration of synergy; however, critically ill patients have many risk factors that render them more susceptible to the nephrotoxicity of aminoglycosides. The use of a quinolone if the organism is susceptible with a β-lactam is an alternative that bypasses the inherent nephrotoxicity of the aminoglycoside. Polymyxin B has rarely been coaxed out of retirement; it has retained activity to most isolates but is only used when no other antimicrobial agents are available because of its potential nephrotoxicity. There are instances when an isolate of *P. aeruginosa* may be resistant to imipenem yet sensitive to meropenem (65).

D. *Enterobacter*

Therapy of infections caused by *Enterobacter* with the β-lactams has been associated with the emergence of resistance during therapy. A recent optimistic study documented the efficacy of a new fourth generation cephalosporin, cefepime, in the treatment of ceftazidime-resistant *Enterobacter* species, citing the lower affinity cefepime for the chromosomal β-lactamase and higher permeability across the outer membrane of the organism (66). Unfortunately, a subsequent report confirmed the emergence of resistance to cefepime during therapy for a susceptible *Enterobacter* (67,68). The question, therefore, has been raised as to whether ceftazidime-resistant, cefepime-sensitive strains of *Enterobacter* are truly sensitive because these seemingly susceptible strains were actually resistant when tested with a higher inoculum (by agar dilution using 10^7 instead of 10^4) (68,69). Consequently, it was concluded that the drug should not be used in high-density infections, such as pneumonia and abscess, because the rapid emergence of resistance would be likely. The guidelines for combination therapy for pneumonia caused by *P. aeruginosa* are also applicable for this organism.

E. *Acinetobacter Baumannii* (*Calcoaceticus* var. *Anitratus*)

Similar to cases with *P. aeruginosa*, nosocomial ventilator-associated pneumonia caused by *Acinetobacter* is associated with a high mortality rate. In a study of 48 patients (70), pneumonia caused by these two organisms have a mortality rate of 71.4% compared to other pathogens (40.7%), with the observation that this rate was in excess of that observed for the underlying disease; however, the impact of antimicrobial therapy was not discussed.

Nosocomial isolates of *Acinetobacter* are frequently multidrug resistant and empirical therapy should be initiated based on the institution's endemic sensitivity pattern for this pathogen. The carbopenems have been effective against the organism, although resistance has been reported (71,72). Of the aminoglycosides, amikacin is most active (72). The ability of *Acinetobacter* to induce β-lactamase production has been described, rendering the use of extended-spectrum cephalosporins ineffective, despite in vitro evidence of susceptibility. In vitro synergy has been shown for fluoroquinolones with aminoglycosides (or β-lactams) and for imipenem and aminoglycoside in aminoglycoside-resistant isolates, but whether these studies are applicable to the clinical arena must be studied further.

In severe nosocomial pneumonia caused by *Acinetobacter* resistant to the carbopenem and the aminoglycosides, some clinical studies suggest that sulbactam is effective (73), but emergence of resistance may limit its usefulness; the organism has retained its susceptibility to polymyxin B.

Usually, combination therapy is recommended for patients with severe infection; the rationale is more intuitive and based on in vitro studies on synergy and disturbing reports of the emergence of resistance while on therapy rather than on information based on clinical trials.

F. *Stenotrophomonas*

Nosocomial pneumonia caused by *Stenotrophomonas (Xanthomonas) maltophilia* parallels the use of antibiotic pressure in patients with underlying debilitating chronic diseases, advanced age, and the use of invasive monitoring devices, and is typically associated with imipenem usage (72). Carmeli and Samore (74) report that the emergence of this organism can be traced to the use of either imipenem or ceftazidime.

Stenotrophomonas is also intrinsically resistant to many commonly used antibiotics for aerobic gram-negative pathogens. At its least resistant, the organism is sensitive to trimethoprim–sulfamethoxazole, minocycline, ticarcillin-clavulanic acid, ceftazidime, fluoroquinolones, and chloramphenicol. Treatment with trimethoprim–sulfamethoxazole, a bacteriostatic agent, has been a standard, although its use in the therapy of bacteremia has been disappointing (75). Resistance rapidly develops to antibiotics (other than trimethoprim–sulfamethoxazole) used as monotherapy. In vitro synergy has been shown for strains sensitive to both ticarcillin-clavulanic acid and ofloxacin (76) and therefore may provide a viable substitution to patients with hypersensitivity to trimethoprim–sulfamethoxazole or when the organism is shown to be resistant to this agent.

G. *Burkholderia (Pseudomonas) Cepacia*

Burholderia is a widely distributed organism, which has no virulence for the normal host. The most commonly infected or colonized patients are those with cystic fibrosis in whom necrotizing pneumonia may occur. The ability of the organism to result in nosocomial transmission by contaminated respiratory equipment is well described (78). Antibiotic therapy is similar to the treatment for *S. maltophilia* and is often unsatisfactory because of failures that occur, despite initial in vitro demonstration of susceptibility, when resistance develops during treatment. Agents that show activity include piperacillin, ceftazidime, sulbactam, trimethoprim–sulfamethoxazole, imipenem, chloramphenicol, minocycline, and ciprofloxacin. Imipenem-resistant strains may be sensitive to meropenem (79). Various combinations have shown synergy in vitro but application to clinical cases remains to be studied. The degree of resistance is related to the type of antibiotic therapy and is likely dependent on the duration of hospitalization and prior antibiotic exposure.

H. *Legionella*

In the 1980s, nosocomial legionellosis occurred as outbreaks in tertiary care centers (79). More recently, cases are sporadic and associated with the presence of this organism in the hospital water supply. Two mechanisms are proposed for the acquisition of the infection: (1) inhalation of contaminated aerosols or microaspiration of water (80) and (2) nasogastric tube feedings diluted with tap water containing legionella (81).

Following the original outbreak of legionellosis in 1976, erythromycin emerged as the drug of choice and, in severe cases, the addition of rifampin has been advocated because of its in vitro and in vivo activity (82). The newer macrolides, clarithromycin and azithromycin, have better in vitro activity and increased intracellular and parenchymal concentration as compared to the parent compound (83,84). Because azithromycin is available in a parenteral form and has a remarkably long half-life of about 16 hours, permitting a shorter course of therapy (from 21 days to 10 days), it will likely replace erythromycin as the drug of choice (79). The problems of ototoxicity, severe phlebitis, and gastrointestinal intolerance despite the intravenous route of the parent compound would be avoided. Macrolides and rifampin, however, may have limited use in transplant recipients because of interaction with cyclosporine, resulting in high cyclosporine levels. The quinolones, ciprofloxacin and levofloxacin, also have activity (80,85) and may be used if there are contraindications for the use of the macrolides (Table 6).

I. *Aspergillosis*

Nosocomial *Aspergillus* pneumonia occurs most frequently in patients undergoing cytotoxic chemotherapy who become neutropenic and require treatment

Table 6 Selected Antibiotics Effective in the Treatment of Legionellosis

Antibiotic	Dosage
Azithromycin	500 mg orally or intravenously every 24 hours
Clarithromycin	500 mg orally every 12 hours
Erythromycin	1 g intravenously every 6 hours
Ciprofloxacin	500 mg orally or intravenously every 24 hours
Levofloxacin	400 mg intravenously every 12 hours
	750 mg orally every 12 hours
Doxycycline	100 mg orally or intravenously every 12 hours
Rifampin	300 mg orally or intravenously every 12 hours

Source: Adapted from Ref. 79.

with multiple antibiotics and in recipients of bone marrow or solid organ transplantation (86,87). The mainstay of therapy has been high-dose amphotericin B therapy in the range of 1.0 to 1.5 mg/kg/day, a dose associated with significant toxicities in patients who already have and are at high risk for enhanced nephrotoxicity because of the concomitant use of aminoglycoside, vancomycin, and cisplatin. Saline loading may be helpful in preventing nephrotoxicity (88). Use of mannitol has not been shown to be effective. Premedication with acetaminophen, antihistamines, low-dose hydrocortisone, and meperidine may prevent chills and other systemic adverse reactions.

The lipid formulations of amphotericin B are about 20 times more costly and have been touted as having less nephrotoxicity while other commonly associated side effects are similar. This formulation of amphotericin permits higher doses (3–5 mg/kg) because the lipotrophic properties concentrate well in lymphoid tissue such as liver and spleen; however, the concentration in pulmonary tissue is unclear.

There are three liposomal compounds currently available: amphotericin B lipid complex (ABLC or Abelcet[R]), amphotericin B colloidal dispersion (ABCD or Amphocil[R]), and L-AMB (or AmBisome[R]), all of which have activity against invasive fungal infections including *Aspergillus*. Use of the liposomal formulation of amphotericin B is reserved for patients in whom invasive pulmonary aspergillosis develops in a setting of preexisting azotemia and in patients with severe intolerance to or who experience disease progression on conventional amphotericin therapy (89,90). White et al. (90) studied the use of amphotericin B colloidal dispersion (ABCD) in an open label clinical trial, comparing it retrospectively to treatment with conventional amphotericin B;

the response rate for pulmonary infection was 48.5% (32 of 66 patients) for the former agent compared with 24.2% (48 of 198 patients) for the latter drug, with less drug toxicity. However, study bias included a higher percentage of neutropenic patients in the amphotericin B group.

The imidazole itraconazole has activity against *Aspergillus*, but initial therapy with this agent should be targeted for patients with subacute disease because it requires about 2 weeks to reach steady-state levels (91–94). This antifungal agent may have a role in consolidation therapy after clinical response is evident from amphotericin B in association with recovery from myelosuppression or with immune reconstitution. Denning (93) studied oral itraconazole in patients with pulmonary aspergillosis with a complete response rate of 33% (17 patients) and partial response in 16% (eight patients). Poorest response rates were noted in AIDS patients and those who have undergone bone marrow transplantation. Efficacy is limited by absorption, which requires an acid media and a postprandial state, conditions that are difficult to achieve because there is often concomitant administration of H_2 blockers, antacids, and omiprazole, all of which decrease stomach acidity and, in the seriously ill, gastrointestinal dysfunction is commonplace. The cyclodextrin formulation of itraconazole (currently approved only for oropharyngeal and esophageal candidiasis) along with an eagerly anticipated parenteral solution will increase the bioavailability of this agent. Itraconzole has many drug interactions, notably with cisapride, terfenadine, and astemizaole, all of which may result in life-threatening arrhythmias. It also increases the effect of coumadin, digoxin, cyclosporine, and tacrolimus, the latter two having pharmacological implications in transplant recipients.

Because of the significant mortality rate associated with invasive pulmonary aspergillosis, it is tempting to use combination therapy with itraconazole and amphotericin B, but this approach has not been scrutinized in clinical trials.

XII. DURATION OF THERAPY

The optimal duration of antimicrobial therapy of nosocomial pneumonia is not well established. Generally, a course for 10 to 21 days is recommended, the longer course would be reasonably indicated for those patients with extensive infection involving multiple lobes, highly resistant organisms such as *Acinetobacter* and *P. aeruginosa*, cavitary disease, or malnutrition (16,45). Because the bioavailability of the quinolones when administered orally is equivalent

Table 7 Selected Antimicrobial Agents in the Therapy of Bacterial Pathogens of Nosocomial Pneumonia with Acquisition Costs[a]

Antimicrobial class	Examples	Pathogens	Common dosages	Cost
Cephamycins	Cefotetan[b]	Second generation cephalosporin with anaerobic activity; possibly, ESBLs	1–2 g q 12 hr	$20–$40
Extended-spectrum penicillins	Cefotaxime[b]	Enteric gram-negative rods, such as *Escherichia coli, Klebsiella*	1–2 g q 8 hr	$25–$50
	Ceftriaxone	As above	1–2 g q 24 hr	$22–$44
	Ceftazidime[b]	Above + *Pseudomonas aeruginosa, Stenotrophomonas*	1–2 g q 8 hr	$29–$48
	Cefepime[b]	Above + *Enterobacter,* streptococci, methicillin-sensitive *Staphylococcus aureus*	1–2 g q 12 hr	$28–$56
β-lactam/β-lactamase inhibitors	Ampicillin/sulbactam[b]	ESBPs, enteric gram-negative rods, possibly *Acinetobacter*	1.5–3.0 g q 6 hr	$27–$54
	Ticarcillin/clavulinate[b]	ESBPs, enteric gram-negative rods, *Pseudomonas aeruginosa, Stenotrophomonas* (used with ofloxacin)	3.1 g q 6 hr	$45
	Piperacillin/tazobactam[b]	ESBPs, enteric gram-negative rods, *P. aeruginosa*	3.375 g q 6 hr	$50
Monobactam	Aztreonam[b]	Aerobic gram-negative rods; no gram-positive coverage or anaerobic coverage	1–2 g q 8 hr	$42–$84

Carbopenem	Imipenem[b]	Polymicrobial infections, aerobic gram-negative rods, including *Acinetobacter, Enterobacter*	500 mg q 6 hr	$90
	Meropenem[b]	Above + *Burkholderia*	1 g q 8 hr	$112
Quinolone	Ciprofloxacin[b]	Aerobic gram-negative rods, including *P. aeruginosa*	400 mg q 12 hr/ 500 mg PO b.i.d.	$36/$5
	Travofloxacin[c]	Above + anaerobes and gram-positive bacteria	300 mg q 24 hr/ 200 mg PO	$45/$6
Aminoglycosides	Amikacin[b]	Aerobic gram-negative rods; most active against *Acinetobacter*	500 mg q 12 hr (example)	$13
	Gentamicin[b]	Aerobic gram-negative rods; most active against *Serratia*	120 mg q 8 hr (example)	$3
	Tobramycin[b]	Aerobic gram-negative rods; most active against *P. aeruginosa*	120 mg q 8 hr (example)	$7
Macrolides	Azithromycin[c]	Legionella	500 mg q 24 hr	$18
Rifampin[c]		Used in synergy: legionella, possibly, methicillin-resistant *S. aureus*	300 mg q 12 hr/ PO	$126/$1
Trimethoprim/ sulfamethoxazole[b]	Septra[R], Bactrim[R]	*Stenotrophomonas, Burkholderia*	15 mL q 8 hr	$6

[a] Acquisition costs per day for a tertiary care community hospital including various discounts and infusion costs.
[b] Dosage has to be modified in renal failure.
[c] Dosing has to be modified in hepatic failure.

to the intravenous route, oral therapy may be possible provided absorption can be assured.

In the treatment of invasive pulmonary aspergillosis, there is no set duration of therapy as eradication of this organism is dependent on the host immune response. For example, those patients treated for invasive disease during the neutropenic phase of induction chemotherapy for acute leukemia who, after recovery from myelosuppression, has a normal chest X-ray, should have antifungal therapy reinstituted when that patient undergoes consolidation therapy if neutropenia is anticipated.

XIII. NEW ANTIBIOTICS ON THE HORIZON

Several new agents that will be released for use in the near future deserve mention. Of the newer quinolones, trovafloxacin and clinafloxacin have enhanced activity against gram-positive pathogens (including MRSA) and anaerobic bacteria when compared with ciprofloxacin while retaining ciprofloxacin's aerobic gram negative activity. These agents may have utility as a single agent for the treatment of nosocomial pneumonia.

Quinupristin/dalfopristin and oxazolidinones have bactericidal activity against staphylococci including the methicillin resistant strains. These would be a welcome addition to the antimicrobial arsenal should adequate clinical trials prove their efficacy.

XIV. SUMMARY

The choice of empirical antibiotic therapy for nosocomial pneumonia is dependent of various factors, the more important being the severity of illness of the patient, prior antibiotic exposure, onset of infection, and resident pathogens in the institution. Antibiotic choice should incorporate an understanding of the pharmacokinetics and pharmacodynamics of antimicrobial agents, the resistance mechanisms of various bacteria, and the ecological impact that antibiotic use has on the institution. Once the pathogen has been identified, it is incumbent on the clinician to narrow the antibiotic spectrum because there are numerous reports linking the use of antimicrobial agents and the emergence of antimicrobial resistance (95–99). Monotherapy is appropriate in most instances from a standpoint of cost and unnecessary antibiotic exposure, except an infections caused by *P. aeruginosa*, *Acinetobacter*, or other highly resistant organisms. Table 7 summarizes the various antimicrobial agents available for the treatment of pathogens associated with nosocomial pneumonia and provides cost information.

Refinement in the diagnosis of nosocomial pneumonia, especially ventilator-associated pneumonia, will certainly decrease the use of unnecessary antimicrobial therapy. An aging population, reliance on invasive devices, use of chemotherapy for malignancies, and immunosuppressives for transplant recipients all create highly susceptible targets for this nosocomial complication. The development of effective antimicrobial agents has not kept pace with the emergence of highly resistant organisms. Arguably, antibiotic literacy and the judicious use of antibiotics are paramount to winning the conflict between the host and microbe.

REFERENCES

1. Gold HS, Moellering RC Jr. Antimicrobial-drug resistance. N Engl J Med 1996; 335:1445–1453.
2. *Staphylococcus aureus* with reduced susceptibility to vancomycin-United States, MMWR 1997; 46:765–766.
3. Update: *Staphylococcus aureus* with reduced susceptibility to vancomycin-United States. MMWR 1997; 46:813–814.
4. Leclerq R, Derlot E, Weber M, Duval J, Courvalin P. Transferable vancomycin and teicoplanin resistance in *Enterococcus faecium*. Antimicrob Agents Chemother 1989; 33:10–15.
5. Noble WC, Virani Z, Cree RGA. Co-transfer of vancomycin and other resistance genes from *Enterococcus faecalis* NCTC 12201 to *Staphylococcus aureus*. FEMS Microbiol Lett 1992; 93:195–198.
6. Data provided by Jonathan Edwards M.S., Statistical Support Section, National Nosocomial Infection Surveillance System, Centers for Disease Control and Prevention. 1998.
7. Fraimow HS, Abrutyn E. Pathogens resistant to antimicrobial agents: epidemiology, molecular mechanisms, and clinical management. Infect Dis Clin North Am 1995; 9(3):497–530.
8. Segal-Maurer S, Urban C, Rahal JJ Jr. Current perspectives on multidrug-resistant bacteria: epidemiology and control. Infect Dis Clin North Am 1996; 10: 939–957.
9. Itokazu GS, Quinn JP, Bell-Dixon C, Kahan FM, Weinstein RA. Antimicrobial resistance rates among aerobic gram-negative recovered from patients in intensive care units: evaluation of a national postmarketing surveillance program. Clin Infect Dis 1996; 23:779–784.
10. Tenover FC, Hughes JM. The challenges of emerging infectious disease: devel-

opment and spread of multiply-resistant bacterial pathogens. JAMA 1996; 275(4):300–304.

11. Jacoby GA. Extended-spectrum β-lactamases and other enzymes providing resistance to oxyimino-β-lactams. Infect Dis Clin North Am 1997; 11:875–887.

12. Ebert SC. Pharmacokinetic and pharmacodynamic considerations in antibiotic selection for different pneumonia settings. Infect Dis Clin Pract 1997; 6:S43–S48.

13. Moore RD, Lietman PS, Smith CR. Clinical response to aminoglycoside therapy: importance of the ratio of peak concentration to minimum inhibitory concentration. J Infect Dis 1987; 155:93–97.

14. Daikos GL, Jackson GG, Lolans VT, Livermore DM. Adaptive resistance to aminoglycoside antibiotics from first-exposure down-regulation. J Infect Dis 1990; 162:414–420.

15. Ferriols-Lisart R, Alós-Almiñana M. Effectiveness and safety of once-daily aminoglycosoides: a meta-analysis. Am J Health Syst Pharm 1996; 53:1141–1150.

16. Campbell GD Jr, Niederman MS, Broughton WA, Craven DE, Fein AM, Fink MP, Gleeson K, Hornick DB, Lynch JP III, Mandell LA, Mason CM, Torres A, Wunderink RG. Hospital-acquired pneumonia in adults: diagnosis, assessment of severity, initial antimicrobial therapy, and preventative strategies: a consensus statement. Am J Respir Crit Care Med 1995; 153:1711–1725.

17. Fink MP, Snydman DR, Niederman MS, Leeper KV Jr, Johnson RH, Heard SO, Wunderink RG, Caldwell JW, Schentag JJ, Siami GA, Zameck RL, Haverstock DC, Reinhart HH, Echols RM, the Severe Pneumonia Study Group. Treatment of severe pneumonia in hospitalized patients: results of a multicenter, randomized, double-blind trial comparing intravenous ciprofloxacin and imipenem-cilastatin. Antimicrob Agents Chemother 1994; 38:547–557.

18. Schelf WM, Mandell GL. Nosocomial pneumonia: pathogenesis and recent advances in diagnosis and therapy. Rev Infect Dis 1991; 13:S743–S751.

19. Arbo MDJ, Syndman DR. Monotherapy is appropriate for nosocomial pneumonia in the intensive care unit. Semin Respir Infect 1993; 8(4):259–267.

20. Lynch JP. Combination antibiotic therapy is appropriate for nosocomial pneumonia in the intensive care unit. Semin Respir Infect 1993; 8(4):268–284.

21. Andrews R, Fasoli R, Scoggins WG, Algozzine GJ, Spann RW, Sundaresh KV, Nathers JAL, Babb R, Kuppinger M, Cooper B. Combined aztreonam and gentamicin therapy for pseudomonal lower respiratory tract infections. Clin Ther 1994; 16:236–252.

22. Croce MA, Fabian TC, Stewart RM, Pritchard FE, Minard G, Trenthem L, Kudsk KA. Empiric monotherapy versus combination therapy of nosocomial pneumonia in trauma patients. J Trauma 1993; 35:303–311.

23. Cometta A, Baumgartner JD, Lew D, et al. Prospective randomized comparison of imipenem monotherapy with imipenem plus netilmicin for treatment of severe infections in nonneutropenic patients. Antimicrob Agents Chemother 1994; 38:1309–1313.

24. Ali MZ, Goetz MB. A meta-analysis of the relative efficacy and toxicity of single daily dosing versus multiple daily dosing aminoglycosides. Clin Infect Dis 1997; 24:796–809.

25. Nordstrom L, Ringberg H, Cronberg S, Tjernstrom O, Walder M. Does administration of an aminoglycoside in a single daily dose affect its efficacy and toxicity? J Antimicrob Chemother 1990; 25:159–173.

26. Gilbert DN. Minireview: once-daily aminoglycoside therapy. Antimicrob Agents Chemother 1991; 35(3):339–405.

27. Hatala R, Dinh T, Cook DJ. Once-daily aminoglycoside dosing in immunocompetent adults: a meta-analysis. Ann Intern Med 1996; 124:717–725.

28. Nicolau DP, Freeman CD, Belliveau PP, Nightingale CH, Ross JW, Quintiliani R. Experience with a once-daily aminoglycoside program administered to 2,184 adult patients. Antimicrob Agents Chemother 1995; 39(3):650–655.

29. Barza M, Ioannidis JPA, Cappelleri JC, Lau J. Single or multiple daily doses of aminoglycosides: a meta-analysis. BMJ 1996; 312:338–345.

30. Craig WA, Redington J, Ebert S. Effect of dosage regimen on in vivo synergy of antibiotic combinations against *Pseudomonas aeruginosa*. In: Einhorn J, Nord CE, Norrby SR, eds. Recent Advances in Chemotherapy. Washington, DC: American Society for Microbiology 1994:470–471.

31. DeBroc ME. Influence of dosage schedules on renal cortical accumulation of amikacin and tobramycin in man. J Antimicobr Chemother 1991; 27(supp C): 41–47.

32. Traynor AM, Nafziger AN, Bertino JS. Aminoglycoside dosing weight correction factors for patients of various body sizes. Antimicrob Agents Chemother 1995; 39:545–548.

33. Bertino JS, Rotschafer JC. Editorial response: single daily dosing of aminoglycosides—a concept whose time has not yet come. Clin Infect Dis 1997; 24:820–823.

34. Honeybourne D. Antibiotic penetration into lung tissue. Thorax 1994; 49:104–106.

35. Ramsey BW, Dorkin HL, Eisenberg JD, Gibson RL, Harwood IR, Kravitz RM, Schidlow DV, Wilmott RW, Astley SJ, McBurnie MA, Wentz KM, Smith AL. Efficacy of aerosolized tobramycin in patients with cystic fibrosis. N Engl J Med 1993; 328:1740–1746.

36. LeConte P, Potel G, Peltier P, Horeau D, Caillon J, Juvin ME, et al. Lung distribution and pharmacokinetics of aerosolized tobramycin. Am Rev Respir Dis 1993; 147:1279–1282.

37. Baran D, de Vuyst P, Ooms HA. Concentrations of tobramycin given by aerosol in the fluid obtained by bronchoalveolar lavage. Respir Med 1990; 84:203–204.

38. Crosby SS, Edwards WAD, Brennan C, Dellinger EP, Bauer LA. Systemic absorption of endotracheally administered aminoglycosides in seriously ill patients with pneumonia. Antimicrob Agents Chemother 1987; 31(6):850–853.

39. Odio W, Vanlaer E, Klastersky J. Concentrations of gentamicin in bronchial

secretions after intramuscular and endotracheal administration. J Clin Pharmacol 1975; 15:518–524.

40. Klastersky J, Carpentier-Meunier F, Kahan-Coppens L, Thijs JP. Endotracheally administered antibiotics for gram-negative bronchopneumonia. Chest 1979; 75: 586–591.

41. Brown RB, Kruse JA, Counts GW, Russell JA, Christou NV, Sands ML, the Endotracheal Tobramycin Study Group. Double-blind study of endotracheal to-bramycin in the treatment of gram-negative bacterial pneumonia. Antimicrob Agents Chemother 1990; 34(2):269–272.

42. Feeley TW, du Moulin GC, Hedley-Whyte J, Bushnell LS, Gilbert JP, Feingold DS. Aerosol polymyxin and pneumonia in seriously ill patients. N Engl J Med 1975; 293:471–475.

43. Makhoul IR, Merzbach D, Lichtig C, Berant M. Antibiotic treatment of experi-mental *Pseudomonas aeruginosa* pneumonia in guinea pigs: comparison of aero-sol and systemic administration. J Infect Dis 1993; 168:1296–1299.

44. Nicolau DP, Nightingale CH, Quintiliani R. Continuous infusion β-lactams: a pharmacodynamic approach. Infect Dis Clin Pract 1996; 5(7):432–434.

45. Quintiliani R, Nicolau DP, Nightingale CH. Pharmacokinetic and pharmacody-namic principles in antibiotic usage. In: Infectious Diseases and Antimicrobial Therapy of the Ears, Nose and Throat. Philadelphia: WB Saunders, 1997:48–55.

46. Niederman MS. Principles of antibiotic use and the selection of empiric therapy for pneumonia. In: Fishman AP, Elias JA, Fishman JA, Grippi MA, Kaiser LR, Senior RM, eds. Fishman's Pulmonary Disease and Disorders. 3rd ed. New York: McGraw-Hill, 1998:1939–1957.

47. Pennington JE. Nosocomial respiratory infections. In: Mandell GL, Bennett JE, Dolin R, eds. Mandell, Douglas and Bennett's Principles and Practice of Infec-tious Disease. 4th ed. New York: Churchill Livingstone, 1995:2599–2616.

48. Schleupner CJ, Cobb DK. A study of the etiologies and treatment of nosocomial pneumonia in a community-based teaching hospital. Infect Control Hosp Epide-miol 1992; 13:515–525.

49. Prodhom GP, Leuenberger P, Koerfer J, Blum A, Chiolero R, Schaller. MD, Perret C, Spinnler O, Blondel J, Siegrist H. Nosocomial pneumonia in mechani-cally ventilated patients receiving antacid, ranitidine, or sucralfate as prophylaxis for stress ulcer: a randomized controlled trial. Ann Intern Med 1994; 120:653–662.

50. Baker AM, Meredith JW, Haponik EF. Pneumonia in intubated trauma patients: microbiology and outcomes. Am J Respir Crit Care Med 1996; 153:343–349.

51. Mayhall CG. Nosocomial pneumonia: diagnosis and prevention. Infect Dis Clin North Am 1997; 11:427–457.

52. Bartlett JG. Anaerobic bacterial infections of the lung. Chest 1987; 91:901–908.

53. Dore P, Robert R, Grollier G, Rouffineau J, Lanquetot H, Charriere JM, Fauchere JL. Incidence of anaerobes in ventilator-associated pneumonia with use of a pro-tected specimen brush. Am J Respir Crit Care Med 1996; 153:1292–1298.

54. Rello J, Torres A, Ricart M, Valles J, Gonzalez J, Artigas A, Rodriguez-Roisin

R. Ventilator-associated pneumonia by *Staphyloccus aureus*: comparison of methicillin-resistant and methicillin sensitive episodes. Am J Respir Crit Care Med 1994; 150:1545–1549.

55. Acar JF, Goldstein EW, Duval J. Use of rifampin for the treatment of serious staphylococcal and gram-negative bacillary infections. Rev Infect Dis 1983; 5(S):502–506.

56. Faville RJ, Zaske DE, Kaplan El, et al. *Staphylococcus aureus* endocarditis: combined therapy with vancomycin and rifampin. JAMA 1984; 240:1963.

57. Markowitz N, Quinn EL, Saravolatz L. Trimethoprim-sulfamethoxazole compared with vancomycin for the treatment of *Staphylococcus aureus* infections. Ann Intern Med 1992; 117:390–398.

58. Wong-Beringer A, Lee NP, Hindler J, Pegues DA. Treatment outcome of extended-spectrum β-lactamase (ESBL) producing *Escherichia coli* and *Klebsiella pneumoniae* bacteremia. In: Abstracts (J-8) of the 37th Interscience Conference on Antimicrobial Agents and Chemotherapy. Toronto, Ontario, Canada: American Society for Microbiology, 1997.

59. Martinez-Martinez L, Hernandez-Alles S, Alberti S, et al. In vivo selection of porin-deficient mutants of *Klebsiella pneumoniae* with increased resistance to cefoxitin and expanded-spectrum cephalosporins. Antimicrob Agents Chemother 1996; 40:342.

60. Taylor GD, Buchanan-Chell M, Kirkland T, Mckenzie M, Wiens R. Bacteremic nosocomial pneumonia. A 7-year experience in one institution. Chest 1995; 108: 786–788.

61. Fagon JY, Chastre J, Domart Y, Trouillet JL, Pierre J, Carne C, Gibert C. Nosocomial pneumonia in patients receiving continuous mechanical ventilation. Am Rev Respir Dis 1989; 139:877–884.

62. Fagon JY, Chastre J, Hance A, Montravers P, Novara A, Gibert C. Nosocomial pneumonia in ventilated patients: a cohort study evaluating attributable mortality and hospital stay. Am J Med 1993; 94:281–288.

63. Rello J, Jubert P, Valles J, Artigas A, Rue M, Niederman MS. Evaluation of outcome for intubated patients with pneumonia due to *Pseudomonas aeruginosa*. Clin Infect Dis 1996; 23:973–978.

64. Hilf M, Yu VL, Sharp J, Zuravleff JJ, Korvick JA, Muder RR. Antibiotic therapy for *Pseudomonas aeruginosa* bacteremia: outcome correlations in a prospective study of 200 patients. Am J Med 1989; 87:540–546.

65. Iaconis JP, Pitkin DH, Sheikh W, Nadler HL. Comparison of antibacterial activities of meropenem and six other antimicrobials against *Pseudomonas aeruginosa* isolates from North American studies and clinical trials. Clin Infect Dis 1997; 24(suppl 2):S191–196.

66. Sanders WE Jr, Tenney JH, Kessler RE. Efficacy of cefepime in the treatment of infections due to multiply resistant *Enterobacter* species. Clin Infect Dis 1996; 23:454–461.

67. Medeiros AA. Editorial response: relapsing infection due to *Enterobacter* species: lessons of heterogeneity. Clin Infect Dis 1997; 25:341–342.

68. Limaye AP, Gautom RK, Black D, Fritsche TR. Rapid emergence of resistance to cefepime during treatment. Clin Infect Dis 1997; 25:339–340.

69. Johnson CC, Livornese L, Gold MJ, Pitsakis PG, Taylor S, Levison ME. Activity of cefepime against ceftazidime-resistant gram-negative bacilli using low and high inocula. J Antimicrob Chemother 1995; 35:765–773.

70. Fagon J-Y, Chastre J, Hance AJ, Montravers P, Novara A, Gibert C. Nosocomial pneumonia in ventilated patients: a cohort study evaluating attributable mortality and hospital stay. Am J Med 1993; 94:281–288.

71. Norrby SR, Faulkner KL, Newell PA. Differentiating meropenem and imipenem/cilastatin. Infect Dis Clin Pract 1997; 6:291–303.

72. Fang FC, Madinger N. Resistant nosocomial gram negative bacillary pathogens: *Acinetobacter baumannii*, *Xanthomonas maltophilia*, and *Pseudomonas cepacia*. Curr Clin Top Infect Dis 1996; 16:52–83.

73. Levin AS, Manrique AEI, Medeiros EAS, Cursino R, Santos CR, Sielfeld ME, Boulos M, Costa SF. Treatment of severe infection by multiresistant *Acinetobacter baumannii* with ampicillin/sulbactam—preliminary report. In: Abstracts of the 37th Interscience Conference on Antimicrobial Agents and Chemotherapy. Toronto, Ontario, Canada: American Society for Microbiology, 1997.

74. Carmeli Y, Samore MH. Comparison of treatment with imipenem vs. ceftazidime as a predisposing factor for nosocomial acquisition of *Stenotrophomonas maltophilia*: a historical cohort study. Clin Infect Dis 1997; 24:1131–1134.

75. Papadakis KA, Vartivarian SE, Anaissie EJ, Samonis G. *Xanthomonas maltophilia* bacteremia in cancer patients: an analysis of 44 episodes. Clin Infect Dis 1994; 19:558.

76. Tesoro EP, Jung R, Messick CR, Martin SJ, Pendland SL. In vitro evaluation of antibiotic combinations against hospital-acquired isolates of *Stenotrophomonas* (*Xanthomonas*) *maltophilia*. In: Abstracts (E-141) of the 37th Interscience Conference on Antimicrobial Agents and Chemotherapy. Toronto, Ontario, Canada: American Society for Microbiology, 1997.

77. Burdge DR, Nakielna EM, Noble MA. Case-control and vector studies of nosocomial acquisition of *Pseudomonas cepacia* in adult patients with cystic fibrosis. Infect Control Hosp Epidemiol 1993; 14:127–130.

78. Iaconis J, Tabinowski A, Nadler H, Sheikh W. Lack of cross-resistance between imipenem-resistant *Pseudomonas cepacia* isolates and meropenem. In: Abstracts of the 33rd Interscience Conference on Antimicrobial Agents and Chemotherapy. Washington, DC: American Society for Microbiology, 1993.

79. Stout JE, Yu VL. Legionellosis. N Engl J Med 1997; 337:682–687.

80. Edelstein PH. Legionnaires' disease. Clin Infect Dis 1993; 16:741–747.

81. Venezia RA, Agresta MD, Hanley EM, Erquhart K, Schoonmaker D. Nosocomial legionellosis associated with aspiration of nasogastric feedings diluted in tap water. Infect Control Hosp Epidemiol 1994; 15:529–533.

82. Baltch Al, Smith RP, Ritz W. Inhibitory and bactericidal activities of levofloxacin, ofloxacin, erythromycin, and rifampin used singly and in combination against *Legionella pneumophila*. Antimicrob Agents Chemother 1995; 39:1661–1666.

83. Yu VL. Legionella infection. In: Neu HC, Young LS, Zinner SH, eds. The New Macrolides, Azalides, and Streptogramins. New York: Marcel Dekker, 1993: 141–146.

84. Kutzman I, Soldo I, Schonwald S, Culig J. Azithromycin for treatment of community acquired pneumonia caused by *Legionella pneumophila*: a retrospective study. Scand J Infect Dis 1995; 27:503–505.

85. Stout JE, Arnold B, Ta CA, Yu VL. Activity of ciprofloxacin, ofloxacin, and levofloxacin against *Legionella pneumophila*, serogroup 1, by broth, dilution and intracellular penetration. In: Program and Abstracts of the 32nd Infectious Disease Society of America Annual Meeting, Orlando, FL. Washington, DC: American Society of Microbiology, October 7–9, 1994.

86. Walsh TJ, Hiemenz JW, Anaissie E. Recent progress and current problems in treatment of invasive fungal infections in neutropenic patients. Infect Dis Clin North Am 1996; 10:365–400.

87. Houston SH, Sinnott JT. Management of the transplant recipient with pulmonary infection. Infect Dis Clin North Am 1995; 9:965–985.

88. Branch RA. Prevention of amphotericin B-induced renal impairment: a review on the use of sodium supplementation. Arch Intern Med 1988; 148:2389.

89. Hospenthal DR, Byrd JC, Weiss RB. Successful treatment of invasive aspergillosis complicating prolonged treatment-related neutropenia in acute myelogenous leukemia with amphotericin B lipid complex. Med Pediatr Oncol 1995; 25:119–122.

90. White MH, Anaissie EJ, Kusne S, Wingard JR, Hiemenz JW, Cantor A, Gurwith M, Du Mond C, Mamelok RD, Bowden RA. Amphotericin B colloidal dispersion vs. amphotericin B as therapy for invasive aspergillosis. Clin Infect Dis 1997; 24:635–642.

91. Kaufmann CA. Role of azoles in antifungal infections. Clin Infect Dis 1996; 22(2);S148–S153.

92. Denning DW, Lee JY, Hostetler JS, Kauffman CA, Galgiani JN, Sugar AM, Gallis H, Dismukes WE. NIAID mycoses study group multicenter trial on oral itraconzaole therapy for invasive aspergillosis. Am J Med 1994; 97:135–144.

93. Denning DW. Diagnosis and management of invasive aspergillosis. In: Remington JS, Swartz M, eds. Current Clinical Topics in Infectious Disease. Boston: Blackwell Science, 1996; 16:277–299.

94. Walsh TJ, Hiemenz JW, Anaissie E. Recent progress and current problems in treatment of invasive fungal infections in neutropenic patients. Infect Dis Clin North Am 1996; 10(2):365–393.

95. Shlaes DM, Gerding DN, John JF Jr, Craig WA, Bornstein DL, Duncan RA, Eckman MR, Farrer WE, Greene WH, Lorian VL, Levy S, McGowan JE Jr, Paul SM, Ruskin J, Tenover FC, Watanakunakorn C. Society for Healthcare Epidemiology of America and Infectious Disease Society of America Joint Committee on the Prevention of Antimicrobial Resistance: Guidelines for the Prevention of Antimicrobial Resistance in Hospitals. Clin Infect Dis 1997; 25:584–599.

96. Jacobson KL, Cohen SH, Inciardi JF, King JK, Lippert WE, Iglesias T, Van-Couwenberghe CJ. The relationship between antecedent antibiotic use and resis-

tance to extended-spectrum cephalosporins in group I β-lactamase-producing organisms. Clin Infect Dis 1995; 21:1107–1113.

97. Archibald LK, Edwards JR, Mathema BB, Pryor ER, McGowan JE Jr, Culver DH, Gaynes RP, Project ICARE Hospitals. Imipenem-resistant *Pseudomonas aeruginosa* in selected intensive care units in the United States. In: Abstracts (J206) of the 37th Interscience Conference on Antimicrobial Agents and Chemotherapy. Toronto, Ontario, Canada: American Society for Microbiology, 1997.

98. Conus P, Francioli P. Relationship between ceftriaxone use and resistance of *Enterobacter* species. J Clin Pharm Ther 1992; 17:303–305.

99. Cornoado VG, Edwards JR, Culver DH, Gaynes RP. Ciprofloxacin resistance among nosocomial *Pseudomonas aeruginosa* and *Staphylococcus aureus* in the United States. Infect Control Hosp Epidemiol 1995; 16:71–75.

5

Selective Decontamination of the Digestive Tract

MARC J. M. BONTEN

University Hospital Utrecht
Utrecht, The Netherlands

ROBERT A. WEINSTEIN

Cook County Hospital
and Rush Medical College
Chicago, Illinois

I. INTRODUCTION

In intensive care units (ICUs), pneumonia is the most frequent nosocomial infection (1–3) and occurs most often as ventilator-associated pneumonia (VAP) in patients on mechanical ventilation. The overall incidence of VAP in different studies varies between 10% and 85%, depending on the patient population and the criteria used to establish the diagnosis. Ventilator-associated pneumonia has been associated with an attributable mortality rate ranging from 13% to 47% (4–7), although this is not a consistent finding (8–10).

According to the time of diagnosis, VAP can be subdivided into early-onset (diagnosed within the first 4 days of ventilation) and late-onset disease (diagnosed after more than 4 days of ventilation) (11). Early-onset VAP is usually caused by community-acquired bacteria colonizing the upper respiratory tract before hospital admission (e.g., *Streptococcus pneumoniae*, *Haemophilus influenzae*, and *Staphylococcus aureus*); these are presumably aspirated into the lungs at, or shortly after, the onset of acute illness that necessitates ICU admission. A correlation between colonization of the upper respiratory tract with Enterobacteriaceae, *Pseudomonas aeruginosa*, and *S. aureus*, the so-called "potential pathogenic microorganisms" (ppmo) and the heightened risk of nosocomial late-onset VAP has been firmly established (10,12). The patient's intestinal and oropharyngeal flora have been assumed to be important sources of bacterial strains, which, after aspiration, cause infection of the lower respiratory tract.

Among the many strategies developed to prevent VAP, selective decontamination of the digestive tract (SDD) is the most extensively studied. However, the data on the benefits of SDD are inconclusive, and SDD has never become a routine infection control strategy in the United States (13–16). Moreover, in The Netherlands, where SDD was first applied in intensive care patients in 1983, only 13% of all ICUs used SDD in 1996, mostly in selected groups of ventilated patients (17).

II. SELECTIVE DECONTAMINATION: THE CONCEPT

Before the application of SDD as a prophylaxis strategy in mechanically ventilated ICU patients, SDD had been applied with some success for prophylaxis of bacterial sepsis and febrile episodes among granulocytopenic patients (18,19). The full protocol of SDD, as originally promoted for mechanically ventilated patients, included four elements: (1) selective eradication of microorganisms from the intestine, the stomach, and the oropharynx by topical nonabsorbale antibiotics; (2) systemic prophylaxis during the first days of ICU admission; (3) a high standard of hygiene in the ICU to prevent exogenous cross infections; and (4) extensive microbiological surveillance to distinguish the type of infection, to monitor compliance and efficacy of treatment, and to detect emergence of resistant microorganisms (20). Surveillance may include collection of specimens (e.g., "rectal swabs") solely for the purpose of detecting emergence of resistant strains.

A. Topical Decontamination of the Digestive Tract

Selective decontamination of the digestive tract is based on the concept of "colonization resistance." Studies in mice revealed that the autochthonous intestinal flora protects against colonization with exogenous flora introduced with food (21). Although the responsible protective bacteria have never been identified exactly, the anaerobic flora has been assumed to be the source of colonization resistance, together with processes that mechanically clear microorganisms from the intestinal tract (e.g., peristalsis, salivary flow) and agents that influence bacterial adherence (e.g., mucus, secretory IgA). Eradication of the anaerobic flora by antibiotics allows overgrowth and colonization with exogenous flora, especially with microorganisms such as Enterobacteriaceae, Pseudomonadaceae, *S. aureus*, and yeasts (ppmo). As a result, the risk for infection with these microorganisms increases. Using topical antimicrobial agents, SDD aims to selectively eradicate ppmo from the intestine without disturbing the presumably protective anaerobic flora. These antimicrobials, therefore, should be nonabsorbable, should be active against ppmo, and should spare the anaerobic flora. Colistin and aminoglycosides meet these requirements and are generally used in SDD regimens. This regimen has excellent activity against Enterobacteriaceae, such as *Klebsiella* species, *Enterobacter* species, and *P. aeruginosa*, because dual colistin and aminoglycoside resistance is uncommon in these bacteria. The combined use of the two drug classes theoretically should delay selection of resistant gram-negative bacilli; the aminoglycoside also ensures activity against *Proteus* species and *Serratia marcescens*, which are typically resistant to colistin. To prevent overgrowth with yeasts, an antifungal (amphotericin B in the original description) has been a component of the SDD regimen.

Gastric colonization with ppmo is a common finding in mechanically ventilated patients (22,23), and colonization at this site has been presumed to have an etiological role in the development of VAP (24). The putative role of the stomach as a reservoir for microorganisms is based on observations of higher rates of gastric colonization in patients with VAP as compared to unaffected controls (22) and on observations that bacteria causing VAP had been isolated from gastric aspirates before the onset of pneumonia (11). Moreover, several studies suggested that preservation of the intragastric acid milieu, by using sucralfate for stress ulcer prophylaxis instead of antacids or H_2-antagonists, was associated with decreased rates of gastric overgrowth by gram-negative bacilli and reduced incidences of VAP (11,25,26).

Oropharyngeal decontamination was not included in the first protocol of SDD in mechanically ventilated patients. However, gastrointestinal decontamination alone did not influence the incidence of respiratory tract infections among multiple trauma patients when compared to a historical control group (27). Addition to the SDD regimen of an oropharyngeal paste containing topical antibiotics resulted in successful decontamination of the oropharynx and a reduction of late-onset respiratory tract infections (27).

B. Systemic Prophylaxis

The use of the combination of intestinal and oropharyngeal decontamination still did not significantly reduce the overall incidence of respiratory tract infections (27), because a large proportion of respiratory tract infections occurred within the first 4 days of mechanical ventilation, before decontamination was established. These cases of early-onset pneumonia were caused by pathogens that had already contaminated patients' lower respiratory tract in the period shortly before, or after, ICU admission, and therefore could not be eradicated by intestinal and oropharyngeal decontamination. Addition of 3 to 7 days (28) of systemic prophylaxis to the SDD regimen resulted in a further reduction of the early-onset infections (27), presumably as a result of preemptive therapy of incubating pneumonia.

III. GENERAL CRITIQUES TO THE CONCEPT OF SDD

As mentioned earlier, SDD was initially applied to granulocytopenic patients. Granulocytopenia and derangement of the protective properties of mucosal surfaces by aggressive chemotherapy or radiotherapy presumably allows intestinal bacteria to translocate. These patients consequently suffer from fever and septic episodes, which are attributed to bacteria or bacterial products that enter the circulation by way of damaged intestinal or oropharyngeal mucosa. The relevance of this mechanism among nongranulocytopenic ICU patients is uncertain. In addition, the importance of gastric colonization in the development of respiratory tract colonization and infections also is controversial (29,30). Although the possibility of the gastropulmonary route of colonization and infection does exist, its relative importance in the pathogenesis of VAP has been questioned (10,31–36). For example, analysis of sequences of colonization of bacteria causing VAP has not unequivocally revealed that the stomach is an important source or reservoir of these bacteria (29). In addition, data to support the pneumonia prophylactic effect of using sucralfate instead of antacids or H_2-antagonists for stress ulcer prevention are not conclusive (29). Finally, the importance of intestinal colonization as a source of pathogens causing VAP has not been demonstrated.

IV. CLINICAL STUDIES

Since 1984, more than 40 original studies on SDD, four meta-analyses, and several extensive reviews (37–40) have been performed. As shown in Tables 1 to 5, many of the studies differed in the regimens of SDD applied, the populations under study, the methods used for diagnosing VAP, endpoints (e.g., all VAP, late-onset VAP only, VAP caused by gram-negative bacilli, mortality rate), and the study design.

A. The Full SDD Regimen

The full SDD regimen (including oropharyngeal and intestinal decontamination and systemic prophylaxis) was studied at least 21 times (Table 1), including six studies with a double-blind, placebo-controlled design (41–46). The reported incidences of VAP among patients receiving SDD ranged from 0% (47,48) to 55% (43), and the incidences ranged from 4% (44,49) to 85% (28) among control patients. In all but two studies (46,50), VAP was diagnosed based on a combination of clinical, radiographical and microbiological criteria only. It has been demonstrated repeatedly that this combination of criteria has a low specificity for VAP (51–54). As a result, many patients given the diagnosis of VAP in fact only may have had tracheobronchitis or just colonization of the upper respiratory tract. Moreover, the use of topical antibiotics in the oropharynx may sterilize culture samples from tracheal aspirates (55), thus invalidating the microbiological criteria for VAP.

Beneficial effects on the incidence of VAP were reported from nine studies (28,48,50,56–61), but not from any of the double-blind studies. However, in one of the six double-blind studies, patients given SDD had a significantly lower incidence of early-onset VAP, with similar incidences of late-onset VAP (45). Furthermore, beneficial effects of SDD seemed to be related particularly to the incidence of VAP among control patients. The incidences among controls ranged from 12% (50) to 85% (28) when SDD significantly prevented VAP, and ranged from 4% (44,49) to 24% (46) when no significant effect was found. The lack of beneficial effects of SDD in five placebo-controlled, double-blind studies might have been due to the purposeful use of systemic prophylaxis in control patients (41–44,46).

Selective decontamination of the digestive tract was associated with a significantly lower mortality rate in 4 (45,59,61,62) of 20 studies. In another analysis, SDD seemed to be beneficial in terms of mortality rate for surgical patients only when successful decontamination could be achieved (63). How-

Table 1 Characteristics of Studies Using the Full Regimen of SDD in Critically Ill Patients

Reference, year	Design	No of patients (SDD vs Ctr)	Patient group	SDD regimen O	E	S	Diagnosis VAP	Incidence of VAP SDD n (%)	Ctr n (%)	p value	Mortality SDD n (%)	Ctr n (%)	p value
Stoutenbeek, 1984 (20)	Cons, HC	63 vs 59	T	PTA	PTA	CFX[a]	Clinical	35 (59)	5 (8)	<0.001	0 (0)	(8)	ns
Ledingham, 1988 (58)	Cons, HC	163 vs 161	Mix	PTA	PTA	CFX 96 h	Clinical	Early[b] 121 (74) Late[b] 3 (3)	Early[b] 109 (68) Late[b] 18 (19)	ns ns	39 (24)	39 (24)	ns
Kerver, 1988 (28)	P, R	49 vs 47	T/S	PTA	P (200 mg), TA	CFX 120–168 h	Clinical	6 (12)	40 (85)	<0.001	14 (29)	15 (32)	ns
Ulrich, 1989 (61)	P, R	48 vs 52	Mix	PNA	PNA	Trim unknown	Clinical	7 (15)	26 (50)	<0.001	15 (31)	28 (54)	<0.02
McClelland, 1990 (56)	Cons, HC	15 vs 12	Mix	PTA	PTA	CFX 96 h	Clinical	1 (7)	6 (50)	<0.05	6 (40)	5 (42)	ns
Blair, 1991 (57)	P, R, PC	126 vs 130	Mix	PTA	PTA	CFX 96 h	Clinical	12 (10)	45 (35)	0.002	24 (15)	32 (19)	ns
Fox, 1991 (62)	Cons, HC	12 vs 12	CS	PTA	PTA	CEP[c] 96 h	NA	NA	NA	NA	2 (17)	8 (66)	<0.05
Hartenauer, 1991 (60)	P, Cons, CO, C	99 vs 101	Mix	PTA	PTA	CFX[c] 96 h	Clinical	10 (10)	46 (45)	<0.01	34 (34)	46 (46)	ns
Aerdts, 1991 (48)	P, R	17 vs 39	Mix	PTA	P (200 mg), NA	CFX 120 h	Clinical	0 (0)	10 (26)	<0.05	(12)	6 (15)	ns
Mackie, 1992 (59)	Cons, HC	31 vs 33	B	PTA	PTA	CFX 96 h	Clinical	2 (7)	9 (27)	<0.05	1 (3)	7 (21)	<0.05
Hammond, 1992 (44)	P, R, DB, PC	114 vs 125	Mix	PTA	PT, A (100 mg)	CFX[c] 72 h	Clinical	8 (7)	8 (6)	ns	21 (18)	21 (17)	ns
Winter, 1992 (50)	P, R, PC, HC	91 vs 92	Mix	PTA	PTA	CFX 72 h	Clinical	4 (4)	11 (12)	<0.05	33 (36)	40 (43)	ns
Cockerill, 1992 (49)	P, R, PC	75 vs 75	Mix	PGNys	P G Nys	CFX 72 h	Bronchoscopy	4 (5)	3 (4)	ns	8 (11)	14 (29)	ns
Jacobs, 1992 (47)	P, R	36 vs 43	Mix	PTA	PTA	CFX 96 h	Clinical	0 (0)	4 (10)	ns	14 (39)	23 (53)	ns

Reference	Design	No. patients	Patient group	Oropharyngeal	Enteral	Systemic	VAP def.	SDD	Control	p	SDD	Control	p
Rocha, 1992 (45)	P, R, DB, PC	47 vs 54	Mix	PTA	PTA	CFX 96 h	Clinical	Early 1 (2) Late 6 (15)	Early 18 (33) Late 7 (13)	<0.05	10 (21)	24 (44)	<0.05
Hammond, 1993 (41)	P, R, DB, PC	13 vs 20	N	PTA	PTA	CFX[c] 72 h	Clinical	2 (15)	1 (5)	ns	2 (15)	3 (15)	ns
Ferrer, 1994 (46)	P, R, DB, PC	39 vs 41	Mix	PTA	PTA	CFX[c] 96 h	Bronchoscopy	7 (18)	10 (24)	ns	12 (31)	11 (27)	ns
Hammond, 1994 (43)	P, R, DB, PC	11 vs 11	T	PTA	PTA	CFX[c] 72 h	Clinical	6 (55)	1 (9)	ns	NA	NA	NA
Hammond, 1995 (42)	P, R, DB, PC	59 vs 76	Mix #	PTA	PTA	CFX 72 h	Clinical	1 (2)	7 (9)	ns	5 (8)	11 (14)	ns
Luiten, 1995 (89)	P, R, C	50 vs 52	AP	PTA	P (200 mg), NA	CFX	NA	NA	NA	NA	11 (50)	18 (52)	ns
Verwaest, 1997 (95)	P, R, C	Gr 1: 193 Gr 2: 200 Ctr: 185	Mix	Gr 1: OA Gr 2: PTA	Gr 1: OA Gr 2: PTA	Gr 1: O, 96 h Gr 2: CFX, 96 h	Clinical	Gr 1: 22 (7) Gr 2: 31 (7)	40 (11)	ns	Gr 1: 34 (18) Gr 2: 31 (16)	31 (17)	ns

[a] Until colonization free.

[b] Total infectious episodes rather than incidence of VAP.

Abbreviations: Design: C = controlled; CO = crossover model; Cons = consecutive patients; DB = double-blind; HC = historical controls; P = prospective; PC = placebo-controlled; R = randomized.

Patient groups: B = burns; CS = cardiac surgical; Mix = mixed; N = neurological; S = surgical; SAP = severe acute pancreatitis; T = trauma; # = with infection on admission.

SDD regimen: E = enteral solution; O = oropharyngeal paste; S = systemic prophylaxis.

Oropharyngeal paste: A = amphotericin B; G = gentamicin; N = norfloxacin; Nys = nystatin; O = ofloxacin; P = polymixin; T = tobramycin; all 2%, all q6h.

Enteral solution: A = amphotericin B (500 mg); G = gentamicin (80 mg); N = norfloxacin (50 mg); Nys = nystatin (2.10^6 U); O = ofloxacin (200 mg); P = polymixin (100 mg); T = tobramycin (80 mg); all q6h, except O (q12h).

Systemic prophylaxis: CEP = cephadrin; CFX = cefotaxime; O = ofloxacin; Trim = trimethoprim.

Incidence of VAP: early = early-onset; late = late-onset.

NA = not analyzed; ns = not statistically significant.

[c] Control patients also received systemic prophylaxis.

Table 2 Characteristics of Studies Using SDD Without Systemic Prophylaxis in Critically Ill Patients

Reference, year	Design	No of patients (SDD vs Ctr)	Patient group	SDD regimen O	SDD regimen E	Diagnosis VAP	Incidence of VAP SDD n (%)	Incidence of VAP Ctr n (%)	p value	Mortality SDD n (%)	Mortality Ctr n (%)	p value
Unertl, 1987 (64)	P, R	19 vs 20	Mix	PGA #	PG	Clinical	1 (19)	9 (45)	<0.01	NA	NA	NA
Flaherty, 1990 (66)	Cons, AR Ctr: sucralfate[a]	51 vs 56	CS	PGNys	PGNys	Clinical	1 (2)	5 (9)	ns	0 (0)	1 (2)	ns
Gastinne, 1992 (65)	P, R, DB, PC	220 vs 225	Mix	PTA	PTA	Clinical Bronchoscopy recommended	26 (12)	33 (15)	ns	75 (34)	67 (30)	ns
Korinek, 1993 (69)	P, R, PC, DB	63 vs 60	N	PGA V(4%)	PGA	Bronchoscopy	15 (24)	25 (42)	<0.04	8 (13)	11 (18)	ns
Wiener, 1995 (67)	P, R, DB, PC	30 vs 31	Med	PGNys	PGNys	Protected catheter	8 (27)	8 (26)	ns	11 (37)	15 (48)	ns
Quinio, 1996 (68)	P, R, PC, DB	76 vs 72	T	PGA	PGA	Clinical	19 (25)	37 (51)	<0.01	13 (17)	10 (14)	ns

[a] Control patients received sucralfate for stress ulcer prophylaxis.

Abbreviations: Design: AR = alternate randomization; Cons = consecutive patients; DB = double-blind; P = prospective; PC = placebo-controlled; R = randomized.

Patient groups: CS = cardiac surgical; Med = medical; Mix = mixed; N = neurological; T = trauma.

Oropharyngeal paste: A = amphotericin B; G = gentamicin; Nys = nystatin; P = polymixin; T = tobramycin, all 2%; PGA# = P (25 mg); G (40 mg); A (300 mg), all q6h.

Enteral solution: A = amphotericin B (500 mg); G = gentamicin (80 mg); Nys = nystatin (2.10^6 U); P = polymixin (100 mg); T = tobramycin (80 mg), all q6h.

Table 3 Characteristics of Studies Using Intestinal Decontamination in Critically Ill Patients

Reference, year	Design	No of patients (SDD vs Ctr)	Patient group	Enteral solution	Overall incidence of infections			Mortality		
					SDD n (%)	Ctr n (%)	p value	SDD n (%)	Ctr n (%)	p value
Hunefeld, 1989 (70)	P, R	102 vs 102	S	PTA[a]	NA	NA	NA	64 (63)	94 (92)	<0.01
Brun-Buisson, 1989 (73)	P, R	36 vs 50	Med	PNalNeo	12 (33)	17 (34)	ns	8 (22)	12 (24)	ns
Godard, 1990 (71)	P, R	97 vs 84	Mix	PTA Ctr: A	Early-onset 54 (56) Late-onset 24 (26)	Early-onset 49 (58) Late-onset 29 (35)	ns ns	12 (12)	15 (18)	ns
Cerra, 1990 (72)	P, R, DB, PC	25 vs 21	S	NNys	12 (48)	15 (71)	0.08	13 (52)	10 (48)	ns

[a] SDD patients also received cefotaxin (2 g, q8h, 72 h).

Abbreviations: Design: DB = double-blind; P = prospective; PC = placebo-controlled; R = randomized.

Patient groups: Med = medical; Mix = mixed; S = surgical.

Enteral solution: A = amphotericin B (500 mg); Nys = nystatin (2.10^6 U); P = polymixin (100 mg); PNalNeo = polymixin (50 mg). nalidixic acid (1 g), neomycin (80 mg); T = tobramycin (80 mg), all q6h; N = norfloxacin 500 mg q8h.

Table 4 Characteristics of Studies Using Oropharyngeal Decontamination in Critically Ill Patients

Reference, year	Design	Patient group	No of patients (SDD vs Ctr)	Oropharyngeal paste #	Diagnosis of VAP	Incidence of VAP			Mortality		
						SDD n (%)	Ctr n (%)	p value	SDD n (%)	Ctr n (%)	p value
Rodriguez, 1990 (75)	P, R	Mixed	13 vs 15	PTA	Clinical	0 (13)	11 (75)	<0.001	4 (30)	5 (33)	ns
Pugin, 1991 (74)	P, R, PC, DB	Mixed	25 vs 27	PNV	Clinical	4 (16)	21 (78)	<0.0001	7 (28)	7 (26)	ns
Abele-Horn, 1997 (76)	P, R	Mixed	58 vs 33	PTA[a]	Clinical	Early 0 (0) Late 13 (22)	Early (33) Late 14 (47)	<0.001 <0.05	11 (19)	5 (17)	ns

[a] All SDD-patients also received cefotaxime (2g, q8h, 72h) systematically for 3 days.

Abbreviations: Design: DB = double-blind; P = prospective; PC = placebo-controlled; R = randomized.

Oropharyngeal paste #: A = amphotericin B; P = polymixin; T = tobramycin; all 2%, all q6h; PNV = polymyxin B (38 mg); neomycin (250 mg); vancomycin (250 mg), q4h.

Incidence of VAP: early = early-onset; late = late-onset.

Table 5 Characteristics and Outcomes of Four Meta-Analyses of SDD

	Vandenbroucke-Grauls (83)	SDD Trialists' (82)	Heyland (85)	Kollef (84)
Year	1991	1993	1994	1994
No. of trials	11	22	25	16
Design of trials				
Prospective	6	22	25	16
Historical control	6[a]	0	0	0
Randomized	6	22	25	14
Double-blind	0	10	10	5
Crossover	2	0	0	2
No. of patients	1489	4142	3395	2270
Outcome measures	Odds ratio (95% CI)	Odds ratio (95% CI)	Relative risk (95% CI)	Risk difference (95% CI)
Pneumonia	0.21 (0.15–0.29)[b] 0.12 (0.08–0.19)[c]	0.37 (0.31–0.43)	0.46 (0.39–0.56)	0.15 (0.12–0.17)
Mortality	0.91 (0.67–1.23)[b] 0.70 (0.45–1.09)[c]	0.90 (0.79–1.04)	0.87 (0.79–0.97)	0.02 (−0.02–0.05)

[a] One study had both a historical and a randomized control group.
[b] Odds ratios of studies with historical control groups.
[c] Odds ratios of studies with randomized control groups.

ever, this observation was not determined by a randomized study, but rather in an observational cohort study in which predicted mortality rates were computed from the APACHE II scores on admission (63).

B. SDD Without Systemic Prophylaxis

The effects of SDD of the oropharynx, stomach, and intestine, but without systemic prophylaxis, were studied at least six times (64–69), including four studies with a placebo-controlled, double-blind design (65,67–69) (see Table 2). Significant lower incidences of VAP in SDD-treated patients were reported from two placebo-controlled, double-blind studies in trauma and neurosurgical patients (68,69). However, again the beneficial effects of SDD seemed to be influenced by the baseline incidence of VAP. The incidences among control patients ranged from 42% (69) to 51% (68) when SDD was beneficial, and the incidences ranged from 9% (66) to 26% (67) when not. In none of the individual studies did SDD result in a significantly lower mortality rate.

C. Gastrointestinal Decontamination Only

Four studies applied only gastric and intestinal decontamination, once in combination with systemic administration of cefotaxim (see Table 3) (70–73). The incidence of VAP was only determined in one study (71) in which bacterial VAP was not diagnosed with quantitative cultures of protected specimen brush in any of the patients receiving intestinal decontamination as compared to 8 (10%) ($p < 0.05$) of the control patients. However, SDD failed to reduce the overall rate of infections (71). In another study, SDD was applied to control an outbreak of intestinal colonization and infection with multiresistant gram-negative bacilli (73). Although SDD was successful in controlling the outbreak, intestinal decontamination did not change the overall rates of nosocomial infections. A lower mortality rate in patients receiving SDD was reported from the one study in which patients also received cefotaxim prophylaxis (70).

D. Oropharyngeal Decontamination

Two studies determined the effects of oropharyngeal decontamination alone, and one determined the effect of oropharyngeal decontamination and systemic prophylaxis on the incidence of VAP (see Table 4) (74–76). Only one of these studies used a placebo-controlled, double-blind study design (74). Although significant reductions in the incidence of VAP were reported in all three studies, the incidences of VAP in control patients were very high when compared to other study populations: 47% (76), 75% (75), and 78% (74). Despite the enormous effects of oropharyngeal decontamination on the incidences of VAP in all three studies, no reduction in mortality rate was found.

E. Systemic Prophylaxis Only

The first attempt to prevent pneumonia with systemic antibiotic prophylaxis is credited to Lepper and coworkers, who administered a variety of systemic antibiotics, singly or in combination, to 72 tracheostomized poliomyelitis patients, and failed to significantly diminish rates of tracheal colonization or pneumonia (77). Petersdorf et al. found no detectable benefit of systemic antibiotic prophylaxis among 62 comatose ICU patients in 1957 (78). In a subsequent randomized double-blind, placebo-controlled study, the same investigators administered oral chloramphenicol to 72 acute heart failure patients and placebo to 78 control patients, without influencing the incidence of pneumonia or mortality rates (79). Problems with selection of resistant pathogens causing pneumonia were reported in two of these studies using systemic antibiotic prophylaxis (77,78). Because of these disappointing results, attempts at preventing VAP with systemic prophylaxis were abandoned for some years. Thirty years later, 570 ICU patients were randomized to receive either 24 hours of penicillin G, cefoxitin, or no antibiotics for prophylaxis of early-onset pneumonia (80). The incidences of early onset pneumonia were 6.1% for patients receiving antibiotics and 7.2% for control subjects (80). More recently, Sirvent and coworkers demonstrated in a prospectively randomized, but not double-blind or placebo-controlled study, that two doses of intravenous cefuroxime (1500 mg) resulted in a reduction in the incidence of early-onset VAP from 36% to 16% in comatose intensive care patients (81). The incidence of late-onset VAP was not decreased statistically (14% versus 8% in patients receiving prophylaxis), and mortality rates were 20% for patients receiving prophylaxis and 14% for control subjects (81).

F. Meta-analyses

In addition to the results of the many comparative trials, four meta-analyses of SDD have been performed (see Table 5) (82–85). The results of these meta-analyses are comparable: SDD results in a decreased incidence of respiratory tract infections caused by aerobic gram-negative bacteria, but has hardly any influence on mortality rates. The investigators of three of four meta-analyses concluded, therefore, that the routine use of SDD was not justified (83–

85). However, it has been argued that metaanalyses should not be used to decide whether to implement a specific clinical practice, but rather to create a hypothesis and to lead to the design of prospective randomized trials with enough patients to test this hypothesis (86,87). In the three largest metaanalyses, the estimated reduction in mortality rate varied from 2% to 13% (82,84,85). This means that, with an assumed baseline mortality rate of 20% and conventional levels of significance, a trial of 8100 patients per group would be needed to demonstrate a 10% risk reduction in mortality rate (85). In another analysis, mortality rates of all SDD-treated patients included in one of the metaanalyses (82) were analyzed as a function of baseline risk of death at study entry, which was represented by the mortality rates of control patients (88). This study suggested that SDD was associated with decreased mortality rates only in populations with a high (>40%) mortality risk at study entry. This is in contrast to the more widely held opinion that SDD cannot be beneficial in patients with severe underlying disease, who have a grim prognosis, independent from the development of VAP. This latter view is supported by the results of two other studies that suggested that the maximum benefit of SDD could be expected in patients with midrange APACHE II scores on admission (47,57). For example, Blair et al. found a reduction of nosocomial pneumonia and mortality rate only in patients with APACHE II scores of 10 to 19 (57).

V. MEASURING EFFECTS OF SDD IN SPECIFIC PATIENT POPULATIONS

In intensive care, SDD was originally applied to trauma patients receiving mechanical ventilation. During the following years, almost all other groups of ventilated intensive care patients have been studied. Most studies included mixed populations of surgical, medical, neurological, and trauma patients, thereby hampering extrapolation of the beneficial effects of SDD to a specific patient group. Only three studies were performed in trauma patients exclusively (20,43,68), and significant reductions in the incidence of VAP were reported from all three. However, historical controls served as a control group in one study (20) and only 22 patients were randomized in another trial (43). Two double-blind, placebo-controlled studies included neurological patients only (41,69). In the larger of these two studies, which included 123 patients, the incidence of VAP in patients receiving SDD without systemic prophylaxis was 24%, compared with an incidence of 42% in control patients (69). In the other study, in which both patient groups received systemic prophylaxis, only 13 patients received SDD, with an incidence of VAP of 15%, and VAP developed in only 1 of 20 control patients (5%) (41). Three studies included only medical intensive care patients, and SDD was not beneficial in any of them (65,67,73). Although these findings may suggest that SDD should not be used in medical patients, the potential benefits of SDD may have been diminished because of modifications of the original regimen. In two studies, which were placebo-controlled and double-blinded, systemic prophylaxis was not included (65,67), and in the remaining study, only the gastrointestinal tract was decontaminated (73). In addition, the high rates of abnormal results on baseline chest radiographs and the common use of empirical systemic antibiotics for the frequent ''undifferentiated'' fevers in medical ICU patients confound the performance and interpretation of controlled trials of SDD in these patients (67).

Selective decontamination of the digestive tract has been used in several other specific patient groups. The incidence of VAP decreased in burn patients (59), and SDD applied to patients with acute pancreatitis reduced the incidence of gram-negative infections, the average number of laparotomies per patient, and mortality rate (89). Moreover, SDD has been shown to reduce postoperative infections caused by gram-negative bacteria during the first 10 days after elective esophageal resection (90). In this study, decontamination and systemic prophylaxis were started before surgery and oropharyngeal and intestinal decontamination were continued thereafter. In patients with liver disease, the combination SDD reduced the risk of infection but not the length of stay in the unit for patients with fulminant liver failure (91). SDD reduced the incidence of pulmonary infections but not of the development of organ system failures in patients undergoing elective liver transplantation (92), and long-term selective intestinal decontamination with norfloxacin effectively prevented the recurrence of spontaneous bacterial peritonitis in cirrhotic patients (93).

VI. RESISTANCE CONCERNS

Besides clinical efficacy, several other concerns, particularly selection of antibiotic-resistant strains, may influence the applicability of SDD on a routine basis. For example, the use of colistin and an aminoglycoside in the SDD regimen may permit overgrowth and infection with several gram-positive bacteria, such as *Enterococcus faecalis* and coagulase-negative staphylococci, which are often resistant to these agents. Antibiotic resistance of gram-negative bacteria and the occurrence or selection of resistant gram-positive microorganisms were monitored in specific surveillance cultures in many SDD studies (Table 6). No evidence of increased incidence of resistant bacteria was

Table 6 Methods of Surveillance and Reported Resistance Problems in SDD Trials

Reference, year	Antibiotics used		Method of monitoring changes in antibiotic resistance	Comments
	Topical	Systemic		
Unertl, 1987 (64)	PGA	—	Surveillance ETr daily Pathogens cultured from clinical specimens	No evidence of increased resistance
Kerver, 1988 (28)	PTA	CFX	Surveillance of O, ETr, R, U thrice weekly Pathogens cultured from clinical specimens	No evidence of increased resistance
Ledingham, 1988 (58)	PTA	CFX	Surveillance of O, ETr, G, U, R thrice weekly Pathogens cultured from clinical specimens	No evidence of increased resistance
Ulrich, 1989 (61)	PNA	Trim	Surveillance of O, R, ETr, U twice weekly Pathogens cultured from clinical specimens	*Enterococcus faecalis* and CNSt, the most frequent pathogens N-res increased in SDD surveillance cultures for CNSt, enterococci, and *Pseudomonas*
Hunefeld, 1989 (70)	PTA	CFX	Surveillance of O, R, ETr three times weekly Pathogens cultured from clinical specimens	No evidence of increased resistance
Brun-Buisson, 1989 (73)	PNalNeo	—	Surveillance of R every 4 days Pathogens cultured from clinical specimens	Selection of SDD-resistant strains (32% vs 58%; $p = 0.02$), especially staphylococci, enterococci, and fungi
Flaherty, 1990 (66)	PGNys	—	Surveillance of O, R weekly, and G every 3 days Pathogens cultured from clinical specimens	No evidence of increased resistance Most resistant microorganisms were *Proteus* and *Morganella* sp., intrisically resisant to polymixin
Rodriguez-Roldan, 1990 (75)	PTA	—	Surveillance O, G, ETr every 3 days Pathogens cultured from clinical specimens	No evidence of increased resistance
Hartenauer, 1991 (60)	PTA	CFX	Surveillance of O, R, ETr, U twice weekly Pathogens cultured from clinical specimens	No evidence of increased resistance to PTA during the first week of SDD for gram-negative bacteria, and no evidence of increased resistance of CNSt

Study			Methods	Results
Blair, 1991 (57)	PTA	CFX	Surveillance of O, ETr, G, U, R twice weekly / Pathogens cultured from clinical specimens	Increasing T resistance of gram-negative bacteria (21% vs 43%)
Mackie, 1992 (59)	PTA	CFX	Surveillance of W, ETr, U, G twice weekly / Pathogens cultured from clinical specimens	No evidence of increased resistance
Cerra, 1992 (72)	NNys	—	Surveillance of Etr, U, B twice weekly / Pathogens cultured from clinical specimens	No evidence of increased resistance / Trend toward increased intestinal colonization with enterococci, without affecting infection rates
Cockerill, 1992 (49)	PGNys	CFX	Surveillance of O, R every 3 days until negative and Etr, U twice weekly	No evidence of increased resistance
Rocha, 1992 (45)	PTA	CFX	Surveillance of O, R, ETr, G, twice weekly / Pathogens cultured from clinical specimens	CFX-res: 38% (SDD patients) to 15% ($p < 0.001$) of isolates / T-res: 38% (SDD patients) to 9% ($p < 0.001$) of isolates / Resistance especially in *Staphylococcus aureus* and *Acinetobacter* spp.
Gastinne, 1992 (65)	PTA	—	No surveillance / Pathogens cultured from clinical specimens	A trend toward an increased rate of staphylococcal pneumonia in SDD patients (7% vs 3%, $p = 0.06$)
Hammond, 1992 (44)	PTA	CFX	Surveillance of O, R, ETr, G, U, W twice weekly and 3 days after discharge from intensive care unit / Pathogens cultured from clinical specimens	No data on antibiotic resistance / Selection of methicillin-resistant CNSt in SDD-treated patients; no evidence of selection of enterocci
Winter, 1992 (50)	PTA	CZA	Surveillance of O, ETr, R thrice weekly / Pathogens cultured from clinical specimens	No evidence of increased resistance
Korinek, 1993 (69)	PGA	—	Surveillance of O, ETr, G on days 3, 6, 12 / Pathogens cultured from clinical specimens	No evidence of increased resistance
Hammond, 1994 (43)	PTA	CFX	Surveillance of O, ETr, G, U, R thrice weekly	Increased colonization rates of oropharynx, stomach and intestine of MRSA in SDD patients

Table 6 Continued

Reference	Antibiotics used		Method of monitoring changes in antibiotic resistance	Comments
	Topical	Systemic		
Wiener, 1995 (67)	PGNys	—	Surveillance of O, R, G every 4–7 days Pathogens cultured from clinical specimens	A trend toward more frequent infections with G-resistant enterococci in SDD patients (4 of 30 vs 1 of 31; $p = 0.2$)
Abele-Horn, 1996 (76)	PTA	CFX	Surveillance of O, R, ETr, G, U, W twice weekly Isolated pathogens	No evidence of increased resistance
Quinio, 1996 (68)	PGA	—	Pathogens cultured from clinical specimens	Selection of methicillin-resistant CNSt in some SDD-treated patients, no evidence of increased resistance
Verwaest, 1997 (95)	PTA/O	CFX	Pathogens cultured from clinical specimens	Pathogens causing infections in SDD-treated patients were more likely to be resistant to O (Enterobacteriaceae, nonfermenters), T (Enterobacteriaceae), and to oxacillin (S. aureus)

Abbreviations: Antibiotics: A = amphotericin B; CZA = ceftazidime; G = gentamicin; N = norfloxacin; Nal = nalidixic acid; Neo = neomycin; Nys = nystatin; O = ofloxacin; P = polymixin; T = tobramycin; CFX = cefotaxime; O = ofloxacin; Trim = trimethoprim.
Surveillance: Etr = endotracheal aspirate; G = gastric aspirate; O = oropharynx; R = rectal swab; U = urine; W = wound swab.

reported from 11 studies (28,49,50,58–60,64,69,70,75,76) or from an observational analysis after 2 years' experience with SDD (94). In contrast, overgrowth and even infections resulting from gram-positive bacteria, resistant to the antibiotics used for SDD, have been reported in several SDD trials (43–45,61,65,67,68,72,73,95–98), as were increased colonization and infection rates resulting from gram-negative–resistant bacteria (45,57,61,95). In a matched cohort analysis, patients receiving an oropharyngeal paste and a solution containing colistin, tobramycin, and amphotericin B without systemic prophylaxis had more frequent tracheal colonization and infection with *E. faecalis* (97). In another report, SDD with amphotericin B, colistin, and norfloxacin was associated with five cases of endocarditis caused by *E. faecalis* (98). Especially concerning are the reports that SDD may select for colonization and infection with methicillin-resistant staphylococci (43,44,68,96). The potential effects of SDD on development of resistance in fungi or of vancomycin resistance in staphylococci are concerning, but theoretical at present.

VII. INTERACTION OF CONTROL AND DECONTAMINATED PATIENTS

An important unsolved question in studies of SDD is whether the presence of heavily colonized control patients, studied next to decontaminated patients, adversely affects the ability to demonstrate potential beneficial results of SDD, because of cross infections. Conversely, a reduction in the number of contagious patients by applying SDD might reduce the acquisition, colonization, and infection incidence in the control group (20). As a result, the beneficial effects of SDD might appear less in controlled trials, because of the overall lower infection rate. Hurley addressed this question by comparing possible cross-infection rates in SDD trials with historic and concurrent controls, but did not find evidence to support this assumption (99). In another trial, patients were studied in two identical ICU wards. In ward one, patients were randomly assigned to receive topical antimicrobial prophylaxis of the oropharynx and stomach. In the second ward, none of the patients received topical prophylaxis. In the second part of the study, all patients in ward one were studied without prophylaxis. Colonization of oropharynx and trachea was lowest in patients receiving prophylaxis and was significantly lower in patients undergoing treatment next to those receiving prophylaxis than in patients undergoing treatment in a ward where no prophylaxis was given (100), supporting the idea that randomized trials might underestimate the benefit of SDD.

Table 7 Results of Costs Analyses in Studies Using SDD

Author, year	Calculated costs of SDD per patient	Costs of treatment of infections per patient (exclusive SDD)		Authors' conclusion on cost analysis
		SDD	Ctr	
Hunefeld, 1989 (70) Gastinne, 1992 (65)	157.31 DM per day $66.50 per day	123.10 DM per day $593 ± $1015	172.25 DM per day $577 ± $1051	"There was no substantial difference between the two groups in terms of the total charges of systmeic antibiotics."
Hammond, 1992 (44)	$500 (total)	$400	$250	"SDD adds substantially to the cost of ICU care."
Cockerill, 1992 (49)	$212 (total)	NA	NA	"Savings from decreasing infection should be substantial."
Rocha, 1992 (45)	$20 per day	$10 per day	$20 per day	"The average cost of the total antibiotics/patient/day was greater in the SDD-group, though the final cost was similar in both groups."
Korinek, 1994 (69)	$70 per day	$418 ± $464 per treated pt $19,258 (total charge)	$361 ± $450 per treated patient $10,670 (total charge)	"SDD is cost-effective due to the reduction of length of stay in the survivor group."
Wiener, 1995 (67)		$780.90	$518.38	"Costs of therapeutic antibiotics were similar for SDD and control patients."
Quinio, 1996 (68)	$5.25 per day	$62 per day $33,127 (total charge)	$75 per day $62,117 (total charge)	"Overall, a 42% savings in antibiotic expenditure was obtained in the SDD group."
Abele-Horn, 1997 (76)	102.11 DM per day during day 1–3, $2.75 DM per day thereafter	76.61 DM per day	106.63 DM per day	"The total cost of antibiotic use was reduce by SOD."

VIII. COST-BENEFIT ANALYSES

A formal cost-benefit analysis of SDD, including the costs of administration and preparation of SDD antibiotics, durations and costs of ICU care, costs of additional antibiotic therapy, costs of non-ICU hospitalization, costs of surveillance and of surveillance cultures, and patient outcome has never been performed. Nine studies, however, analyzed associated costs of antibiotic use (Table 7). The costs for the daily administration of SDD medication varied considerably, depending on the antibiotics used and the country of study origin. The authors of three studies concluded that the use of SDD reduced antibiotic expenditure (68,69,76).

IX. CONCLUSION

Based on the available data, there is still no basis for the routine use of SDD in an intensive care unit. In this we concur with two recently published statements on the prevention of nosocomial pneumonia. The Hospital Infection Control Practices Advisory Committee from the Centers for Disease Control and Prevention concluded that ''currently available data do not justify the routine use of SDD for prevention of nosocomial pneumonia in ICU patients'' (101). The American Thoracic Society categorized SDD among the regimens with unproven value for prevention of hospital-acquired pneumonia (102). The growing number of publications reporting overgrowth and infections resulting from gram-positive bacteria, especially methicillin-resistant *S. aureus* (MRSA) and enterococci, discourage its routine use in mechanically ventilated ICU patients. This is particularly important for countries such as the United States, where colonization with MRSA and vancomycin-resistant enterococci probably is endemic in many ICUs (1,103–106) and where SDD may provide a selective growth advantage for these resistant bacteria. In addition, the absence of any effects on mortality rates or costs should limit widespread use of SDD.

However, prevention of VAP still is an important goal for intensive care medicine. Although the relative importance of endogenous and exogenous sources of bacteria causing VAP has not been elucidated, optimal compliance with infection control measures, such as handwashing, to minimize the occurrence of cross infection and a rational use of antimicrobials remain cornerstones of infection prevention in the ICU (107). In addition, several alternative strategies have been developed; these aim to interrupt the gastropulmonary route of colonization or to prevent aspiration of oropharyngeal secretions and show promising results (108–112). Future large randomized and, preferably, double-blind studies are needed to demonstrate the clinical values of these measures and to determine whether there is yet a role for SDD in combination with other measures for select patient populations (e.g., trauma or transplant surgery).

REFERENCES

1. Emori TG, Gaynes RP. An overview of nosocomial infections, including the role of the microbiology laboratory. Clin Microbiol Rev 1993; 6:428–442.
2. Vincent JL, Bihari DJ, Suter PM, et al. The prevalence of nosocomial infection in intensive care units in Europe. Results of the European prevalence of infection in intensive care (EPIC) study. JAMA 1995; 274:639–644.
3. Bergmans DCJJ, Bonten MJM, Gaillard CA, et al. Indications for antibiotic use in ICU patients: a one-year prospective surveillance. J Antimicrob Chemother 1997; 39:527–535.
4. Gross PA, van Antwerpen C. Nosocomial infections and hospital deaths. A case-control study. Am J Med 1983; 75:658–662.
5. Leu HS, Kaiser DL, Mori M, Woolson RF, Wenzel RP. Hospital-acquired pneumonia: attributable mortality and morbidity. Am J Epidemiol 1989; 129:1258–1267.
6. Rello J, Jubert P, Valles J, Artigas A, Rué M, Niederman MS. Evaluation of outcome for intubated patients with pneumonia due to *Pseudomonas aeruginosa*. Clin Infect Dis 1996; 23:973–978.
7. Fagon JY, Chastre J, Hance AJ, Montravers P, Novara A, Gibert C. Nosocomial pneumonia in ventilated patients: a cohort study evaluating attributable mortality and hospital stay. Am J Med 1993; 94:281–288.
8. Craven DE, Kunches LM, Kilinsky V, Lichtenberg DA, Make BJ, McCabe WR. Risk factors for pneumonia and fatality in patients receiving continuous mechanical ventilation. Am Rev Respir Dis 1986; 133:792–796.
9. Torres A, Aznar R, Gatell JM, et al. Incidence, risk, and prognosis factors of nosocomial pneumonia in mechanically ventilated patients. Am Rev Respir Dis 1990; 142:523–528.
10. Bonten MJM, Bergmans DCJJ, Ambergen AW, et al. Risk factors for pneumonia, and colonization of respiratory tract and stomach in mechanically ventilated ICU patients. Am J Respir Crit Care Med 1996; 154:1339–1346.
11. Prod'hom G, Leuenberger P, Koerfer J, et al. Nosocomial pneumonia in mechanically ventilated patients receiving antacid, ranitidine, or sucralfate as prophylaxis for stress ulcer: a randomised controlled trial. Ann Intern Med 1994; 120:653–662.

12. Papazian L, Bregeon F, Thirion X, et al. Effect of ventilator-associated pneumonia on mortality and morbidity. Am J Respir Crit Care Med 1996; 154:91–97.

13. Craven DE. Use of selective decontamination of the digestive tract: is the light at the end of the tunnel red or green? Ann Intern Med 1992; 117:609–611.

14. Craven DE. Prevention of hospital-acquired pneumonia: measuring effect in ounces, pounds and tons. Ann Intern Med 1995; 122:229–231.

15. Fink MP. Selective digestive decontamination: a gut issue for the nineties. Crit Care Med 1992; 20:559–562.

16. Weinstein RA. Selective intestinal decontamination—an infection control measure whose time has come? Ann Intern Med 1989; 110:853–855.

17. Bonten MJM, Weinstein RA. Selective decontamination of the digestive tract: a measure whose time has passed? Curr Opin Infect Dis 1996; 9:270–275.

18. Dekker AW, Rozenberg-Arska M, Verhoef J. Infection prophylaxis in acute leukemia: a comparison of ciprofloxacin with trimethoprim-sulfamethoxazole and colistin. Ann Intern Med 1987; 106:7–12.

19. Guiot HFL, van Furth R. Partial antibiotic decontamination. BMJ 1977; 1:800–802.

20. Stoutenbeek CP, van Saene HKF, Miranda DR, Zandstra DF. The effect of selective decontamination of the digestive tract on colonization and infection rate in multiple trauma patients. Intens Care Med 1984; 10:185–192.

21. van der Waaij D. Colonization resistance of the digestive tract: clinical consequences and implications. J Antimicrob Chemother 1982; 10:263–270.

22. Torres A, El-Ebiary M, González J, et al. Gastric and pharyngeal flora in nosocomial pneumonia acquired during mechanical ventilation. Am Rev Respir Dis 1993; 148:352–357.

23. du Moulin GC, Paterson DG, Hedley-Whyte J, Lisbon A. Aspiration of gastric bacteria in antacid-treated patients: a frequent cause of postoperative colonisation of the airway. Lancet 1982; i:242–245.

24. Heyland D, Mandell LA. Gastric colonization by gram-negative bacilli and nosocomial pneumonia in the intensive care unit patient: evidence for causation. Chest 1992; 101:187–193.

25. Driks MR, Craven DE, Celli BR, et al. Nosocomial pneumonia in intubated patients given sucralfate as compared with antacids or histamine type 2 blockers: the role of gastric colonisation. N Engl J Med 1987; 317:1376–1382.

26. Cook DJ, Reeve BK, Guyatt GH, et al. Stress ulcer prophylaxis in critically ill patients; resolving discordant meta-analyses. JAMA 1996; 275:308–314.

27. Stoutenbeek CP, van Saene HKF, Miranda DR, Zandstra DF, Langrehr D. The effect of oropharyngeal decontamination using topical nonabsorbable antibiotics on the incidence of nosocomial respiratory tract infections in multiple trauma patients. J Trauma 1987; 27:357–364.

28. Kerver AJH, Rommes JH, Mevissen-Verhage EAE, et al. Prevention of colonization and infection in critically ill patients: a prospective randomized study. Crit Care Med 1988; 16:1087–1093.

29. Bonten MJM, Gaillard CA, de Leeuw PW, Stobberingh EE. Role of coloniza-

tion of the upper intestinal tract in the pathogenesis of ventilator-associated pneumonia. Clin Infect Dis 1997; 24:309–319.

30. Niederman MS, Craven DE. Editorial response: devising strategies for preventing nosocomial pneumonia—should we ignore the stomach? Clin Infect Dis 1997; 24:320–323.

31. Bonten MJM, Gaillard CA, van Tiel FH, Smeets HGW, van der Geest S, Stobberingh EE. The stomach is not a source for colonization of the upper respiratory tract and pneumonia in ICU patients. Chest 1994; 105:878–884.

32. Bonten MJM, Gaillard CA, van der Geest S, et al. The role of intragastric acidity and stress ulcer prophylaxis on colonization and infection in mechanically ventilated patients. A stratified, randomized, double blind study of sucralfate versus antacids. Am J Respir Crit Care Med 1995; 152:1825–1834.

33. Apte NM, Karnad DR, Medhekar TP, Tilve GH, Morye S, Bhave GG. Gastric colonization and pneumonia in intubated critically ill patients receiving stress ulcer prophylaxis: a randomized, controlled trial. Crit Care Med 1992; 20:590–593.

34. Reusser P, Zimmerli W, Scheidegger D, Marbet GA, Buser M, Gyr K. Role of gastric colonization in nosocomial infections and endotoxemia: a prospective study in neurosurgical patients on mechanical ventilation. J Infect Dis 1989; 160:414–421.

35. de Latorre FJ, Pont T, Ferrer A, Rossello J, Palomar M, Planas M. Pattern of tracheal colonization during mechanical ventilation. Am J Respir Crit Care Med 1995; 152:1028–1033.

36. Martínez-Pellús AJ, Ruiz J, Garcia J, et al. Role of selective digestive decontamination in the prevention of nosocomial pneumonia: is gastric decontamination necessary? Intens Care Med 1992; 18:218–221.

37. Duncan RA, Steger KA, Craven DE. Selective decontamination of the digestive tract: risks outweigh benefits for intensive care unit patients. Semin Respir Infect 1993; 8:308–324.

38. Hamer DH, Barza M. Prevention of hospital-acquired pneumonia in critically ill patients. Antimicrob Agents Chemother 1993; 37:931–938.

39. Verhoef J, Verhage EAE, Visser MR. A decade of experience with selective decontamination of the digestive tract as prophylaxis for infections in patients in the intensive care unit: what have we learned? Clin Infect Dis 1993; 17:1047–1054.

40. Flaherty JP, Weinstein RA. Infection control and pneumonia prophylaxis strategies in the intensive care unit. Semin Respir Infect 1990; 5:191–203.

41. Hammond JMJ, Potgieter PD. Neurologic disease requiring long-term ventilation. The role of selective decontamination of the digestive tract in preventing nosocomial infection. Chest 1993; 104:547–551.

42. Hammond JMJ, Potgieter PD. Is there a role for selective decontamination of the digestive tract in primarily infected patients in the ICU? Anaesth Intens Care 1995; 23:168–174.

43. Hammond JMJ, Potgieter PD, Saunders GL. Selective decontamination of the

digestive tract in multiple trauma patients—is there a role? Results of a prospective, double-blind, randomized trial. Crit Care Med 1994; 22:33–39.

44. Hammond JMJ, Potgieter PD, Saunders GL, Forder AA. Double-blind study of selective decontamination of the digestive tract in intensive care. Lancet 1992; 340:5–9.

45. Rocha LA, Martin MJ, Pita S, et al. Prevention of nosocomial infection in critically ill patients by selective decontamination of the digestive tract: a randomized, double blind, placebo-controlled study. Intens Care Med 1992; 18:398–404.

46. Ferrer M, Torres A, González J, et al. Utility of selective digestive decontamination in mechanically ventilated patients. Ann Intern Med 1994; 120:389–395.

47. Jacobs S, Foweraker JE, Roberts SE. Effectiveness of selective decontamination of the digestive tract in an ICU with a policy encouraging a low gastric pH. Clin Intens Care 1992; 3:52–58.

48. Aerdts SJA, van Dalen R, Clasener HAL, Festen J, van Lier HJJ, Vollaard EJ. Antibiotic prophylaxis of respiratory tract infection in mechanically ventilated patients: a prospective, blinded, randomized trial of the effect of a novel regimen. Chest 1991; 100:783–791.

49. Cockerill FR III, Muller SR, Anhalt JP, et al. Prevention of infection in critically ill patients by selective decontamination of the digestive tract. Ann Intern Med 1992; 117:545–553.

50. Winter R, Humphreys H, Pick A, MacGowan AP, Willatts SM, Speller DCE. A controlled trial of selective decontamination of the digestive tract in intensive care and its effect on nosocomial infection. J Antimicrob Chemother 1992; 30: 73–87.

51. Torres A, Puig de la Bellacasa J, Xaubet A, et al. Diagnostic value of quantitative cultures of bronchoalveolar lavage and telescoping plugged catheters in mechanically ventilated patients with bacterial pneumonia. Am Rev Respir Dis 1989; 140:306–310.

52. Fagon JY, Chastre J, Hance AJ, Domart Y, Trouillet JL, Gibert C. Evaluation of clinical judgment in the identification and treatment of nosocomial pneumonia in ventilated patients. Chest 1993; 103:547–553.

53. Chastre J, Fagon JY, Trouillet JL. Diagnosis and treatment of nosocomial pneumonia in patients in intensive care units. Clin Infect Dis 1995; 21:S226–S237.

54. Chastre J, Fagon JY. Invasive diagnostic testing should be routinely used to manage ventilated patients with suspected pneumonia. Am J Respir Crit Care Med 1994; 150:570–574.

55. Gastinne H, Wolff M, Lachatre G, Boiteau R, Savy FP. Antibiotic levels in bronchial tree and in serum during selective digestive decontamination. Intens Care Med 1991; 17:215–218.

56. McClelland P, Murray AE, Williams PS, et al. Reducing sepsis in severe combined acute renal and respiratory failure by selective decontamination of the digestive tract. Crit Care Med 1990; 18:935–939.

57. Blair P, Rowlands BJ, Lowry K, Webb H, Armstrong P, Smilie J. Selective

decontamination of the digestive tract: a stratified, randomized, prospective study in a mixed intensive care unit. Surgery 1991; 110:303–310.

58. Ledingham IMA, Eastaway AT, McKay IC, Alcock SR, McDonalds JC, Ramsay G. Triple regimens of selective decontamination of the digestive tract, systemic cefotaxime, and microbiological surveillance for prevention of acquired infection in intensive care. Lancet 1988; i:785–790.

59. Mackie DP, van Hertum WAJ, Schumburg T, Kuijper EC, Knape P. Prevention of infection in burns: preliminary experience with selective decontamination of the digestive tract in patients with extensive injuries. J Trauma 1992; 32: 570–575.

60. Hartenauer U, Thülig B, Diemer W, et al. Effect of selective flora suppression on colonization, infection, and mortality in critically ill patients: a one-year, prospective consecutive study. Crit Care Med 1991; 19:463–473.

61. Ulrich C, Harinck-de Weerd JE, Bakker NC, Jacz K, Doornbos L, de Ridder VA. Selective decontamination of the digestive tract with norfloxacin in the prevention of ICU-acquired infections: a prospective randomized study. Intens Care Med 1989; 15:424–431.

62. Fox MA, Peterson S, Fabri BM, van Saene HKF, Williets T. Selective decontamination of the digestive tract in cardiac surgical patients. Crit Care Med 1991; 19:1486–1490.

63. Tetteroo GWM, Wagenvoort JHT, Mulder PGH, Ince C, Bruining HA. Decreased mortality rate and length of hospital stay in surgical intensive care unit patients with successful selective decontamination of the gut. Crit Care Med 1993; 21:1692–1698.

64. Unertl K, Ruckdeschel G, Selbmann HK, et al. Prevention of colonization and respiratory infections in long-term ventilated patients by local antimicrobial prophylaxis. Intens Care Med 1987; 13:106–113.

65. Gastinne H, Wolff M, Delatour F, Faurisson F, Chevret S. A controlled trial in intensive care units of selective decontamination of the digestive tract with nonabsorbable antibiotics. N Engl J Med 1992; 326:594–599.

66. Flaherty JP, Nathan C, Kabins SA, Weinstein RA. Pilot trial of selective decontamination for prevention of bacterial infection in an intensive care unit. J Infect Dis 1990; 162:1393–1397.

67. Wiener J, Itokazu G, Nathan C, Kabins SA, Weinstein RA. A randomized, double-blind, placebo-controlled trial of selective decontamination in a medical-surgical intensive care unit. Clin Infect Dis 1995; 20:861–867.

68. Quinio B, Albanèse J, Bues-Charbit M, Viviand X, Martin C. Selective decontamination of the digestive tract in multiple trauma patients. Chest 1996; 109: 765–772.

69. Korinek AM, Laisne MJ, Nicolas MH, Raskine L, Deroin V, Sanson-Lepors MJ. Selective decontamination of the digestive tract in neurosurgical intensive care unit patients: a double-blind, randomized, placebo-controlled study. Crit Care Med 1993; 21:1466–1473.

70. von Hunefeld G. Klinische Studie zur selektiven Darmdekolonisation bei 204

langzeitbeatmeten abdominal- und unfallchirurgischen Intensivpatienten. Anaesthesiol Reanimat 1989; 14:131–153.

71. Godard J, Guillaume C, Reverdy ME, et al. Intestinal decontamination in a polyvalent ICU: a double-blind study. Intens Care Med 1990; 16:307–311.

72. Cerra FB, Maddaus MA, Dunn DL, et al. Selective gut decontamination reduces nosocomial infections and length of stay but not mortality or organ failure in surgical intensive care unit patients. Arch Surg 1994; 127:163–169.

73. Brun-Buisson C, Legrand P, Rauss A, et al. Intestinal decontamination for control of nosocomial multiresistant gram-negative bacilli: study of an outbreak in an intensive care unit. Ann Intern Med 1989; 110:873–881.

74. Pugin J, Auckenthaler R, Lew DP, Suter PM. Oropharyngeal decontamination decreases incidence of ventilator-associated pneumonia: a randomized, placebo-controlled, double-blind clinical trial. J Am Med Assoc 1991; 265:2704–2710.

75. Rodríguez-Roldán JM, Altuna-Cuesta A, López A, et al. Prevention of nosocomial lung infection in ventilated patients: use of an antimicrobial pharyngeal nonabsorbable paste. Crit Care Med 1990; 18:1239–1242.

76. Abele-Horn M, Dauber A, Bauernfeind A, et al. Decrease in nosocomial pneumonia in ventilated patients by selective oropharyngeal decontamination. Intens Care Med 1996; 23:187–195.

77. Lepper MH, Kofman S, Blatt N. Effect of eight antibiotics used singly and in combination on the tracheal flora following tracheostomy in poliomyelitis. Antibiotics Chemother 1954; 4:829–843.

78. Petersdorf RG, Curtin JA, Hoeprich PD, et al. A study of antibiotic prophylaxis in unconscious patients. N Engl J Med 1957; 257:1001–1009.

79. Petersdorf RG, Merchant RK. A study of antibiotic prophylaxis in patients with acute heart failure. N Engl J Med 1959; 260:565–575.

80. Mandelli M, Mosconi P, Langer M, Cigada M. Prevention of pneumonia in an intensive care unit: a randomized multicenter clinical trial. Crit Care Med 1989; 17:501–505.

81. Sirvent JM, Torres A, El-Ebiary M, Castro P, de Batlle J, Bonet A. Protective effect of intravenously administered cefuroxime against nosocomial pneumonia in patients with structural coma. Am J Respir Crit Care Med 1997; 155:1729–1734.

82. Selective Decontamination of the Digestive Tract Trialists' Collaborative Group. Meta-analysis of randomised controlled trials of selective decontamination of the digestive tract. BMJ 1993; 307:525–532.

83. Vandenbroucke-Grauls CMJE, Vandenbroucke JP. Effect of selective decontamination of the digestive tract on respiratory tract infections and mortality in the intensive care unit. Lancet 1991; 338:859–862.

84. Kollef MH. The role of selective digestive tract decontamination on mortality and respiratory tract infections: a meta-analysis. Chest 1994; 105:1101–1108.

85. Heyland DK, Cook DJ, Jaeschke R, Griffith L, Lee HN, Guyatt GH. Selective

decontamination of the digestive tract: an overview. Chest 1994; 105:1221–1229.

86. Villar J, Carroli G, Belizán JM. Predictive ability of meta-analyses of randomised controlled trials. Lancet 1995; 345:772–776.

87. Borzak S, Ridker PM. Discordance between meta-analyses and large-scale randomized, controlled trials. Examples from the management of acute myocardial infarction. Ann Intern Med 1995; 123:873–877.

88. Sun X, Wagner DP, Knaus WA. Does selective decontamination of the digestive tract reduce mortality for severely ill patients? Crit Care Med 1996; 24: 753–755.

89. Luiten EJT, Hop WCJ, Lange JF, Bruining HA. Controlled clinical trial of selective decontamination for the treatment of severe acute pancreatitis. Ann Surg 1995; 222:57–65.

90. Tetteroo GWM, Wagenvoort JHT, Castelein A, Tilanus HW, Ince C, Bruining HA. Selective decontamination to reduce gram-negative infections. Lancet 1990; 335:704–707.

91. Rolando N, Gimson A, Wade J, Philpott-Howard J, Casewell M, Williams R. Prospective controlled trial of selective parenteral and enteral antimicrobial regimen in fulminant liver failure. Hepatology 1993; 17:196–201.

92. Bion JF, Badger I, Crosby HA, et al. Selective decontamination of the digestive tract reduces gram-negative pulmonary colonization but not systemic endotoxemia in patients undergoing elective liver transplantation. Crit Care Med 1994; 22:40–49.

93. Ginés P, Rimola A, Planas R, et al. Norfloxacin prevents spontaneous bacterial peritonitis recurrence in cirrhosis: results of a double-blind, placebo-controlled trial. Hepatology 1990; 12:716–724.

94. Hammond JMJ, Potgieter PD. Long-term effects of selective decontamination on antimicrobial resistance. Crit Care Med 1995; 23:637–645.

95. Verwaest C, Verhaegen J, Ferdinande P, et al. Randomized, controlled trial of selective digestive decontamination in 600 mechanically ventilated patients in a multidisciplinary intensive care unit. Crit Care Med 1997; 25:63–71.

96. Kaufhold A, Behrendt W, Kräuss T, van Saene HKF. Selective decontamination of the digestive tract and methicillin-resistant *Staphylococcus aureus* (letter). Lancet 1992; 339:1411–1412.

97. Bonten MJM, Gaillard CA, van Tiel FH, van der Geest S, Stobberingh EE. Colonization and infection with *Enterococcus faecalis* in intensive care units: the role of antimicrobial agents. Antimicrob Agents Chemother 1995; 39:2783–2786.

98. Sijpkens YWJ, Buurke EJ, Ulrich C, van Asselt GJ. *Enterococcus faecalis* colonisation and endocarditis in five intensive care patients as late sequelae of selective decontamination. Intens Care Med 1995; 21:231–234.

99. Hurley JC. Prophylaxis with enteral antibiotics in ventilated patients: selective decontamination or selective cross-infection? Antimicrob Agents Chemother 1995; 39:941–947.

100. Bonten MJM, Gaillard CA, Johanson WG Jr, et al. Colonization in patients receiving and not receiving topical antimicrobial prophylaxis. Am J Respir Crit Care Med 1994; 150:1332–1340.

101. Tablan OC, Anderson LJ, Arden NH, et al. Guideline for prevention of nosocomial pneumonia. Part I. Issues on prevention of nosocomial pneumonia, 1994. Infect Control Hosp Epidemiol 1994; 15:588–627.

102. American Thoracic Society. Hospital-acquired pneumonia in adults: diagnosis, assessment of severity, initial antimicrobial therapy, and preventative strategies. A consensus statement. Am J Respir Crit Care Med 1996; 153:1711–1725.

103. Morris JG Jr, Shay DK, Hebden JN, et al. Enterococci resistant to multiple antimicrobial agents, including vancomycin. Establishment of endemicity in a University Medical Center. Ann Intern Med 1995; 123:250–259.

104. Bonten M, Hayden MK, Nathan C, et al. Epidemiology of colonisation of patients and environment with vancomycin-resistant enterococci. Lancet 1996; 348:1615–1619.

105. Wells CL, Juni BA, Cameron SB, et al. Stool carriage, clinical isolation, and mortality during an outbreak of vancomycin-resistant enterococci in hospitalized medical and/or surgical patients. Clin Infect Dis 1995; 21:45–50.

106. Slaughter S, Hayden MK, Nathan C, et al. A comparison of the effect of universal use of gloves and gowns with that of glove use alone on acquisition of vancomycin-resistant enterococci in a medical intensive care unit. Ann Intern Med 1996; 125:448–456.

107. Doebbeling BN, Stanley GL, Sheetz CT, et al. Comparative efficacy of alternative hand-washing agents in reducing nosocomial infections in intensive care units. N Engl J Med 1992; 327:88–93.

108. Valles J, Artigas A, Rello J, et al. Continuous aspiration of subglottic secretions in preventing ventilator-associated pneumonia. Ann Intern Med 1995; 122: 179–186.

109. Orozco-Levi M, Torres A, Ferrer M, et al. Semirecumbent position protects from pulmonary aspiration but not completely from gastroesophageal reflux in mechanically ventilated patients. Am J Respir Crit Care Med 1995; 152:1387–1390.

110. Torres A, Serra-Batlles J, Ros E, et al. Pulmonary aspiration of gastric contents in patients receiving mechanical ventilation: the effect of body position. Ann Intern Med 1992; 116:540–543.

111. Montecalvo MA, Steger KA, Farber HW, et al. Nutritional outcome and pneumonia in critical care patients randomized to gastric versus jejunal feedings. Crit Care Med 1992; 20:1377–1387.

112. Heyland D, Bradley C, Mandell LA. Effect of acidified enteral feedings on gastric colonization in the critically ill patients. Crit Care Med 1992; 20:1388–1394.

6

Immunoprophylaxis and Immunomodulation for Prevention of Nosocomial Pneumonia

WALTER W. WILLIAMS

Centers for Disease Control
and Prevention
Atlanta, Georgia

NANCY H. ARDEN

Baylor University School of Medicine
Houston, Texas

JAY C. BUTLER

Centers for Disease Control
and Prevention
Anchorage, Alaska

I. BACKGROUND

Pneumonia is the second most common nosocomial infection in the United States and is associated with substantial morbidity and mortality (1). Most patients who have nosocomial pneumonia are infants, young children, and persons 65 years of age or older; persons who have severe underlying disease, immunosuppression, depressed sensorium, or cardiopulmonary disease; and persons who have undergone thoracoabdominal surgery. Although patients receiving mechanically assisted ventilation do not represent a major proportion of patients who have nosocomial pneumonia, they are at highest risk for acquiring the infection (1).

Traditional preventive measures for nosocomial pneumonia include decreasing aspiration by the patient, preventing cross contamination or colonization from the hands of health care workers (HCWs), appropriate disinfection or sterilization of respiratory therapy devices, education of hospital staff and patients, and the focus of this chapter, use of available immunizing agents to protect against particular infections.

II. ETIOLOGY, CURRENTLY LICENSED AND NEW IMMUNIZING AGENTS

Bacteria have been the most frequently isolated pathogens, comprising more than 70% of isolates from sputum and tracheal aspirates obtained from patients who had pneumonia at hospitals participating in the National Nosocomial Infection Surveillance (NNIS) System (1). Most bacterial nosocomial pneumonias occur by aspiration of bacteria colonizing the oropharynx or upper gastrointestinal tracts of patients. Although aerobic gram-negative bacilli are recovered infrequently or are found in low numbers in pharyngeal cultures of healthy persons, the likelihood of colonization substantially increases among persons with conditions that are common among hospitalized patients (1). Thus, *Pseudomonas aeruginosa*, *Enterbacter* sp., *Klebsiella pneumoniae*, *Escherichia coli*, *Serratia marcescens*, and *Proteus* sp., are the predominant organisms isolated from patients with nosocomial pneumonia. However, in patients in whom pneumonia develops within less than 5 days of hospitalization, *Streptococcus pneumoniae*, *Haemophilus influenzae*, and *Staphylococcus aureus* are more frequently isolated than gram-negative bacilli (2). Most *H. influenza* recovered from adults are nontypable strains, and nosocomial transmission of *H. influenzae* type b infection among adults has been documented rarely (3). Among residents of long-term care facilities, *S. pneumoniae* is the most common cause of bacterial pneumonia, although gram-negative bacilli are also important agents (4,5). Outbreaks of *S. pneumoniae* among hospitalized patients and residents of long-term care facilities have been observed occasionally (6,7).

Viruses, also, can be an important and often unappreciated cause of nosocomial pneumonia, causing as many as 20% of endemic nosocomial pneumonia infections (1). Nosocomial respiratory viral infections have exogenous sources and usually follow community outbreaks occurring during particular times of the year (8–15). A number of viruses—adenoviruses, influenza virus, measles virus, parainfluenza viruses, respiratory syncytial virus (RSV), rhinoviruses, and varicella-zoster virus—can cause nosocomial pneumonia. Adenoviruses, influenza viruses, parainfluenza viruses, and RSV reportedly have accounted for most cases (70%) of nosocomial pneumonias caused by viruses (1).

Of the many bacterial and viral etiological agents of nosocomial pneumonia, licensed vaccines are available against *S. pneumoniae*, *H. influenzae* type b, *Bordetella pertussis*, influenza virus, measles virus, and varicella-zoster virus. In general, recommendations for using influenza and pneumococcal vaccines target those who are at increased risk for illness and death associated with influenza and pneumococcal infections (16,17). Although *S. pneumoniae* and influenza are not the leading causes of the illness, many patients in whom nosocomial pneumonia develops are in the high-risk groups for whom influenza and pneumococcal vaccination is routinely recommended (1,16,17).

Because *S. pneumoniae* and influenza viruses contribute to the morbidity and mortality associated with nosocomial pneumonia and vaccines against these infections are available and recommended for routine use in those at highest risk, this chapter focuses on use of vaccines against these diseases and current work on passive immunization.

Other vaccines (e.g., meningococcal and adenovirus vaccines) are indicated only in special situations or for certain populations (18,19). Vaccines against *H. influenzae* type b and pertussis are not recommended or licensed for routine vaccination of adults. Although no licensed vaccines are yet available against RSV or parainfluenza, basic research is underway to develop vaccines and therapeutic agents for these respiratory pathogens (20). Advances have also been made in developing vaccines against *P. aeruginosa* and *P. (Burkholderia) cepacia*. Vaccine preparations have been tested in various animal model systems and small phase I/II studies. These vaccine preparations include several surface proteins, high molecular weight polysaccharides, mucoid exopolysaccharides, an outer membrane protein (protein F), and a low molecular weight octavalent O-polysaccharide-toxin A conjugate (20). Work is also underway to improve the effectiveness of licensed inactivated influenza virus vaccine using novel vaccine delivery systems (e.g., microencapsulation, liposomes) or more conventional adjuvants, and to develop new live, attenuated, and peptide-based influenza vaccines (20). In addition, significant advances recently have been made with respect to several different multivalent pneumococcal conjugate vaccines (20,21). Table 1 summarizes the indications, schedule, and major precautions for use of influenza and pneumococcal vaccines.

Table 1 Immunizing Agents and Immunization Schedules

Generic name	Primary schedule and booster(s)	Indications	Major precautions and contraindications	Special considerations
Influenza vaccine (inactivated whole-virus and split).	Annual vaccination with current vaccine. Either whole- or split-virus vaccine may be used intramuscularly (IM)	Persons with high-risk medical conditions and/or ≥65 years of age and their care providers and household contacts.	History of anaphylactic hypersensitivity following egg ingestion or other exposure to egg protein (e.g., occupational exposure).	No evidence exists of maternal or fetal risk when vaccine is given during pregnancy. Influenza vaccination is recommended for women who will be in the second and third trimesters of pregnancy during the influenza season because of increased risk for hospitalization.
Pneumococcal polysaccharide vaccine (23 valent).	One dose IM or subcutaneously; revaccination recommended for those at highest risk ≥5 years after the first dose.	Adults who are at increased risk of pneumococcal disease and its complications because of underlying health conditions; older adults, especially those age ≥65 who are healthy.	The safety of vaccine in pregnant women has not been evaluated; it should not be administered during pregnancy unless the risk of infection is high. Previous recipients of any type of pneumococcal polysaccharide vaccine who are at highest risk for fatal infection or antibody loss may be revaccinated ≥5 years after the first dose.	

III. VACCINATION WITH PNEUMOCOCCAL POLYSACCHARIDE VACCINE

A. Pneumococcal Polysaccharide Vaccine

The currently available pneumococcal vaccines, manufactured by both Merck and Company, Inc. (Pneumovax® 23) and Lederle Laboratories (Pnu-Immune® 23), include 23 purified capsular polysaccharide antigens of *S. pneumoniae* (serotypes 1, 2, 3, 4, 5, 6B, 7F, 8, 9N, 9V, 10A, 11A, 12F, 14, 15B, 17F, 18C, 19A, 19F, 20, 22F, 23F, and 33F). The 23 capsular types in the vaccine represent at least 85% to 90% of the serotypes that cause invasive pneumococcal infections among children and adults in the United States (22–24). The six serotypes that most frequently cause invasive drug-resistant pneumococcal infection in the United States (serotypes 6B, 9V, 14, 19A, 19F, and 23F) are represented in the 23-valent vaccine (25,26). Pneumococcal capsular polysaccharide antigens induce type-specific antibodies that enhance opsonization, phagocytosis, and killing of pneumococci by leukocytes and other phagocytic cells. After vaccination, an antigen-specific antibody response, indicated by a two-fold or greater increase in serotype-specific antibody, develops within 2 to 3 weeks in greater than or equal to 80% of healthy young adults (27); however, immune responses may not be consistent among all 23 serotypes in the vaccine. The levels of antibodies that correlate with protection against pneumococcal disease have not been clearly defined. Children vaccinated with pneumococcal polysaccharide vaccine are not significantly less likely to be colonized with *S. pneumoniae* than are those who are not vaccinated (28).

B. Risk Factors and Target Groups for Vaccination

Children younger than 2 years old and adults 65 years of age or older are at increased risk for pneumococcal infection; however, T-cell independent antigens such as polysaccharides produce limited antibody responses in children younger than age 2 years, and clinical trials of the pneumococcal capsular polysaccharide vaccines among young children have demonstrated limited or no evidence of efficacy (29–31). Persons who have certain underlying medical conditions also are at increased risk for development of pneumococcal infection or experiencing severe disease and complications as are those who have decreased responsiveness to polysaccharide antigens or rapid decline in serum antibody. As many as 91% of adults who have invasive pneumococcal infection have at least one of the underlying medical conditions mentioned below, including age greater than or equal to 65 years (32–35).

C. Recommendations for Vaccine Use

The vaccine is both cost effective and protective against invasive pneumococcal infection when administered to immunocompetent persons aged 2 years or older. Therefore, all persons in the following categories should receive the 23-valent pneumococcal polysaccharide vaccine (Table 2). If earlier vaccination status is unknown, persons in these categories should be given pneumococcal vaccine.

1. Persons Aged 65 Years or Older

All persons in this category should receive the pneumococcal vaccine, including previously unvaccinated persons and persons who have not received vaccine within 5 years (and were younger than 65 years of age at the time of vaccination). All persons who have unknown vaccination status should receive one dose of vaccine.

2. Persons Aged 2 to 64 Years Who Have Chronic Illness

Persons aged 2 to 64 years who are at increased risk for pneumococcal disease or its complications if they become infected should be vaccinated. Persons at increased risk for severe disease include those with chronic illness such as chronic cardiovascular disease (e.g., congestive heart failure [CHF] or cardiomyopathies), chronic pulmonary disease (e.g., chronic obstructive pulmonary disease [COPD] or emphysema, and asthma that occurs with chronic bronchitis, emphysema, or long-term use of systemic corticosteroids), diabetes mellitus, alcoholism, chronic liver disease (cirrhosis) (36–39), or cerebrospinal fluid leaks.

3. Persons Aged 2 to 64 Years Who Have Functional or Anatomical Asplenia

Persons aged 2 to 64 years who have functional or anatomical asplenia (e.g., sickle cell disease or splenectomy) also should be vaccinated. These persons are at highest risk for pneumococcal infection, because this condition leads to reduced clearance of encapsulated bacterial from the bloodstream. Persons with such a condition should be informed that vaccination does not guarantee protection against fulminant pneumococcal disease, for which the case-fatality rate is 50% to 80%. Asplenic patients with unexplained fever or manifestations of sepsis should receive prompt medical attention, including evaluation and treatment for suspected bacteremia. Chemoprophylaxis also should be considered in these patients. When elective splenectomy is being planned, pneumococcal vaccine should be administered at least 2 weeks before surgery.

4. Persons Aged 2 to 64 Years Who Are Living in Special Environments or Social Settings

Persons aged 2 to 64 years who are living in environments or social settings in which the risk for invasive pneumococcal disease or its complications is increased (e.g., Alaskan natives and certain Native American populations) should be vaccinated. In addition, because of recently reported outbreaks of pneumococcal disease (40), vaccination status should be assessed for residents of nursing homes and other long-term-care facilities.

5. Immunocompromised Persons

Persons who have conditions associated with decreased immunological function that increase the risk for severe pneumococcal disease or its complications should be vaccinated. Although the vaccine is not as effective for immunocompromised patients as it is for immunocompetent persons, the potential benefits and safety of the vaccine justify its use.

The risk for pneumococcal infection is high for persons who have decreased responsiveness to polysaccharide antigens or increased rate of decline in serum antibody concentrations. The vaccine is recommended for persons in these groups, including the following: immunocompromised persons aged greater than or equal to 2 years, including persons with human immunodeficiency virus (HIV) infection, leukemia, lymphoma, Hodgkin's disease, multiple myeloma, generalized malignancy, chronic renal failure or nephrotic syndrome (37,39), or other conditions associated with immunosuppression (e.g., organ or bone marrow transplantation); and persons receiving immunosuppressive chemotherapy, including long-term systemic corticosteroids (41). If earlier vaccination status is unknown, immunocompromised persons should be administered pneumococcal vaccine.

When cancer chemotherapy or other immunosuppressive therapy is being considered (e.g., for patients with Hodgkin's disease or those who undergo organ or bone marrow transplantation), the interval between vaccination and initiation of immunosuppressive therapy should be at least 2 weeks. Vaccination during chemotherapy or radiation therapy should be avoided because of poor immune responsiveness.

Table 2 Recommendations for the Use of Pneumococcal Vaccine

Groups for which vaccination is recommended	Strength of recommendation[a]	Revaccination[b]
Immunocompetent persons[c]		
Persons aged ≥65 years	A	Second dose of vaccine if patients received vaccine ≥5 years previously and were aged <65 years at the time of vaccination.
Persons aged 2–64 years with chronic cardiovascular disease,[d] chronic pulmonary disease,[e] or diabetes mellitus	A	Not recommended.
Persons aged 2–64 years with alcoholism, chronic liver disease,[f] or cerebrospinal fluid leaks	B	Not recommended.
Persons aged 2–64 years with functional or anatomical splenia[g]	A	If patient is aged >10 years: single revaccination ≥5 years after previous dose. If patient is aged ≤10 years: consider revaccination 3 years after previous dose.

Person age 2–64 years living in special environ-ments or social settings[h]	C	Not recommended.

Immunocompromised persons[c]

Immunocompromised persons aged ≥2 years, includ-ing those with human immunodeficiency virus, leukemia, lymphoma, Hodgkin's disease, multiple myeloma, generalized malignancy, chronic renal failure, or nephrotic syndrome; those receiving im-munosuppressive chemotherapy (including cortico-steroids); and those who have received an organ or bone marrow transplant.	C	Single revaccination if ≥5 years have elapsed since receipt of first dose. If patient is aged ≤10 years: consider revaccination 3 years after previous dose.

[a] The following categories reflect the strength of evidence supporting the recommendations for vaccination: A, strong epidemiological evidence and substantial clinical benefit support the recommendation for vaccine use; B, moderate evidence supports the recommendation for vaccine use; C, effectiveness of vaccination is not proven, but the high risk for disease and the potential benefits and safety of the vaccine justify vaccination.

[b] Strength of evidence for all revaccination recommendations is "C."

[c] If earlier vaccination status is unknown, patients in this group should be administered pneumococcal vaccine.

[d] Including congestive heart failure and cardiomyopathies.

[e] Including chronic obstructive pulmonary disease and emphysema.

[f] Including cirrhosis.

[g] Including sickle cell disease and splenectomy.

[h] Including Alaskan natives and certain Native American populations.

D. Vaccine Administration

Pneumococcal vaccine is administered intramuscularly or subcutaneously as one 0.5-mL dose. Pneumococcal vaccine may be administered at the same time as influenza vaccine (by separate injection in the other arm) without an increase in side effects or decreased antibody response to either vaccine (42,43). Pneumococcal vaccine also may be administered concurrently with other vaccines.

E. Side Effects and Adverse Reactions

Pneumococcal polysaccharide vaccine generally is considered safe based on clinical experience since 1977, when the pneumococcal polysaccharide vaccine was licensed in the United States. Mild, local side effects (e.g., pain at the injection site, erythema, and swelling) develop in approximately half of persons who receive pneumococcal vaccine. These reactions usually persist for less than 48 hours. Moderate systemic reactions (e.g., fever and myalgias) and more severe local reactions (e.g., local induration) are rare. Intradermal administration may cause severe local reactions and is inappropriate. Severe systemic adverse effects (e.g., anaphylactic reactions) rarely have been reported after administration of pneumococcal vaccine (34,37). Pneumococcal vaccination has not been causally associated with death or neurological illness (e.g., Guillain-Barré syndrome) among vaccine recipients.

F. Vaccine Efficacy, Effectiveness, and Cost Effectiveness

Several clinical trails have been conducted evaluating the efficacy of vaccine against pneumonia and pneumococcal bacteremia. In addition, multiple case-control and serotype prevalence studies have provided evidence for pneumococcal vaccine effectiveness against invasive disease (23,44–55).

1. Efficacy Against Nonbacteremic Pneumococcal Disease

Pneumococcal capsular polysaccharide vaccine was shown to be effective at preventing pneumococcal pneumonia in young American military recruits (47) and in otherwise healthy South African gold miners (44,46). However, it is not clear whether data from these trials can be generalized to nonepidemic situations in the United States, where most pneumococcal disease in adults occurs in the elderly or in persons with chronic medical conditions. Vaccine efficacy for nonbacteremic pneumonia was not demonstrated for these populations in two postlicensure randomized, controlled trials (RCTs) conducted in the United States (49,51). However, these studies may have lacked sufficient statistical power to detect a difference in the incidence of laboratory-confirmed, nonbacteremic pneumococcal pneumonia between the vaccinated and nonvaccinated study groups (56). A metaanalysis evaluating pneumococcal vaccine efficacy by combining the results of nine randomized, controlled trials also did not demonstrate a protective effect for nonbacteremic pneumonia among persons in high-risk groups (57). The ability to evaluate vaccine efficacy in these studies is limited because of the lack of specific and sensitive diagnostic tests for nonbacteremic pneumococcal pneumonia.

2. Effectiveness Against Invasive Disease

Effectiveness in case-control studies generally has ranged from 56% to 81% (50,53–55). A serotype prevalence study based on CDC's pneumococcal surveillance system demonstrated a 57% (95% confidence interval [CI] = 45%–66%) overall protective effectiveness against invasive infections caused by serotypes included in the vaccine among persons at least 6 years of age (23). Vaccine effectiveness of 65% to 84% also was demonstrated among specific patient groups (e.g., persons who have diabetes mellitus, coronary vascular disease, congestive heart failure, chronic pulmonary disease, and anatomical asplenia). Effectiveness in immunocompetent persons aged 65 years old and older was 75% (95% CI = 57%–85%). Vaccine effectiveness could not be confirmed for certain groups of immunocompromised patients (e.g., those with sickle cell disease, chronic renal failure, immunoglobulin deficiency, Hodgkin's disease, non-Hodgkin's lymphoma, leukemia, or multiple myeloma). However, this study could not accurately measure effectiveness in each of these groups because of the minimal numbers of unvaccinated patients with these illnesses. In an earlier study, vaccinated children and young adults aged 2 to 25 years who had sickle cell disease or who had undergone splenectomy experienced significantly less bacteremic pneumococcal disease than patients who were not vaccinated (58). A metaanalysis of nine randomized controlled trials of pneumococcal vaccine concluded that pneumococcal vaccine is efficacious in reducing the frequency of bacteremic pneumococcal pneumonia among adults in low-risk groups (57). However, the vaccine is not effective in preventing disease caused by non-vaccine serotype organisms (54).

3. Cost Effectiveness

In a recent cost-effectiveness analysis based on efficacy of the pneumococcal polysaccharide vaccine for prevention of only pneumococcal bacteremia and meningitis among persons at least 65 years old, vaccination of elderly persons was shown to be cost saving (59). Thus, the vaccine compares favorably with other standard preventive practices.

G. Revaccination

1. Duration of Immunity

Following pneumococcal vaccination, serotype-specific antibody levels decline after 5 to 10 years and decrease more rapidly in some groups than others (42,60–63), which suggests that revaccination may be indicated to provide continued protection. However, data concerning serological correlates of protection are not conclusive, which limits the ability to precisely define indications for revaccination based on serological data alone. Polysaccharide vaccines, including the currently available pneumococcal vaccine, do not induce T-cell–dependent responses associated with immunological memory. Antibody levels increase after revaccination, but an anamnestic response does not occur (64). The overall increase in antibody levels among elderly persons has been determined to be lower after revaccination than following primary vaccination (65). Long-term follow-up data concerning antibody levels in persons who have been revaccinated are not yet available.

Data from one epidemiological study have suggested that vaccination may provide protection for at least 9 years after receipt of the initial dose (23). Decreasing estimates of effectiveness with increasing interval since vaccination, particularly among the very elderly (i.e., persons 85 years old and older), have been reported (54).

2. Indications for Revaccination

Routine revaccination of immunocompetent persons previously vaccinated with 23-valent polysaccharide vaccine is not recommended. However, revaccination once is recommended for persons at least 2 years old who are at highest risk for serious pneumococcal infection and those who are likely to have a rapid decline in pneumococcal antibody levels, provided that 5 or more years have elapsed since receipt of the first dose of pneumococcal vaccine. Revaccination 3 years after the previous dose may be considered for children at highest risk for severe pneumococcal infection who would be 10 years old or younger at the time of revaccination. These children include those with functional or anatomical asplenia (e.g., sickle cell disease or splenectomy) and those with conditions associated with rapid antibody decline after initial vaccination (e.g., nephrotic syndrome, renal failure, or renal transplantation). Revaccination is contraindicated for persons who had a severe reaction (e.g., anaphylactic reaction or localized arthus-type reaction) to the initial dose they received.

Persons at highest risk and those most likely to have rapid declines in antibody levels include persons with functional or anatomical asplenia (e.g., sickle cell disease or splenectomy), HIV infection, leukemia, lymphoma, Hodgkin's disease, multiple myeloma, generalized malignancy, chronic renal failure, nephrotic syndrome, or other conditions associated with immunosuppression (e.g., organ or bone marrow transplantation), and those receiving immunosuppressive chemotherapy (including long-term systemic corticosteroids). If vaccination status is unknown, patients in these categories should be administered pneumococcal vaccine.

Persons 65 years old and older should be administered a second dose of vaccine if they received the vaccine 5 or more years previously and were younger than 65 years at the time of primary vaccination. Elderly persons with unknown vaccination status should be administered one dose of vaccine.

The need for subsequent doses of pneumococcal vaccine is unclear and will be assessed when additional data become available. Because data are insufficient concerning the safety of pneumococcal vaccine when administered three or more times, revaccination following a second dose is not routinely recommended.

3. Adverse Reactions Following Revaccination

Early studies have indicated that local reactions (i.e., arthus-type reactions) among adults receiving the second dose of 14-valent vaccine within 2 years after the first dose are more severe than those occurring after initial vaccination (37,66). However, subsequent studies have suggested that revaccination after intervals of greater than or equal to 4 years is not associated with an increased incidence of adverse side effects (37,67,68). Although severe local reactions may occur following a second dose of pneumococcal vaccine, the rate of adverse reactions is no greater than the rate after the first dose. No data are available to allow estimates of adverse reaction rates among persons who received more than two doses of pneumococcal vaccine.

H. Persons with Uncertain Vaccination Status

To help avoid the administration of unnecessary doses, every patient should be given a record of the vaccination. However, providers should not withhold vaccination in the absence of an immunization record or complete medical record. The patient's verbal history should be used to determine prior vaccination status. When indicated, vaccine should be administered to patients who are uncertain about their vaccination history.

I. Antimicrobial Resistance

The impact of antimicrobial resistance on mortality rate is not clearly defined. Emerging antimicrobial resistance further emphasizes the need for preventing pneumococcal infections by vaccination. Strains of drug-resistant *S. pneumoniae* have become increasingly common in the United States and in other parts of the world (26,69). In some areas, as many as 35% of pneumococcal isolates have been reported to have intermediate-level (minimum inhibitory concentration [MIC] = 0.1–1.0 µg/mL) or high-level (MIC ≥ to 2 µg/mL) resistance to penicillin (CDC, unpublished data; 25,70,71). Many penicillin-resistant pneumococci are also resistant to other antimicrobial drugs (e.g., erythromycin, trimethoprim-sulfamethoxazole, and extended-spectrum cephalosporins). Penicillin resistance and multidrug resistance can make choosing optimal empirical antimicrobial therapy for suspected cases of meningitis, pneumonia, and otitis media difficult (72). Treating infections with nonsusceptible organisms may require the use of expensive alternative antimicrobial agents and may result in prolonged hospitalization and increased medical costs. The impact of antimicrobial resistance on mortality rate is not clearly defined.

IV. VACCINATING WITH INACTIVATED VACCINE FOR INFLUENZA A AND B

A. Inactivated Influenza Vaccine

Each year's influenza vaccine contains three virus strains (usually two type A and one type B) representing the influenza viruses that are likely to circulate in the northern hemisphere during the upcoming winter (17). The vaccine is made from highly purified, egg-grown viruses that have been made noninfectious (inactivated). Whole-virus, subvirion, and purified surface-antigen preparations are available.

B. Recommendations for the Use of Influenza Vaccine

Influenza vaccine is strongly recommended for any person aged 6 months or older, who—because of age or underlying medical condition—is at increased risk for complications of influenza. Health care workers and others (including household members) in close contact with persons in high-risk groups also should be vaccinated. In addition, influenza vaccine may be administered to any person who wishes to reduce the chance of becoming infected with influenza (17).

Although the current influenza vaccine can contain one or more of the antigens administered in previous years, annual vaccination with the current vaccine is necessary because immunity declines in the year following vaccination. Because the previous year's vaccine differs from the current vaccine each year, supplies of vaccine from prior years should not be administered to provide protection for the current influenza season.

Two doses administered at least 1 month apart may be required for satisfactory antibody responses among previously unvaccinated children younger than 9 years old; however, studies of vaccines similar to those being used currently have indicated little or no improvement in antibody response when a second dose is administered to adults during the same season (73,78).

During recent decades, data on influenza vaccine immunogenicity and side effects have been obtained for intramuscularly administered vaccine (74–78). Because recent influenza vaccines have not been adequately evaluated when administered by other routes, the intramuscular route is recommended. Adults and older children should be vaccinated in the deltoid muscle and infants and young children in the anterolateral aspect of the thigh (79).

C. Target Groups for Special Vaccination Programs

Groups at increased risk for influenza-related complications include the following:

- Persons 65 years old and older
- Residents of nursing homes and other chronic care facilities that house persons of any age who have chronic medical conditions
- Adults and children who have chronic disorders of the pulmonary or cardiovascular systems, including children with asthma
- Adults and children who have required regular medical follow-up or hospitalization during the preceding year because of chronic metabolic diseases (including diabetes mellitus), renal dysfunction, hemoglobinopathies, or immunosuppression (including immunosuppression caused by medications)
- Children and teenagers (aged 6 months to 18 years) who are receiv-

ing long-term aspirin therapy and therefore might be at risk for developing Reye's syndrome after influenza
* Women who will be in the second or third trimester of pregnancy during the influenza season

Persons who are clinically or subclinically infected can transmit influenza virus to persons at high risk whom they care for or live with. Some persons at high risk (e.g., the elderly, transplant recipients, and persons with AIDS) can have a low antibody response to influenza vaccine (74,75,78,80–83). Efforts to protect these members of high-risk groups against influenza might be improved by reducing the likelihood of influenza exposure from their caregivers. Therefore, the following groups should be vaccinated:

* Physicians, nurses, and other personnel in both hospital and outpatient care settings
* Employees of nursing homes and chronic care facilities who have contact with patients or residents
* Providers of home care to persons at high risk (e.g., visiting nurses and volunteer workers)
* Household members (including children) of persons in high-risk groups

D. Vaccination of Persons Infected with Human Immunodeficiency Virus

Limited information exists regarding the frequency and severity of influenza illness among HIV-infected persons, but reports suggest that symptoms might be prolonged and the risk for complications increased for some HIV-infected persons (84,85). Influenza vaccine has produced protective antibody titers against influenza in vaccinated HIV-infected persons who have minimal AIDS-related symptoms and high $CD4^+$ T-lymphocyte cell counts (78,80–82). In patients who have advanced HIV disease and low $CD4^+$ T-lymphocyte cell counts, however, influenza vaccine may not induce protective antibody titers (78,80–82); a second dose of vaccine does not improve the immune response for these persons (78). Because influenza can result in serious illness and complications and because influenza vaccination may result in protective antibody titers, vaccination will benefit many HIV-infected patients (17).

E. Simultaneous Administration of Other Vaccines

The target groups for influenza and pneumococcal vaccination overlap considerably. For persons at high risk who have not previously been vaccinated with pneumococcal vaccine, health care providers should strongly consider administering pneumococcal and influenza vaccines concurrently (17). Both vaccines can be administered at the same time at different sites without increasing side effects (16). However, influenza vaccine is administered each year, whereas pneumococcal vaccine is not (16,17).

F. Side Effects and Adverse Reactions

Because influenza vaccine contains only noninfectious viruses, it cannot cause influenza. Respiratory disease after vaccination represents coincidental illness unrelated to influenza vaccination. The most frequent side effect of vaccination is soreness at the vaccination site that lasts up to 2 days (86–88). These local reactions generally are mild and rarely interfere with the ability to conduct usual daily activities. In addition, two types of systemic reactions have occurred:

1. Fever, malaise, myalgia, and other systemic symptoms can occur following vaccination and most often affect persons who have had no exposure to the influenza virus antigens in the vaccine (e.g., young children). These reactions begin 6 to 12 hours after vaccination and can persist for 1 or 2 days.
2. Immediate—presumably allergic—reactions (e.g., hives, angioedema, allergic asthma, and systemic anaphylaxis) rarely occur after influenza vaccination. These reactions probably result from hypersensitivity to some vaccine component; most reactions likely are caused by residual egg protein.

G. Immunogenicity, Vaccine Effectiveness, and Cost Effectiveness

1. Immunogenicity

In most vaccinated children and young adults, high postvaccination hemagglutination-inhibition antibody titers develop. These antibody titers are protective against illness caused by strains similar to those in the vaccine or the related variants that may emerge during outbreak periods. In elderly persons and persons with certain chronic diseases, lower postvaccination antibody titers may develop than in healthy young adults, and thus they may remain susceptible to influenza-related upper respiratory tract infection (17,74–76,89). However, even if influenza illness develops despite vaccination, the vaccine can be effective in preventing lower respiratory tract involvement or other secondary complications, thereby reducing the risk for hospitalization and death (90–95).

2. Vaccine Effectiveness

The effectiveness of influenza vaccine in preventing or attenuating illness varies, depending primarily on the age and immunocompetence of the vaccine recipient and the degree of similarity between the virus strains included in the vaccine and those that circulate during the influenza season (17,89–97). When a good match exists between vaccine and circulating viruses, influenza vaccine has been shown to prevent illness in approximately 70% to 90% of healthy persons younger than 65 years (89). In these circumstances, studies also have indicated that the effectiveness of influenza vaccine in preventing hospitalization for pneumonia and influenza among elderly persons living in settings other than nursing homes or similar chronic care facilities ranges from 30% to 70%. Among elderly persons residing in nursing homes, influenza vaccine can be 50% to 60% effective in preventing hospitalization and pneumonia and 80% effective in preventing death, even though efficacy in preventing influenza illness may often be in the range of 30% to 40% (90–95).

3. Cost Effectiveness

Influenza vaccination of persons 65 years of age and older can save money and improve health (98,99). Influenza vaccination has been shown to be cost saving for healthy working adults (96) and can reduce direct costs and be cost saving in high-risk elderly populations in managed care settings (91,100).

H. Timing of Influenza Vaccination Activities

Beginning each September (when vaccine for the upcoming influenza season becomes available), persons at high risk who are seen by health care providers for routine care, planning elective surgery, or as a result of hospitalization should be offered influenza vaccine (17). Opportunities to vaccinate persons at high risk for complications of influenza should not be missed.

The optimal time for organized vaccination campaigns for persons in high-risk groups is usually the period from October through mid-November.

In the United States, influenza activity generally peaks between late December and early March. High levels of influenza activity infrequently occur in the contiguous 48 states before December. Administering vaccine too far in advance of the influenza season should be avoided. Vaccination programs can be undertaken as soon as current vaccine is available if regional influenza activity is expected to begin earlier than December.

V. PASSIVE IMMUNIZATION

A. Preparations and Indications

Immunoglobulin (Ig) intended for intramuscular administration has been primarily used for passive immunization against hepatitis A and measles following exposure and in some patients with immunoglobulin deficiency. It is not indicated for routine prophylaxis of bacterial or viral pneumonia in healthy patients. Currently, eight preparations of intravenous immunoglobulin (IVIg) are commercially available for passive immunization in the United States (101). Because of the successful use of immune and hyperimmune globulin against bacterial sepsis in animal models, there has been renewed interest in their potential use in immunocompromised high-risk patients (34). Administration of immunoglobulins has not had a place in the prophylaxis of influenza, because influenza does not have a viremic stage in pathogenesis, and pooled human antibodies would be lacking in appropriate specificity (102). Okuno et al., however, in a mouse model, have demonstrated protection from the lethal effect of a mouse-adapted strain of influenza A virus by a monoclonal antibody with cross-neutralizing activity among influenza A subtypes (103).

B. Pneumococcal and Other Bacterial Infections

Often those least likely to respond to pneumococcal vaccination are persons who are at greatest risk for invasive disease. Intramuscular or intravenous immunoglobulin administration may be useful for preventing pneumococcal infection in children with congenital or acquired immunodeficiency diseases, including those with HIV infection, who have recurrent, serious bacterial infections, that is, two or more serious bacterial infections (e.g., bacteremia, meningitis, or pneumonia) in a 1-year period (16). Intravenous immunoglobulin given monthly can reduce the occurrence of pneumococcal infections in adults with lymphoma (104). Standard immunoglobulin decreased the incidence of pneumonia, especially pneumonia resulting from gram-negative bacteria, in high-risk postsurgical patients (105). A human hyperimmune globulin termed bacterial polysaccharide immunoglobulin prepared from plasma donors immunized with *Haemophilus influenzae* type b (Hib), pneumococcal, and meningococcal vaccines, provided significant protection from invasive Hib infection during infancy (106,107). Oral administration of a polyvalent bacterial lysate has reduced mortality rate after infection with *S. pneumoniae* or influenza A in mice (108). Human polyvalent intravenous immunoglobulin given intravenously or intranasally in treated mice led to more antibodies to pneumolysin than in controls and greater resistance to reinfection (109). These findings suggest that local passive immunotherapy may be an effective means of treating certain pneumonias and may promote acquired resistance to reinfection. Although the results of these trials are promising, continuous use of intravenous immunoglobulin for prophylaxis can be expensive, and cost-effectiveness studies suggest that using intravenous immunoglobulin prophylaxis would be extremely expensive for each quality-adjusted life-year saved (110). Data are inadequate to evaluate the utility of intravenous immunoglobulin administration in the prevention of pneumococcal disease among HIV-infected adults.

VI. STRATEGIES FOR IMPLEMENTING PNEUMOCOCCAL AND INFLUENZA VACCINE RECOMMENDATIONS

The most effective strategy to optimally decrease the risk for pneumococcal infections and influenza, including cases that are acquired nosocomially, is to ensure that all persons for whom pneumococcal and influenza vaccination is recommended are identified and vaccinated in every setting where they receive care (16,17). Vaccination should ideally occur in a timely fashion before high-risk individuals are admitted to hospitals for inpatient care and the risk for nosocomial pneumonia increases. Successful vaccination programs have combined education for health care workers, publicity and education targeted toward potential recipients, a plan for identifying persons at high risk (usually by medical record review), and efforts to remove administrative and financial barriers that prevent persons from receiving the vaccine.

Barriers to achieving high pneumococcal and influenza vaccination levels among adults include (1) missed opportunities to vaccinate adults during contacts with health care providers in offices, outpatient clinics, and hospitals; (2) lack of vaccine delivery systems in the public and private sectors that can reach adults in different settings (e.g., health care, workplace, and college or university settings); (3) patient and provider fears concerning adverse events following vaccination; and (4) lack of awareness among both patients and providers of the seriousness of pneumococcal disease and influenza and benefits of vaccination (16,17,111,112).

A. Provider-Based Strategies

Provider-based strategies that have proved effective in increasing adult vaccination rates include physician reminder systems and practice-based tracking systems. Physician reminder systems consisting of charts, computers, or preventive health checklists remind physicians to review the need for vaccination for each patient and to administer vaccines to those at risk. Staff in physicians' offices, clinics, health maintenance organizations, and employee health clinics can be instructed to identify and label the medical records of patients who should be vaccinated. Patients in high-risk groups who do not have regularly scheduled visits during autumn should be reminded by mail or telephone of the need for vaccine. The use of preventive health checklists has increased pneumococcal vaccination rates four-fold (113) and from 5% to 42% (114). In one hospital, implementation of a computer reminder system that prompted physicians to review pneumococcal vaccination status before discharge increased pneumococcal vaccination rates from less than 4% to 45% (115).

In practice-based tracking systems, providers identify patients who are at risk and maintain rosters showing the proportion who receive vaccination. Physicians using such a tracking system have administered 30% more influenza vaccine than those not using the system (116).

B. Organizational Strategies

Organizational strategies in health care delivery settings (e.g., standing orders [rather than obtaining individual vaccination orders for each patient] for pneumococcal and influenza vaccination of high-risk patients who are eligible to receive vaccine) are the most effective methods for increasing pneumococcal and influenza vaccination rates among persons at high risk (117). High vaccination coverage rates can be achieved when pneumococcal and influenza vaccination programs are targeted to hospitalized patients at high risk (117). All unvaccinated persons who are at least 65 years old and younger persons (including children) with high-risk conditions who are hospitalized at any time from September through March should be offered and strongly encouraged to receive influenza vaccine before they are discharged. Pneumococcal vaccine should be offered throughout the year. A hospital-based immunization strategy is effective and capable of reaching those patients in whom severe influenza or pneumococcal disease is most likely to develop (118–121). In a New York hospital, instituting standing orders for pneumococcal vaccination of the elderly and at-risk patients increased the pneumococcal vaccination rate from zero to 78% (122). Similar increases were achieved for influenza vaccination in community hospitals in Minnesota (118,123).

Administration of influenza and pneumococcal vaccines should be included in routine clinical practice, and the vaccines, when indicated, should be administered before discharge of hospitalized patients to prevent subsequent admissions for influenza or pneumococcal disease. Eligible patients in high-risk groups can be identified by physicians, infection control practitioners, nurse specialists, and clinical pharmacists. Pneumococcal and influenza vaccination also should be routinely provided for residents of nursing homes and other long-term care facilities, in outpatient facilities providing continuing care to patients at high risk (e.g., hospital specialty care clinics, outpatient rehabilitation programs, hemodialysis centers), and in facilities providing episodic or acute care.

C. Strategies Targeting Health Care Workers

Administrators of all health care facilities should arrange for influenza vaccine to be offered to all personnel before the influenza season. Personnel should be provided with appropriate educational materials and strongly encouraged to receive vaccine. Particular emphasis should be placed on vaccination of persons who care for members of high-risk groups (e.g., staff of intensive care units [including newborn intensive care units], staff of medical/surgical units, and employees of nursing homes and chronic care facilities). Using a mobile cart to take vaccine to hospital wards or other work sites and making vaccine available during night and weekend work shifts can enhance compliance, as can a follow-up campaign early in the course of a community outbreak.

D. Age-Based Strategies

Persons aged 50 to 64 years commonly have chronic illness, and 12% have pulmonary conditions that place them at increased risk for pneumococcal disease (124). However, vaccination levels of those with risk factors are estimated to be low (16). A specific age-based standard should improve vaccination rates among persons with high-risk conditions. Therefore, age 50 years has been established as a time to review the overall immunization status of patients; risk factors that indicate the need to administer pneumococcal vaccine and begin annual influenza vaccination should be evaluated at this visit (124,125). Vaccination status also should be assessed during the adolescent immunization visit at age 11 to 12 years (126). This visit provides an opportunity to review the need for pneumococcal and influenza vaccines; adolescents with high-risk conditions should be vaccinated.

REFERENCES

1. Centers for Disease and Control and Prevention (CDC). Guidelines for prevention of nosocomial pneumonia. MMWR 1997; 46 (No. RR-1):1–79.
2. American Thoracic Society. Hospital-acquired pneumonia in adults: diagnosis, assessment of severity, initial antimicrobial therapy, and preventive strategies. Am J Respir Crit Care Med 1995; 153:1711–1725.
3. Heath TC, Hewitt MC, Jalaudin B, et al. Invasisive *Haemophilus influenza* type b disease in elderly nursing home residents: two related cases. Emerg Infect Dis 1997; 3:178–182.
4. Marrie TJ, Slayter KL. Nursing home-acquired pneumonia—treatment options. Drugs Aging 1996; 8:338–348.
5. Drinka PJ, Gauerke C, Voeks S, et al. Pneumonia in nursing home. J Gen Intern Med 1994; 9:650–652.
6. Berk SL, Gage KA, Holtsclaw-Berk SA, Smith JK. Type 8 pneumococcal pneumonia: an outbreak on an oncology ward. South Med J 1985; 78:159–161.
7. Centers for Disease Control and Prevention. Outbreaks of pneumococcal pneumonia among unvaccinated residents in chronic-care facilities. MMWR 1997; 46:60–62.
8. Balkovic ES, Goodman RA, Rose FB, et al. Nosocomial influenza A(H1N1) infection. Am. J Med Technol 1980; 46:318–320.
9. Van Voris LB, Belshe RB, Shaffer JL. Nosocomial influenza B virus infection in the elderly. Ann Intern Med 1982; 96; 153–158.
10. Pachucki CT, Walsh Pappas SA, Fuller GF, Krause SL, Lentino JR, Schaaf DM. Influenza A among hospital personnel and patients: implications for recognition, prevention, and control. Arch Intern Med 1990; 149:77–80.
11. Hall CB. Nosocomial viral infections: perennial weeds on pediatric wards. Am J Med 1981; 70:670–676.
12. Glezen WP. Viral pneumonia as a cause and result of hospitalization. J Infect Dis 1983; 147:765–770.
13. Wenzel RP, Deal EC, Hendley JO. Hospital-acquired viral respiratory illness on a pediatric ward. Pediatrics 1977; 60:367–371.

14. Hall CB. Hospital-acquired pneumonia in children. Semin Respir Infect 1987; 2:48–56.
15. Glezen WP, Loda FA, Clyde WA Jr, et al. Epidemiologic patterns of acute lower respiratory diseases in pediatric group practice. J Pediatr 1971; 78:397–406.
16. CDC. Prevention of pneumococcal disease: recommendations of the Advisory Committee on Immunization Practices (ACIP). MMWR 1997; 46(No. RR-8): 1–24.
17. CDC. Prevention and control of influenza: recommendations of the Advisory Committee on Immunization Practices (ACIP). MMWR 1997; 46(No. RR-9): 1–25.
18. CDC. Control and prevention of meningococcal disease and control and prevention of serogroup C meningococcal disease: evaluation and management of suspected outbreaks: recommendations of the Advisory Committee on Immunization Practices (ACIP). MMWR 1997; 46(No. RR-5):1–21.
19. Rubin BA, Rorke LB. Adenovirus vaccines. In: Plotkin SA, Mortimer EA Jr, eds. Vaccines. 2nd ed. Philadelphia: WB Saunders, 1994:475–502.
20. National Institutes of Health. Accelerated development of vaccines 1995. Division of Microbiology and Infectious Diseases, National Institute of Allergy and Infectious Diseases, Bethesda, MD: National Institutes of Health; 12–13, 21–23.
21. Kayhty H, Eskola J. New vaccines for the prevention of pneumococcal infections. Emerg Infect Dis 1996; 2:289–298.
22. Robbins JB, Austrian R, Lee CJ, et al. Considerations for formulating the second-generation pneumococcal capsular polysaccharide vaccine with emphasis on the cross-reactive types within groups. J Infect Dis 1983; 148:1136–1159.
23. Butler JC, Breiman RF, Campbell JF, Lipman HB, Broome CV, Facklam RR. Pneumococcal polysaccharide vaccine efficacy: an evaluation of current recommendations. JAMA 1993; 270:1826–1831.
24. Butler JC, Breiman RF, Lipman HB, Hofmann J, Facklam RR. Serotype distribution of *Streptococcus pneumoniae* infections among preschool children in the United States, 1978–1994: implications for development of a conjugate vaccine. J Infect Dis 1995; 171:885–889.
25. Hofmann J, Cetron MS, Farley MM, et al. The prevalence of drug-resistant *Streptococcus pneumoniae* in Atlanta. N Engl J Med 1995; 333:481–486.
26. Butler JC, Hofmann J, Cetron MS, Elliott JA, Facklam RR, Breiman RF. The continued emergence of drug-resistant *Streptococcus pneumoniae* in the United States: an update from the Centers for Disease Control and Prevention's Pneumococcal Sentinel Surveillance System. J Infect Dis 1996; 174:986–993.
27. Musher DM, Luchi M, Watson DA, Hamilton R, Baughn RE. Pneumococcal polysaccharide vaccine in young adults and older bronchitics: determination of IgG responses by ELISA and the effect of adsorption of serum with non-type-specific cell wall polysaccharide. J Infect Dis 1990; 161:728–735.
28. Douglas RM, Hansman D, Miles HB, Paton JC. Pneumococcal carriage and

type-specific antibody. Failure of a 14-valent vaccine to reduce carriage in healthy children. Am J Dis Child 1986; 140:1183–1185.

29. Douglas RM, Paton JC, Duncan SJ, Hansman DJ. Antibody response to pnueumococcal vaccination in children younger than five years of age. J Infect Dis 1984; 149:861–869.

30. Koskela M, Leinonen M, Häivä VM, Timonen M, Mäkelä PH. First and second dose antibody responses to pnuemococcal polysaccharide vaccine in infants. Pediatr Infect Dis 1986; 5:45–50.

31. Leinonen M, Säkkinen A, Kalliokoski R, Luotonen J, Timonen M, Mäkelä PH. Antibody response to 14-valent pneumococcal capsular polysacchride vaccine in pre-school age children. Pediatr Infect Dis 1986; 5:39–44.

32. Breiman RF, Spika JS, Navarro VJ, Darden PM, Darby CP. Pneumococcal bacteremia in Charleston County, South Carolina: a decade later. Arch Intern Med 1990; 150:1401–1405.

33. Plouffe JF, Breiman RF, Facklam RR, Franklin County Pneumonia Study Group. Bacteremia with *Streptococcus pneumoniae* in adults—implications for therapy and prevention. JAMA 1996; 275:194–198.

34. Fedson DS, Musher DM. Pneumococcal vaccine. In: Plotkin SA, Mortimer EA Jr, eds. Vaccines. 2nd ed. Philadelphia: WB Saunders, 1994:517–563.

35. Mufson MA, Oley G, Hughey D. Pneumococcal disease in a medium-sized community in the United States. JAMA 1982; 248:1486–1489.

36. Burman LA, Norrby R, Trollfors B. Invasive pneumococcal infections: incidence, predisposing factors, and prognosis. Rev Infect Dis 1985; 7:133–142.

37. CDC. Recommendations of the Immunization Practices Advisory Committee: pneumococcal polysaccharide vaccine. MMWR 1989; 38:64–68, 73–76.

38. Lipsky BA, Boyko EJ, Inui TS, Koepsell TD. Risk factors for acquiring pneumococcal infections. Arch Intern Med 1986; 146:2179–2185.

39. Musher DM. *Streptococcus pneumoniae*. In: Mandell GL, Bennet JE, Dolin R, eds. Principles and Practice of Infectious Diseases. 4th ed. Churchill Livingstone, 1994:1811–1826.

40. CDC. Outbreaks of pneumococcal pneumonia among unvaccinated residents in chronic-care facilities—Massachusetts, October 1995, Oklahoma, February 1996, and Maryland, May-June 1996. MMWR 1997; 46:60–62.

41. CDC. Recommendations of the Advisory Committee on Immunization Practices (ACIP): use of vaccines and immunoglobulins in persons with altered immunocompetence. MMWR 1993; 42(No. RR-4):1–18.

42. Hilleman MR, Carlson AJ, McLean AA, Vella PP, Weibel RE, Woodhour AF. *Streptococcus pneumoniae* polysaccharide vaccine: age and dose responses, safety, persistence of antibody, revaccination, and simultaneous administration of pneumococcal and influenza vaccines. Rev Infect Dis 1981; 3(suppl):S31–S42.

43. DeStefano F, Goodman RA, Noble GR, McClary GD, Smith SJ, Broome CV. Simultaneous administration of influenza and pneumococcal vaccines. JAMA 1982; 247:2551–2554.

44. MacLeod CM, Hodges RG, Heidelberger M, Bernhard WG. Prevention of pneumococcal pneumonia by immunization with specific capsular polysaccharides. J Exp Med 1945; 82:445–465.

45. Kaufman P. Pneumonia in old age: active immunization against pneumonia with pneumococcus polysaccharide—results of a six year study. Arch Intern Med 1947; 79:518–531.

46. Austrian R, Douglas RM, Schiffman G, et al. Prevention of pneumococcal pneumonia by vaccination. Trans Assoc Am Physicians 1976; 89:184–189.

47. Smit P, Oberholzer D, Hayden-Smith S, Koornhof HJ, Hilleman MR. Protective efficacy of pneumococcal polysaccharide vaccines. JAMA 1977; 238:2613–2616.

48. Riley ID, Tarr PI, Andrews M, et al. Immunisation with a polyvalent pneumococcal vaccine. Lancet 1977; 1:1338–1341.

49. Broome CV. Efficacy of pneumococcal polysaccharide vaccines. Rev Infect Dis 1981; 3(suppl):S82–S96.

50. Shapiro ED, Clemens JD. A controlled evaluation of the protective efficacy of pneumococcal vaccine for patients at high risk of serious pneumococcal infections. Ann Intern Med 1984; 101:325–330.

51. Simberkoff MS, Cross AP, Al-Ibrahim M, et al. Efficacy of pneumococcal vaccine in high-risk patients: results of a Veterans Administration cooperative study. N Engl J Med 1986; 315:1318–27.

52. Forrester HL, Jahnigen DW, LaForce FM. Inefficacy of pneumococcal vaccine in a high-risk population. Am J Med 1987; 83:425–430.

53. Sims RV, Steinmann WC, McConville JH, King LR, Zwick WC, Schwartz JS. The clinical effectiveness of pneumococcal vaccine in the elderly. Ann Intern Med 1988; 108:653–657.

54. Shapiro ED, Berg AT, Austrian R, et al. The protective efficacy of polyvalent pneumococcal polysaccharide vaccine. N Engl J Med 1991; 325:1453–1460.

55. Farr BM, Johnston BL, Cobb DK, et al. Preventing pneumococcal bacteremia in patients at risk: results of a matched case-control study. Arch Intern Med 1995; 155:2336–2340.

56. Spika JS, Fedson DS, Facklam RR. Pneumococcal vaccination—controversies and opportunities. Infect Dis Clin North Am 1990; 4:11–27.

57. Fine MJ, Smith MA, Carson CA, et al. Efficacy of pneumococcal vaccination in adults: a meta-analysis of randomized controlled trials. Arch Intern Med 1994; 154:2666–2677.

58. Ammann AJ, Addiego K, Wara DW, Lubin D, Smith WB, Mentzer WC. Polyvalent pneumococcal-polysaccharide immunization of patients with sickle cell anemia and patients with splenectomy. N Engl J Med 1977; 297:897–900.

59. Sisk JE, Moskowitz AJ, Whang W, et al. Cost effectiveness of vaccination against pneumococcal bacteremia among elderly people. JAMA 1997; 278:1333–1339.

60. Mufson MA, Krause HE, Schiffman G. Long-term persistence of antibody fol-

lowing immunization with pneumococcal polysaccharide vaccine. Proc Soc Exp Biol Med 1983; 173:270–275.

61. Mufson MA, Krause HE, Schiffman G, Hughey DF. Pneumococcal antibody levels one decade after immunization of healthy adults. Am J Med Sci 1987; 293:279–289.

62. Vella PP, McLean AA, Woodhour AF, Weibel RE, Hilleman MR. Persistence of pneumococcal antibodies in human subjects following vaccination. Proc Soc Exp Biol Med 1980; 164:435–438.

63. Kraus C, Fischer S, Ansorg R, Hüttemann U. Pneumococcal antibodies (IgG, IgM) in patients with chronic obstructive lung disease 3 years after pneumococcal vaccination. Med Microbiol Immunol 1985; 174:51–58.

64. Garner CV, Pier GB. Immunologic considerations for the development of conjugate vaccines. In: Cruse JM, Lewis RE, eds. Conjugate Vaccines. Basel, Switzerland: Karger, 1989; 11–17.

65. Mufson MA, Hughey DF, Turner CE, Schiffman G. Revaccination with pneumococcal vaccine of elderly persons 6 years after primary vaccination. Vaccine 1991; 9:403–407.

66. Boroоño JM, McLean AA, Vella PP, et al. Vaccination and revaccination with polyvalent pneumococcal polysacchande vaccines in adults and infants. Proc Soc Exp BioL Med 1978; 157:148–154.

67. Mufson MA, Krause HE, Schiffman G. Reactivity and antibody responses of volunteers given two or three doses of pneumococcal vaccine. Proc Soc Exp Biol Med 1984; 177:220–225.

68. Rigau-Perez JG, Overturf GD, Chan LS, Weiss J, Powars D. Reactions to booster pneumococcal vaccination in patients with sickle cell disease. Pediatr Infect Dis 1983; 2:199–202.

69. Klugman KP. Pneumococcal resistance to antibiotics. Clin Microbiol Rev 1990; 3:171–196.

70. Arnold KE, Leggiadro RJ, Breiman RF, et al. Risk factors for carriage of drug-resistant *Streptococcus pneumoniae* among children in Memphis, Tennessee. J Pediatr 1996; 128:757–64.

71. Duchin JS, Breiman RF, Diamond A, et al. High prevalence of multidrug-resistant *Streptococcus pneumoniae* among children in a rural Kentucky community. Pediatr Infect Dis J 1995; 14:745–750.

72. American Academy of Pediatrics, Committee on Infectious Diseases. Therapy for children with invasive pneumococcal infections. Pediatrics 1997; 99:289–299.

73. Gross PA, Weksler ME, Quinnan GV Jr, Douglas RG Jr, Gaerlan PF, Denning CR. Immunization of elderly people with two doses of influenza vaccine. J Clin Microbiol 1987; 25:1763–1765.

74. Cate TR, Couch RB, Parker D, Baxter B. Reactogenicity, immunogenicity, and antibody persistence in adults given inactivated influenza virus vaccines— 1978. Rev Infect Dis 1983; 5:737–747.

75. Beyer WEP, Palache AM, Baljet M, Masurel N. Antibody induction by influ-

enza vaccines in the elderly: a review of the literature. Vaccine 1989; 7:385–394.

76. La Montagne JR, Noble GR, Quinnan GV, et al. Summary of clinical trials of inactivated influenza vaccine—1978. Rev Infect Dis 1983; 5:723–736.

77. Wright PF, Cherry JD, Foy HM, et al. Antigenicity and reactogenicity of influenza A/USSR/77 virus vaccine in children—a multicentered evaluation of dosage and safety. Rev Infect Dis 1983; 5:758–764.

78. Miotti PG, Nelson KE, Dallabetta GA, Farzadegan H, Margolick J, Clements ML. The influence of HIV infection on antibody responses to a two-dose regimen of influenza vaccine. JAMA 1989; 262:779–783.

79. ACIP. General recommendations on immunization. MMWR 1994; 43(No. RR-1):1–38.

80. Huang KL, Ruben FL, Rinaldo CR Jr, Kingsley L, Lyter DW, Ho M. Antibody responses after influenza and pneumococcal immunization in HIV-infected homosexual men. JAMA 1987; 257:2047–2050.

81. Jackson CR, Vavro CL, Penningron KN, et al. Effect of influenza immunization on immunologic and virologic parameters in HIV+ pediatric patients (abstr). In: Program and Abstracts of the 2nd National Conference: Human Retroviruses and Related Infections. Washington, DC: American Society for Microbiology, 1995.

82. Nelson KE, Clements ML, Miotti P, Cohn S, Polk BF. The influence of human immunodeficiency virus (HIV) infection on antibody responses to influenza vaccines. Ann Intern Med 1988; 109:383–388.

83. Engelhard D, Nagler A, Hardan I, et al. Antibody response to a two-dose regimen of influenza vaccine in allogenic T-cell depleted and autologous AMT recipients. Bone Marrow Transplant 1993; 11:1–5.

84. Safrin S, Rush JD, Mills J. Influenza in patients with human immunodeficiency virus infection. Chest 1990; 98:33–37.

85. Thurn JR, Henry K. Influenza A pneumonitis in a patient infected with the human immunodeficiency virus (HIV). Chest 1989; 95:807–810.

86. Govaert TME, Aretz K, Masurel N, et al. Adverse reactions to influenza vaccine in elderly people: a randomized double blind placebo controlled trial. BMJ 1993; 307:988–990.

87. Margolis KL, Nichol KL, Poland GA, Pluhar RE. Frequency of adverse reactions to influenza vaccine in the elderly: a randomized, placebo-controlled trial. JAMA 1990; 307:988–990.

88. Margolis KL, Poland GA, Nichol KL, et al. Frequency of adverse reactions after influenza vaccination. Am J Med 1990; 88:27–30.

89. Dowdle WR. Influenza immunoprophylaxis after 30 years' experience. In: Nayak DP, ed. Genetic Variation Among Influenza Viruses. New York: Academic Press, 1981:525–534.

90. Patriarca PA, Weber JA, Parker RA, et al. Efficacy of influenza vaccine in nursing homes: reduction in illness and complications during an influenza A(H3N2) epidemic. JAMA 1985; 253:1136–1139.

91. Nichol KL, Margolis KL, Wuorenema J, Sternberg T. The efficacy and cost effectiveness of vaccination against influenza among elderly persons living in the community. N Engl J Med 1994; 331:778–784.

92. Foster DA, Talsma AN, Furumoto-Dawson A, et al. Influenza vaccine effectiveness in preventing hospitalization for pneumonia in the elderly. Am J Epidemiol 1992; 136:296–307.

93. Fedson DS, Wajda A, Nichol JP, et al. Clinical effectiveness of influenza vaccination in Manitoba. JAMA 1993; 270:1956–1961.

94. Barker WH, Mullooly JP. Effectiveness of inactivated influenza vaccine among non-institutionalized elderly persons. In: Kendal AP, Patriarca PA, eds. Options for the control of influenza. New York: Alan R. Liss, 1986:169–182.

95. Arden NH, Patriarca PA, Kendal AP. Experiences in the use and efficacy of inactivated influenza vaccine in nursing homes. In: Kendal AP, Patriarca PA, eds. Options for the control of influenza. New York: Alan R. Liss, 1986:155–168.

96. Nichol KL, Lind A, Margolis KL, et al. The effectiveness of vaccination against influenza in healthy, working adults. N Engl J Med 1995; 333:889–893.

97. Gross PA, Quinnan GV, Rodstein M, et al. Association of influenza immunization with reduction in mortality in an elderly population: a prospective study. Arch Intern Med 1988; 148:562–565.

98. Helliwell BE, Drummond MF. The costs and benefits of preventing influenza in Ontario's elderly. Can J Public Health 1988; 79:175–180.

99. Riddiough MA, Sisk Je, Bell JC. Influenza vaccination:cost-effectiveness and public policy. JAMA 1983; 249:3189–3195.

100. Mullooly JP, Bennet MD, Hornbrook MC, et al. Influenza vaccination programs for elderly persons: cost effectiveness in a health maintenance organization. Ann Intern Med 1994; 121:947–952.

101. Grabenstein JD. ImmunoFacts: Vaccines & Immunologic Drugs. St. Louis: Facts and Comparisons, 1995:212–224.

102. Kilbourne ED. Inactivated influenza vaccines. In: Plotkin SA, Mortimer EA Jr, eds. Vaccines. 2nd ed. Philadelphia: WB Saunders, 1994:565–581.

103. Okuno Y, Matsumoto K, Isegawa Y, Ueda S. Protection against the mouse-adapted A/FM/1/47 strain of influenza A virus in mice by a monoclonal antibody with cross-neutralizing activity among H1 and H2 strains. Virol 1994; 68:517–520.

104. Buckley RH, Schift RI. The use of intravenous immune globulin in immunodeficiency diseases. N Engl J Med 1991; 325:110–117.

105. The Intravenous Immunoglobulin Collaborative Study Group. Prophylactic intravenous administration of standard immune globulin as compared with core-lipopolysaccharide immune globulin in patients at high risk of postsurgical infection. N Engl J Med 1992; 327:234–240.

106. Siber GR, Thompson C, Reid GR, Almeido-Hill J, Zacher B, Wolff M, Santosham M. Evaluation of bacterial polysaccharide immune globulin for the

treatment or prevention of *Haemophilus influenzae* type b and pneumococcal disease. J Infect Dis 1992; 165(suppl 1):S129–S133.

107.   Santosham M, Reid R, Ambrosino DM, Wolff M, Almeido-Hill J, Priehs C, Aspery KM, Garret S, Croll L, Foster S, et al. Prevention of *Haemophilus influenza* type b infections in high-risk infants treated with bacterial polysaccharide immune globulin. N Engl J Med 1987; 317:923–929.

108.   van Daal GJ, So KL, Mouton JW, van't Veen A, Tenbrinck R, Bergmann KC, Lachmann B. Oral immunization with a polyvalent bacterial lysate can reduce mortality by infection with *S. pneumoniae* or influenza A in mice. Pneumologie 1990; 44:1180–1182.

109.   Ramisse F, Binder P, Szatanik M, Alonso JM. Passive and active immunotherapy for experimental pneumococcal pneumonia by polyvalent human immunoglobulin or F(ab')2 fragments administered intranasally. J Infect Dis 1996; 173: 1123–1128.

110.   Weeks JC, Tierney MR, Weinstein MC. Cost effectiveness of prophylactic immune globulin in chronic lymphocytic leukemia. N Engl J Med 1991; 325:81–86.

111.   Williams WW, Hickson MA, Kane MA, Kendal AP, Spika JS, Hinman AR. Immunization policies and vaccine coverage among adults: the risk for missed opportunities. Ann Intern Med 1988; 108:616–625.

112.   CDC. Increasing pneumococcal vaccination rates—United States, 1993. MMWR 1995; 44:741–744.

113.   Cheney C, Ramsdell JW. Effect of medical records' checklists on implementation of periodic health measures. Am J Med 1987; 83:129–136.

114.   Cohen DI, Littenberg B, Wetzel C, Neuhauser D. Improving physician compliance with preventive medicine guidelines. Med Care 1982; 20:1040–1045.

115.   Clancy CM, Gelfman D, Poses RM. A strategy to improve the utilization of pneumococcal vaccine. J Gen Intern Med 1992; 7:14–18.

116.   Buffington J, Bell KM, LaForce FM, et al. A target-based model for increasing influenza immunizations in private practice. J Gen Intern Med 1991; 6:204–209.

117.   Gyorkos TW, Tannenbaum TN, Abrahamowicz M, et al. Evaluation of the effectiveness of immunization delivery methods. Can J Public Health 1994; 85(suppl):S14–S30.

118.   Crose BJ, Nichol K, Peterson DC, Grimm MB. Hospital-based strategies for improving influenza vaccination rates. J Fam Pract 1994; 38:258–261.

119.   Schwartz B, Breiman R. Pneumococcal immunization: from policy to practice (editorial). JAMA 1990; 264:1154–1155.

120.   Fedson DS. Improving the use of pneumococcal vaccine through a strategy of hospital-based immunization: a review of its rationale and implications. J Am Geriatr Soc 1985; 33:142–150.

121.   Fedson DS, Harward MP, Reid RA, Kaiser DL. Hospital-based pneumococcal immunization. Epidemiologic rationale from the Shenandoah study. JAMA 1990; 264:1117–1122.

122. Klein RS, Adachi N. An effective hospital-based pneumococcal immunization program. Arch Intern Med 1986; 146:327–329.
123. Margolis KL, Nichol KL, Wuoernma J, VonSternberg TL. Exporting a successful influenza vaccination program from teaching hospital to a community outpatient setting. J Am Geriatr Soc 1992; 40:1021–1023.
124. CDC. Assessing adult vaccination status at age 50 years. MMWR 1995; 44:561–563.
125. American College of Physicians Task Force on Adult Immunization, Infectious Diseases Society of America. Guide for adult immunization. 3rd ed. Philadelphia: American College of Physicians, 1994:107–114.
126. CDC. Immunization of adolescents: recommendations of the Advisory Committee on Immunization Practices (ACIP), the American Academy of Pediatrics, the American Academy of Family Physicians, and the American Medical Association. MMWR 1996; 45(No. RR-13):1–16.

7

Using Quality Improvement Techniques for the Prevention of Nosocomial Pneumonia

ALICE H. M. WONG

Royal University Hospital
Saskatoon, Saskatchewan, Canada

RICHARD P. WENZEL

Virginia Commonwealth University
Richmond, Virginia

Nosocomial pneumonias are the second most frequently reported hospital-acquired infection, accounting for 16% to 19% of all nosocomial infections and affecting approximately 300,000 patients in the United States each year (1). The overall or crude mortality rate is 30% (90,000 deaths), and the direct or attributable mortality rate is 10% (30,000 deaths). Therefore, one-third of the deaths are directly due to the pneumonia and two-thirds to the underlying diseases (2). Furthermore, the extra length of hospital stay directly attributable to the pneumonias is estimated to be 9 days (2.7 million patient-days per year in the United States). Thus, morbidity rates, mortality rates, and direct costs are great. For these reasons, prevention of nosocomial pneumonias is clearly of great importance.

Specific risk factors such as those related to the host, device, or environment and those related to therapeutic measures such as stress ulcer prophylaxis are discussed elsewhere. This chapter discusses the roles of staff education, quality control (QC), quality assurance (QA), and continuous quality improvement (CQI) on reducing the rates of nosocomial pneumonia. Quality control usually refers to laboratory tests, such as pulmonary function tests, and deals with eliminating variation and errors in the testing process. Quality assurance is a term referring to the activities of people and has been replaced by the

187

term quality assessment, implying measurement and continuous quality improvement employed as a proactive effort in the organization.

To evaluate quality, it is necessary to define what quality means. In the health care setting, Leebov defines quality as ''doing the right things consistently to ensure (1) the best possible clinical outcomes for patients, (2) satisfaction for all of our many customers, (3) retention of talented staff, and (4) sound financial performance'' (3). Improving quality may be achieved in two ways. Reducing variation around a standard (statistical quality control) is one method, and raising the standard is the other (3). Donabedian (4) described three realms useful for approaching the assessment of quality: (1) structure, (2) process, and (3) outcome (Fig. 1). Structure is represented by the characteristics of the setting in which the care is provided. Process consists of all of the activities and interactions that occur in the care of patients, and outcome defines the effects of care on the health and welfare of individuals or populations (5).

In comparing the components of quality control and quality assurance versus continuous quality programs, one might find it helpful to know how to evaluate quality. A primary goal of QA programs is to identify outliers or deviations from a standard with subsequent corrective reaction. Frequently, individuals are identified as being responsible for a problem. However, the goal of CQI is to prevent a problem with quality by searching for problem processes and continually correcting deficiencies; blame for a problem is placed upon the system and not on an individual ''bad apple'' (6). The partici-

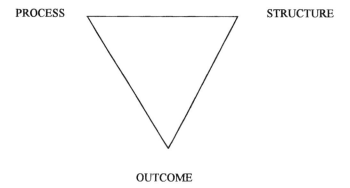

Figure 1   Donabedian's Triad. Avedis Donabedian envisioned an approach to solving problems with delivery of quality health care by focusing separately on the structure, process and outcome of the care administered. (From Ref. 5.)

Table 1 Comparison of Quality Assessment and Continuous Quality Improvement Techniques in the Prevention of Nosocomial Pneumonia

---

Prevention Method

QA: Essentially a surveillance system to determine nosocomial pneumonia rates and to intervene if higher than accepted standard.

CQI: A proactive method with the goal of identifying problem processes that may cause higher nosocomial pneumonia rates. Subsequently there would be attempts to intervene to prevent pneumonia acquisition even if the nosocomial pneumonia rate was less than the accepted standard.

Goal

QA: A static, target rate of nosocomial pneumonia.

CQI: A never-ending attempt to lower the rate of nosocomial pneumonia.

Problem Identification

QA: Problem people.

CQI: Problem processes.

---

pation of all employees is encouraged in the quality improvement process. What better person to ask about problems in the system than the employees who have to deal with them on a daily basis? The goal in a CQI model is a constantly moving target rather than a static standard. Developed by Shewhart and refined by Deming and Juran, these techniques revolutionized Japanese industry (3). Only years later were these principles adopted by US industry. In medicine at large in the United States, the change from an emphasis on QA to CQI methods is supported by the Joint Commission on Accreditation of Hospitals (7). These new standards will have to be met for accreditation, and a remote review of institution-generated data on quality care will replace the intense, on-site review of the Joint Commission. Table 1 compares QA and CQI techniques in nosocomial pneumonia prevention protocols.

I. ORGANIZING A QUALITY IMPROVEMENT COMMITTEE

Traditionally, infection control programs have played a major role in quality assessment. The shift of emphasis from QA to CQI methodology will require their continued involvement. How should an institution organize and implement a CQI program to reduce the occurrence of nosocomial pneumonia (Fig. 2)? The first step is to form a dedicated, multidisciplinary committee to address this issue. Team members should include representatives from respiratory ther-

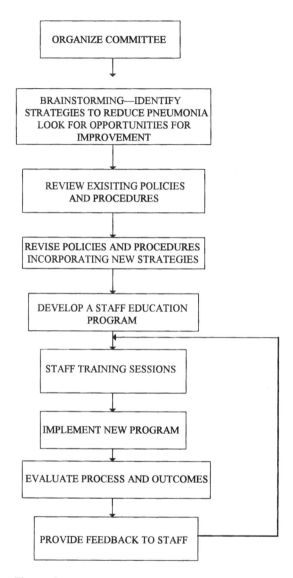

Figure 2 Steps involved in organizing and implementing a continuous quality improvement program.

apy, nursing, intensive care unit (ICU) nurse managers, pulmonary, critical care, infectious diseases, infection control, quality health, internal medicine, and surgery. Ideal characteristics of a committee include members who (1) have a common goal, (2) have complementary skills, and (3) are committed to each others' growth and success (8). This committee should meet at least on a monthly basis. Once the quality improvement team has been assembled, targets for improvement need to be identified.

II. IDENTIFICATION OF OPPORTUNITIES FOR IMPROVEMENT

Brainstorming assists in identifying many ideas as possible opportunities for improvement. This may be aided by drawing flowcharts of all the different processes that impact the development of pneumonia, such as patient positioning and maintenance of and handling of ventilatory equipment at the bedside. Cause and effect diagrams (3), also known as fishbone diagrams, are a visual aid in identifying the relationship between a potential risk factor and the development of nosocomial pneumonia (Fig. 3). Presentation of the relative importance of the risk factors (9) in a table (Table 2) or in the form of a pareto chart (3) helps prioritize efforts. Given that the ICU is a particularly high-risk environment in that mechanical ventilation is associated with a 21 times greater risk of pneumonia, preventive efforts should particularly focus on this area (10).

The Centers for Disease Control and Prevention (CDC) document, "Guideline for Prevention of Nosocomial Pneumonia" (11) provides recommendations of infection control measures that should be implemented (Table 3). Regarding specific practice and process recommendations to prevent nosocomial pneumonia, measures should be directed at known risk factors. These risk factors may be broadly divided into host-, device-, and personnel- or procedure-related factors. Host factors include the presence of underlying lung disease, a depressed level of consciousness, an immunosuppressed state, and recent upper abdominal or thoracic surgery. Device-related factors include the presence of nasogastric and enteral feeding tubes and the requirement for intubation and ventilatory support. In terms of personnel- and procedure-related factors, patient positioning, antibiotic use, specific stress ulcer prophylaxis, and spread of organisms by health care workers' hands are all important issues (11). Next, new policies and procedures must be developed and approved by the committee and presented to administration for approval. These

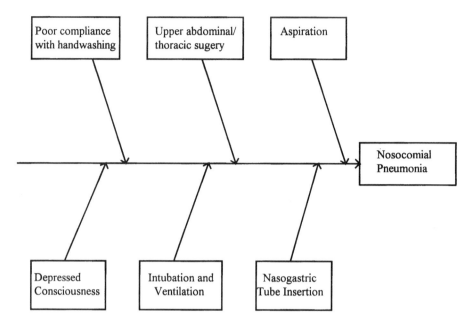

Figure 3 Cause and effect diagram for nosocomial pneumonia. Such simple diagrams allow the CQI team to identify and focus on specific risk factors leading to an
infection. The opportunities for improvement are often more visible.

Table 2 Risk Factors for Nosocomial
Pneumonia

Factor	Odds ratio (range)
Neuromuscular disease	3.9–18
Endotracheal intubation	3.0–12.9
Aspiration	5–10.6
Nasogastric intubation	6.5
Thoracic/upper abdominal surgery	4.3–6
Severity of illness	2.9–6.4
Decreased level of consciousness	9–5.8
Age	2.1–4.6
Intracranial pressure (ICP) monitor	4.2
Prolonged mechanical ventilation	1.2–3.1

Source: Ref. 9.

Table 3 Risk Factors and Suggested Infection Control Interventions

Risk factor	Suggested infection control measure
Host-related	
Chronic obstructive pulmonary disease	Use incentive spirometry, positive end-expiratory pressure, continuous positive airway pressure by mask.
Immunosuppression	Decrease duration of immunosuppression; avoid exposure to potential pathogens.
Depressed consciousness	Administer central nervous system depressents with caution.
Thoracic/upper abdominal surgery	Position patient property; give adequate analgesia, initiate early mobilization
Device-related	
Endotracheal intubation and mechanical ventilation	Apply gentle suctioning of secretions; position head of bed (HOB) up at 30° to 45°; use nonalkalinizing gastric cytoprotective agent for stress bleeding prophylaxis; do not routinely do ventilator circuit change more frequently than every 48 hours, drain and discard inspiratory tubing condensate, or use heat–moisture exchanger if indicated.
Nasogastric tube insertion and enteral feeds	Routinely check tube placement; remove nasogastric tube promptly when no longer required; position HOB up.
Personnel- or procedure-related	
Cross contamination by hands	Educate and train staff, apply adequate hand washing, appropriate gloving, and surveillance for pneumonia; give feedback to staff.
Antibiotic administration	Use antibiotics carefully, especially on high-risk patients such as those in the intensive care unit.

Source: Ref. 11.

changes in policy and procedures can then be incorporated into an educational program for staff. It is important to include accountability in the policies. Which staff members are responsible for a particular aspect of care must be clearly defined.

III. STAFF EDUCATION

There are several factors that must be considered before the presentation of new materials for staff education. The question of who will be responsible for teaching the staff will arise. Ideally, the teaching of the staff should be done by members of the quality improvement committee. It is important that members of the committee consistently support policies in interactions with their peers.

The format of the education program should use a variety of tools. Formats may include brief lectures followed by visual presentation of principles such as the consequences of touching multiple patients without adequate hand-washing. Flow diagrams of processes to be implemented should be reviewed. The goal of staff education is to increase awareness of the links between the care methods and procedures with the risk for nosocomial pneumonia. Active participation of staff in discussing various scenarios is key to maintaining interest. For example, the relationship between particular procedures and practices and the development of nosocomial pneumonia may be illustrated by staging mock scenarios such as a resuscitation attempt. Encouragement of staff participation in identifying breaks in technique will help in emphasizing important points. Possible interventions should be discussed. Depending on the size of the health care institution and the type of patients cared for, it may be necessary to tailor the education program for a particular group of employees.

The employees who are targeted for staff education programs should include nurses (particularly ICU nurses), orderlies, respiratory therapists and physicians. To provide incentives for compliance with the program, proof of attendance may be required as a condition of employment. A centralized record of all employees who have undergone training should be maintained in the quality health or hospital epidemiology department. To provide a measure of the adequacy of the training, a written test could be given before and after the training session. An opportunity for discussion of the materials presented can be made available at the end of the session. The answers to the test questions should be discussed at that time as well.

The staff should be given the chance to evaluate the training session in terms of the content and the usefulness of the format. They should also be encouraged to identify areas of interest that were not covered in the presentation that should be covered in future sessions. Feedback to the staff of the test results should be given with scores of the group rather than with individual scores so that no one feels singled out or threatened. Refresher training should be provided on a yearly basis to ensure that staff members are kept up to date in the case of further changes and that they are reminded of the importance of continuing on with their current practices.

IV. CQI IMPLEMENTATION

What resources are required for program implementation? Administrators clearly have an important role to play in a CQI program because they must ensure the provision of adequate resources to initiate a CQI program. It is folly leading to frustration and failure for a hospital administration to seek improvement in a process and yet fail to provide adequate resources. Resources include adequate personnel and laboratory backup as well as support for instituting new policies and procedures. Posters depicting processes provide a visual reminder of the changes and are sometimes helpful. With the changes, it is anticipated that there may be resistance to change on the part of the staff because more effort will be required on their part, but reinforcement of the benefits that patients may reap as a result of their efforts aid in overcoming this barrier.

V. PROGRAM EVALUATION

A variety of clinical quality indicators may be used to evaluate the efficacy of efforts to prevent nosocomial pneumonia. A clinical indicator may be defined as "a quantitative measure that can be used as a guide to monitor and evaluate the quality of important patient care and support service activities" (12). The indicator measure may be a structure, process, or outcome of care (13). In addition to measuring the rate of nosocomial pneumonia, other indicators could include the appropriateness of antimicrobial utilization or the proportion of staff compliant with handwashing policies. For each clinical quality indicator, a threshold above which a more detailed review is indicated needs to be set (13). However, the quality of the assessment depends on whether accurate benchmark rates are available for comparison (14). With differences in nosocomial pneumonia rates between large and small hospitals (1), it is necessary to account for differences in severity of patient illness and patient mix before meaningful comparisons can be made (15). The latter is essentially an epidemiological problem of controlling for confounding either by stratifying the analysis (infections in intubated versus nonintubated patients) or modeling the data by using logistic regression (16). It may be more reasonable to use previous rates from the institution as benchmark rates and endeavor to improve upon those. If previous rates of nosocomial pneumonia are not available, it becomes necessary to conduct surveillance such that the baseline rate may be determined.

Once the CQI program is implemented, ongoing surveillance provides the data with which to measures its effectiveness (17). A standardized case definition should be used to ensure comparability between different abstractors. The CDC definition (Table 4) for nosocomial pneumonia is commonly used. The case definition differs for ventilated versus nonventilated patients and it depends on the age of the patient (18). Interinstitutional rates cannot be compared without standardization of the case definition. Surveillance for nosocomial pneumonia has typically been the domain of the hospital epidemiology and infection control department. It is a fundamental part of the specialized function of infection control practitioners (19,20).

Active surveillance is the recommended method of case finding (21). Because of the time commitment and cost involved in whole-house surveillance, many institutions perform unit-based surveillance. In this case, reporting by the laboratory or by hospital staff of unusual clusters of nosocomial pneumonia is an additional means by which cases may be found. Infection control practitioners (ICPs), independent of the clinical team, should continue to be the main surveyors for the data. However, QA staff may also be trained in surveillance, and both functions could be integrated into a single program (8). Because ICU patients on ventilators have a greatly increased rate for nosocomial pneumonia (10), it is worthwhile to stratify patients into risk groups with separate rates reported for ventilated and nonventilated patients. The denominators would be ventilator days, not hospital days. The nosocomial pneumonia rates should be calculated by the ICP on a monthly basis and reviewed with the hospital epidemiologist. Reporting of rates should occur to the infection control and the quality improvement committees and hospital administration.

Process surveillance is a vital component of program evaluation. Process surveillance may be defined as the "consistent and quantitative monitoring of practices that directly or indirectly contribute to a health outcome and the use of those data to improve outcomes" (22). In the design of process surveil-

Table 4   Case Definition for Nosocomial Pneumonia Adapted from CDC Criteria

For a diagnosis of nosocomial pneumonia, the following criteria must be met:
1. Rales or dullness to percussion of the chest on physical examination and any of the following
   A. New onset of purulent sputum or change in character of sputum
   B. Organism isolated from blood culture
   C. Pathogen isolated from transtracheal aspirate, bronchial brushing, or biopsy
2. Chest radiograph with new or progressive infiltrate, consolidation, cavitation, or pleural effusion and one of the following:
   A. New onset of purulent sputum or change in character of sputum
   B. Organism isolated from blood culture
   C. Pathogen isolated from transtracheal aspirate, bronchial brushing, or biopsy
   D. Isolation of virus or detection of viral antigen in respiratory secretions
   E. Diagnostic single antibody titer or four-fold increase in paired serum samples for pathogen
   F. Histopathology consistent with pneumonia
3. If patient age is younger than 12 months, any two of the following symptoms or signs: tachypnea, bradycardia, apnea, wheezing, rhonchi, or cough with any of the following:
   A. Increased respiratory sections
   B. New onset of purulent sputum or change in character of sputum
   C. Organism isolated from blood culture
   D. Isolation of pathogen from transtracheal aspirate, bronchial brushing, or biopsy
   E. Isolation of virus or detection of viral antigen in respiratory secretions
   F. Diagnostic single antibody titer or four-fold increase in paired serum samples for pathogen
   G. Histopathology consistent with pneumonia
4. If patient age is younger than 12 months, chest radiograph showing new or progressive infiltrate, cavitation, consolidation, or pleural effusion and any of the following:
   A. Increased respiratory secretions
   B. New onset of purulent sputum or change in character of sputum
   C. Organism isolated from blood culture:
   D. Pathogen isolated from transtracheal aspirate, bronchial brushing, or biopsy
   E. Isolation of virus or detection of viral antigen in respiratory secretions
   F. Diagnostic single antibody titer or four-fold increase in paired serum samples for pathogen
   G. Histology consistent with pneumonia

Source: Ref. 6.

lance activities, there are several factors to consider. The processes that will be monitored need to be prioritized. In the case of preventive efforts for nosocomial pneumonia, it is helpful to examine the relative importance of risk factors to determine where the most effort should be directed. The outcome of the process to be targeted must be clearly identified (19). Examples of processes that impact upon the outcome of nosocomial pneumonia that need to be evaluated include compliance with handwashing, the procedure followed when ventilated patients are suctioned, and how often patients are suctioned. Are patients positioned appropriately with the heads of their beds elevated if their conditions permit? A regular review of compliance with procedure and policy should take place so that interventions may be undertaken before there is a noticeable change in pneumonia rate. Quality improvement in process can only come about if there is a mechanism for the use of the collected data to

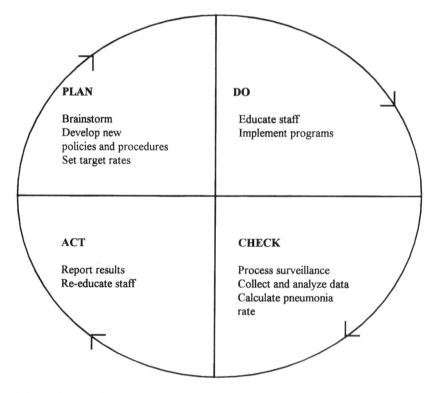

Figure 4   Plan-Do-Check-Act cycle for nosocomial pneumonia.

impact upon clinical practice. Thus, feedback needs to be provided to the caregivers. Feedback may be provided in the form of trend charts on a quarterly basis for pneumonia rates. Trend charts may also be used to depict the compliance rate with infection control interventions (e.g., handwashing). The above steps may be illustrated in a model called the Plan-Do-Check-Act (PDCA) cycle of Shewhart (3). Figure 4 shows an example for nosocomial pneumonia prevention.

VI. THE IMPACT OF CQI PROGRAMS

There are several examples of the effectiveness of the utility of the CQI model in prevention of nosocomial pneumonia. Kelleghan et al. (23) described the impact of CQI upon nosocomial ventilator-associated pneumonia (VAP) in an acute care hospital. A multidisciplinary team was formed whose specific aim was to reduce the incidence of VAP. Ventilator-associated pneumonia was targeted because of its association with a greatly increased risk of death. Despite accounting for only 25% of all nosocomial pneumonias, it accounted for the majority of pneumonia-related deaths. Following a review of policies and procedures and the development of an education program, surveillance was intensified, handwashing practices were surveyed, and periodic feedback was provided for staff. A 57% reduction (15 cases) in VAP over the course of the year was observed (based on baseline measured rate of VAP) despite VAP rates already being below literature based thresholds. The estimated cost saving was $105,000. Over time, the VAP rate increased but with more education and feedback, the rate once again decreased.

Another example of the successful application of CQI principles to reduce the risk of VAP is that of Joiner et al. (24). Using similar methodology as Kelleghan and colleagues (23), a multidisciplinary quality improvement team was formed. A new protocol was developed for the ICU which incorporated "state-of-the-art" care recommendations. Following institution of the protocol, a significant reduction in the mean nosocomial pneumonia rate was realized. The estimated savings were $126,000. A third example of the use of such techniques by McGowan et al. also resulted in a significant reduction in VAP rates (25).

Clearly, the utilization of CQI techniques is effective in reducing the rates of nosocomial pneumonia. In addition to substantial cost savings for the institution, such approaches offer tangible benefits to patients.

REFERENCES

1. Horan TC, White JW, Jarvis WR, Emori TG, Culver DH, Munn VP, Thornsberry C, Olson DR, Hughes JM. Nosocomial infection surveillance, 1984. MMWR 1986; 35:175S–295S.

2. Leu HS, Kaiser KL, Mori M, Woolson RF, Wenzel RP. Hospital acquired pneumonia: attributable mortality and morbidity. Am J Epdemiol 1989; 129:1258–1267.

3. Leebov W. The Quality Quest: A Briefing for Health Care Professionals. Chicago: American Hospital Publishing Inc., 1991.

4. Donabedian A. Quality assessment and assurance: unity of purpose, diversity of means. Inquiry 1988, 25:173–192.

5. Donabedian A. Defining and Measuring the Quality of Health Care. In: Wenzel RP, ed. Assessing Quality Health Care. Perspectives for Clinicians. Baltimore: Williams & Wilkins, 1992:41–64.

6. Berwick DM. Continuous improvement as an ideal in health care. N Engl J Med 1989; 320(1):53–56.

7. O'Leary DS. Accreditation in the quality improvement mold—a vision for tomorrow. QRB 1991; 27:72–77.

8. Wenzel RP. Healthcare reform and the hospital epidemiologist. In: Wenzel RP, ed. Prevention and Control of Nosocomial Infections. 3rd ed. Baltimore: Williams Wilkins, 1997:47–54.

9. Wiblin RT, Wenzel RP. Hospital-acquired pneumonia. Curr Clin Top Infect Dis 1996; 16:194–214.

10. Haley RW, Hootan TM, Culver DH, Stanley RC, Emori TG. Nosocomial infections in U.S. hospitals, 1975–1976. Estimated frequency by selected characteristics of patients. Am J Med 1981; 70:947–959.

11. Tablan OC, Anderson LJ, Arden NH, Breiman RF, Butler JC, McNeil MM, The Hospital Infection Control Practices Advisory Committee. Guideline for prevention of nosocomial pneumonia. Infect Control Hosp Epidemiol 1994; 15(9):588–627.

12. Anonymous. Characteristics of clinical indicators. QRB 1989; 15:330–339.

13. Decker MD, Sprouse MW. Hospitalwide Surveillance Activities. In: Wenzel RP, ed. Assessing Quality Health Care. Perspectives for Clinicians. Baltimore: Williams & Wilkins, 1992:157–192.

14. Gross PA. Striving for benchmark infection rates: progress in control for patient mix. Am J Med 1991; 91(suppl 3B):16S–20S.

15. Salemi C, Morgan JW, Kelleghan SI, Hiebert-Crape B. Severity of illness classification for infection control departments: a study in nosocomial pneumonia. Am J Infect Control 1993; 21(3):117–126.

16. Wenzel RP, Nettleman MD. Principles of applied epidemiology for infection control. In: Mayhall CG, ed. Hospital Epidemiology and Infection Control. Baltimore: Williams & Wilkins 1996:73–80.

17. Morrison AJJ, Kaiser DL, Wenzel RP. A measurement of the efficacy of nosocomial infection control using the 95 percent confidence interval for infection rates. Am J Epidemiol 1987; 126:292–297.
18. Garner JS, Jarvis WR, Emori TG, Horan TC, Hughes JM. CDC definitions for nosocomial infections, 1988. Am J Infect Control 1988; 16:128–140.
19. Haley RW, Gaynes RP, Aber RC, Bennett JV. Surveillance of nosocomial infections. In: Bennet JV, Brachman PS, eds. Hospital Infections. 3rd ed. Boston: Little, Brown, 1992:79–108.
20. Perl TM. Surveillance, reporting, and the use of computers. In: Wenzel RP, ed. Prevention and Control of Nosocomial Infections. 3rd ed. Baltimore: Williams & Wilkins 1997:127–161.
21. Abrutyn E, Talbot GH. Surveillance strategies: a primer. Infect Control 1987; 8(11):459.
22. Baker OG. Process surveillance: an epidemiologic challenge for all health care organizations. Am J Infect Control 1997; 25(2):96–101.
23. Kelleghan SI, Salemi C, Padilla S, McCord M, Mermilliod G, Canola T, Becker L. An effective continuous quality improvement approach to the prevention of ventilator-associated pneumonia. Am J Infect Control 1993; 21(6):322–330.
24. Joiner GA, Salisbury D, Bollin GE. Utilizing quality assurance as a tool for reducing the risk of nosocomial ventilator-associated pneumonia. Am J Med Qual 1996; 11(2):100–103.
25. McGowan H, Mattson S, Silva K, Naylor F, Magee M. Interdepartmental intervention and surveillance for ventilator associated pneumonia in critical care patients; a continuous quality improvement activity. Am J Infect Control 1994; 22(2):111.

8

Neonatal and Pediatric
Intensive Care Unit Patients

MICHAEL T. BRADY

Children's Hospital and The Ohio State University
Columbus, Ohio

I. INTRODUCTION

Nosocomial lower respiratory tract infections (LRI) represent a significant concern to those caring for hospitalized infants and children because of both their frequency and their potential severity. Pneumonia is the second most common nosocomial infections in all patients hospitalized in the United States regardless of age (1,2). Data from the National Nosocomial Infections Surveillance (NNIS) System documents that nosocomial pneumonia is the second most frequent hospital-acquired infection in critically ill infants and children as well (2,3). Many of the significant risk factors for the development of nosocomial pneumonia previously identified in adult patients, such as severe underlying cardiopulmonary disease, immunosuppression, depressed sensorium, and prior thoracoabdominal surgery, are present in pediatric patients and place them similarly at risk for nosocomial lower respiratory tract infections. In addition, there are specific clinical situations that are unique for neonatal and pediatric patients that provide additional risks for severe nosocomial lower respiratory tract infections (Table 1).

Although less information is available concerning the actual frequency and risk factors for nosocomial lower respiratory tract infection in children as compared to adults, there is adequate documentation of its importance, particularly for patients hospitalized within intensive care settings (3–7). Nosoco-

Table 1 Additional Factors that Place Infants and Children at Risk for Nosocomial Respiratory Infections

---

Alterations of barrier defenses
    Congenital anomalies (e.g., cleft palate, tracheoesophageal fistula)
    Uncuffed endotracheal tubes
    Cystic fibrosis and bronchopulmonary disease, resulting in compromised
        mucociliary clearance
    Newborn infants lacking endogenous flora that can block colonization with
        pathogens (e.g., group B streptococcus)
Immunological deficiencies
    Congenital immunodeficiencies (e.g., hypogammaglobulinemia, DiGeorge
        syndrome)
    Young age, resulting in increased susceptibility:
        a. Newborn infants have immature/inexperienced immune system (immaturity
          of immune system is exaggerated in prematurely born infants).
        b. There is less prior experience with many community-acquired respiratory
          infections (e.g., respiratory syncytial virus, influenza).
        c. There is less opportunity to receive protection by immunizations (e.g.,
          neonates or inadequately immunized children).
Increased exposure to potential pathogens
    Higher concentration of patients with highly contagious community-acquired
        viral infections in pediatric health care facilities (infected patients and health
        care workers)
    More intimate contact by health care givers, enhancing transmission (e.g., bottle
        feeding, changing diapers)
    Difficulty maintaining good hygiene in infants and young children (e.g.,
        handwashing, drooling, putting things in mouth)

---

mial pneumonia and tracheitis can have significant clinical consequences, both directly related to the morbidity of the infection, as well as adverse consequences associated with required therapies. Unnecessary exposure to broad-spectrum antibiotics, reintubation, increase in duration of mechanically assisted ventilation, increased length and cost of hospitalization, secondary infections including sepsis, and even death may be directly attributable to nosocomial pneumonia or tracheitis in infants and children. Reducing the impact of hospital-acquired lower respiratory tract infections in pediatric patients requires an understanding of the etiological agents and specific risk factors that are responsible for acquisition of these infections and for designing intervention strategies that specifically meet the needs of infants and children who are hospitalized within intensive care settings.

Newer therapies and respiratory devices have markedly enhanced opportunities to provide life-saving care to critically ill children. High-frequency ventilation (pressure limited, time cycled, jet, or oscillator) allows severely ill infants and children to be adequately ventilated at lower volumes than with conventional mechanical ventilation while improving gas exchange and minimizing barotrauma (8–10). Extracorporeal membrane oxygenation (ECMO) can be used to manage intractable hypoxemia not responsive to mechanical ventilation (11–13). Liquid ventilation offers an opportunity to achieve improved gas exchange for infants with severe surfactant deficiency or severe lung injury (e.g., barotrauma, infection, atelectasis) (14–15). Exogenous surfactant replacement can be given to premature infants and other children who lack adequate surfactant for normal lung function (16–19). These newer modalities are certainly beneficial to the critically ill infant or child. Their effect on the occurrence of nosocomial pneumonia or tracheitis has yet to be clearly defined. However, trials with these newer technologies have not attributed any significant increase in risk for nosocomial LRI in infants or children when compared to those receiving conventional mechanical ventilation. In one study of 80 neonates receiving ECMO, there was only one episode of nosocomial tracheitis and no episodes of pneumonia. The tracheitis occurred while the infant was still on ECMO (20). Most infections reported in ECMO patients are bacterial or fungal infections of ECMO catheters (21). Also, the continuous gas outflow through the larynx that occurs with high-frequency ventilation may prevent pulmonary aspiration and protect against the development of nosocomial pneumonia.

Dexamethasone has been used to diminish the inflammatory injury which contributes to the chronic lung disease in oxygen- and ventilator-dependent neonates with bronchopulmonary dysplasia (BPD) (22,23). The use of corticosteroids in high doses would seem to create an additional risk for infection in these vulnerable children. There does not appear to be any definite increase in risk for the development of nosocomial LRI in dexamethasone-treated neonates (22–25).

II. EPIDEMIOLOGY

Lower respiratory tract infections comprise 6% to 27% of all nosocomial infections detected in a pediatric intensive care setting (3,4,26). The actual frequency of nosocomial pneumonia and tracheitis occurring in hospitalized children varies considerably because of marked differences in patient populations cared for in different facilities. Interhospital variations in use of specific diagnostic methods to establish the presence and etiological agents of nosocomial pneumonia and tracheitis also affect the frequency and accuracy of identifying nosocomial lower respiratory tract infections.

Because of the difficulty in accurately establishing the diagnosis of a hospital-acquired pneumonia or tracheitis in a critically ill child, a standardized approach for defining these infections offers the best opportunity for interhospital comparisons. The Centers for Disease Control and Prevention (CDC) definitions for lower respiratory tract infections in children are included in Tables 2 and 3 (27). However, pneumonia and tracheitis may still be diagnosed and treated in children who do not satisfy these criteria. Also, children who fulfill these criteria may not truly have a nosocomial LRI. This occurs most commonly when the child exhibits a deterioration in his or her underlying pulmonary condition.

In general, the rate of nosocomial infections, including nosocomial respiratory tract infections, varies inversely with age. Hospital-wide nosocomial infection rates (of all types) have been reported as 11.5% for children 23 months of age and younger, 3.6% for children 2 to 4 years of age, and 2.6% for children at least 5 years old (26). Within a pediatric intensive care unit (PICU), nosocomial infection rates were two to three times higher for children 1 month of age or younger compared with children who were at least 2 years old at the time of hospitalization (3).

Nosocomial lower respiratory tract infections may occur in children hospitalized in any area of a hospital. However, the children at greatest risk for nosocomial pneumonia and tracheitis are those cared for in an intensive care setting; these account for >50% of all nosocomial pneumonias (28). Nosocomial lower respiratory tract infection will develop in approximately 2% to 10% of children in a pediatric intensive care unit. Similar but slightly lower proportions apply in infants cared for in neonatal intensive care units.

The majority of information available for assessing the frequency and etiological agents for pediatric nosocomial infections is available from the NNIS from the CDC (2). This standardized system has allowed reporting from approximately 60 pediatric centers. The information collected for nosocomial pneumonia and tracheitis is obtained using ICU-specific denominator data. Ventilator-associated pneumonia rates are calculated using a formula of the number of ventilator-associated pneumonias divided by the number of ventilator-days for patients in the intensive care unit during the surveillance period and then multiplying this number by 1000. This device-associated infection rate is further stratified by birth weight for infants hospitalized in neonatal intensive care units. Because mechanically assisted ventilation appears to be

Table 2 Criteria Used by the National Nosocomial Infections Surveillance System to Define Nosocomial Pneumonia

Infection site: Pneumonia
Definition: Pneumonia must meet at least one of the following criteria:
Criterion 1:   Patient has rales or dullness to percussion on physical examination of the chest
and
at least *one* of the following:
a. New onset of purulent sputum or change in character of sputum[a]
b. Organisms cultured from blood
c. Isolation of an etiological agent from a specimen obtained by transtracheal aspirate, bronchial brushing, or biopsy
Criterion 2:   Patient has a chest radiological examination that shows new or progressive infiltrate, consolidation, cavitation, or pleural effusion[b]
and
at least *one* of the following:
a. New onset of purulent sputum or change in character of sputum[a]
b. Organisms cultured from blood
c. Isolation of an etiological agent from a specimen obtained by transtracheal aspirate, bronchial brushing, or biopsy
d. Isolation of virus from or detection of viral antigen in respiratory secretions
e. Diagnostic single antibody titer (IgM) or four-fold increase in paired sera (IgG) for pathogen
f. Histopathological evidence of pneumonia
Criterion 3:   Patient 1 year of age or younger has at least *two* of the following signs or symptoms:
apnea, tachypnea, bradycardia, wheezing, rhonchi, or cough
and
at least *one* of the following:
a. Increased production of respiratory secretions
b. New onset of purulent sputum or change in character of sputum[a]
c. Organisms cultured from blood or diagnostic single antibody titer (IgM) or four-fold increase in paired sera (IgG) for pathogen
d. Isolation of an etiological agent from a specimen obtained by transtracheal aspirate, bronchial brushing, or biopsy
e. Isolation of virus or detection of viral antigen in respiratory secretions
f. Histopathological evidence of pneumonia

Table 2 Continued

Criterion 4:	Patient 1 year of age or younger has a chest radiological examination that shows new or progressive infiltrate, cavitation, consolidation, or pleural effusion[b]

and

at least *one* of the following:

a. Increased production of respiratory secretions
b. New onset of purulent sputum or change in character of sputum[a]
c. Organisms cultured from blood or diagnostic single antibody titer (IgM) or four-fold increase in paired sera (IgG) for pathogen
d. Isolation of an etiological agent from a specimen obtained by transtracheal aspirate, bronchial brushing, or biopsy
e. Isolation of virus from or detection of viral antigen in respiratory secretions
f. Histopathological evidence of pneumonia

[a] Expectorated sputum cultures are *not* useful in the diagnosis of pneumonia but may help identify the etiological agent and provide useful antimicrobial susceptibility data.
[b] Findings from serial chest radiographs may be more helpful than a single radiograph.
Source: Ref. 27.

the greatest risk factor for the development of a nosocomial lower respiratory tract infection, this device-associated infection rate appears to be optimal for comparisons between centers, as well as for monitoring trends within a hospital or an individual intensive care unit. However, there may still be significant interhospital variability in population characteristics that affects the risks for acquiring and rates of nosocomial infections. The pooled mean for ventilator-associated pneumonia in patients hospitalized in pediatric intensive care units from 58 different pediatric centers in 1996 was 5.9 ventilator-associated cases of pneumonia per 1000 ventilator-days (2). The rate of pneumonia for children hospitalized in an intensive care setting but not on a ventilator was 3.0 cases of pneumonia per 1000 patient-days (2). In the neonatal intensive care unit, the ventilator-associated pneumonia rates per 1000 ventilator-days by birth weight were as follows: $\leq$1000 g, 4.9; 1001–1500 g, 4.2; 1501–2500 g, 3.6; greater than > 2500 g, 2.9 (2).

In 1990, the NNIS pediatric hospitals reported 6.4 lower respiratory tract infections that were not pneumonia per 1000 ventilator-days (29). In children hospitalized in pediatric intensive care settings, the vast majority of these infections of the lower respiratory tract would be tracheitis but not pneumonia. Children's Hospital in Columbus, Ohio, has seen a steady increase in the number of lower respiratory tract infections in PICU patients on mechanically

Table 3 Criteria Used by the National Nosocomial Infections Surveillance System to Define Nosocomial Lower Respiratory Tract Infection Without Pneumonia

Infection site: Bronchitis, tracheobronchitis, bronchiolitis, tracheitis, without evidence of pneumonia

Definition: Tracheobronchial infections must meet at least one of the following criteria:

Criterion 1: Patient has *no* clinical or radiological evidence of pneumonia

and

at least *two* of the following signs or symptoms with no other recognized cause: temperature >38°C, cough, new or increased sputum production, rhonchi, wheezing

and

at least *one* of the following:
a. Positive culture obtained by deep tracheal aspirate or bronchoscopy
b. Positive antigen test on respiratory secretions

Criterion 2: Patient 1 year of age or younger has *no* clinical or radiological evidence of pneumonia

and

patient has at least *two* of the following signs or symptoms with no other recognized cause: temperature >38°C, cough, wheezing, respiratory distress, apnea, bradycardia

and

at least *one* of the following:
a. Organisms cultured from material obtained by deep tracheal aspirate or bronchoscopy
b. Positive antigen test on respiratory secretions
c. Diagnostic single antibody titer (IgM) or four-fold increase in paired sera (IgG) for pathogen

Reporting instruction: Do *not* report chronic bronchitis in a patient with chronic lung disease as an infection unless there is evidence of an acute secondary infection, manifested by change in organism.

Source: Ref. 27.

assisted ventilation diagnosed as tracheitis (Table 4) (30). The proportion of nosocomial infections in PICU patients which are diagnosed as tracheitis has increased from 10.7% in 1991 to 36.6% in 1996 (rates were 5.6 in 1991 and 16.5 in 1996 per 1000 ventilator-days); the proportion of nosocomial infections diagnosed as pneumonia has declined from 14.3% in 1991 to 8.5% in 1996 (rates were 5.6 in 1991 and 3.8 in 1996 per 1000 ventilator-days). It is

Table 4 Annual Frequency of Nosocomial
Pneumonia and Tracheitis in Children
Hospitalized in the PICU at Children's Hospital,
Columbus, OH

Year	Pneumonia (Rate[a])	Tracheitis (Rate[a])
1991	3 (5.6)	3 (5.6)
1992	6 (9.9)	4 (6.6)
1993	2 (2.3)	11 (12.6)
1994	5 (3.0)	16 (9.6)
1995	9 (5.7)	19 (12.0)
1996	6 (3.8)	26 (16.5)

[a] Number of infections per 1000 ventilator-days
Source: Ref. 30.

not clear whether this represents a change in the disease process or a difference in how the diagnosis is defined.

In the neonatal intensive care unit (NICU) setting, it is even more diffi-cult to find data on the true frequency of nosocomial tracheitis. At the occur-rence of nosocomial tracheitis in the NICU has varied considerably from year to year. Since 1992, nosocomial tracheitis has represented 11.5% to 25% of all identified nosocomial infections in the NICU patients (30). The rate of tracheitis for neonates on mechanical ventilation has varied without any spe-cific identifiable pattern, from 3.7 to 10.8 per 1000 ventilator-days.

In pediatric patients, as is the case in adults, aerobic gram-negative ba-cilli are the predominate agents responsible for nosocomial pneumonia and tracheitis (1,26,31). Gram-positive cocci, particularly *Staphylococcus* species, are seen with a slightly lower frequency than gram-negative bacilli in both pneumonia and tracheitis. However, nosocomial acquisition of respiratory vi-ruses, such as respiratory syncytial virus (RSV), influenza, adenovirus, and parainfluenza viruses, are more likely to result in significant lower respiratory tract disease in children when compared to adult patients (32,34). Nosocomial RSV infection results in dramatic increases in morbidity and mortality rates in critically ill children hospitalized for treatment of congenital heart disease, immunocompromised states, bronchopulmonary dysplasia, cystic fibrosis, and asthma (32–34). Mortality rates for nosocomial RSV in patients had been reported to be as high as 37% (4,35). However, this occurred prior to the current era of early and aggressive repair of congenital heart defects. Earlier repair of certain congenital heart lesions and better management of critically ill children in intensive care settings has resulted in reduced mortality rate attributed to nosocomial RSV infection. Even children without underlying heart disease can experience severe disease following hospital acquisition of RSV; mortality rates as high as 1.5% have been noted for nosocomial RSV infection of children without any underlying cardiac defects (4).

Children cared for in intensive care settings infected with the common community virus may be admitted to the hospital because they have symptomatic disease resulting from these viral infections. They may also be admitted for another illness, without exhibiting any respiratory symptoms. Infants with RSV and other respiratory virus infections may initially exhibit apnea, lethargy, and anorexia with or without typical symptoms of rhinnorrhea, cough, tachypnea, or wheezing. Despite a lack of respiratory symptoms, respiratory secretions from these infected children (but lacking respiratory symptoms) have very large concentrations of virus (e.g., 10^5–10^7 virions/mL) (35). Shedding may last for as long as 21 days (mean 7 days) in healthy children and up to 6 weeks in immunosuppressed children (36). Symptomatic as well as asymptomatic RSV-infected children may contaminate equipment, environmental surfaces in the ICU, and hands of personnel, as well as result in transmission to and infection of personnel.

Legionella species are an important and common nosocomial pathogen in adults; but they are rare as a cause of nosocomial infection in children. Immunosuppressed children are most commonly affected when nosocomial *Legionella* is identified (37). It is unclear why children are at such a lower risk compared to hospitalized adults because potable water at facilities caring for children frequently contains some level of *Legionella* contamination.

Lower respiratory tract disease may develop in neonates while hospitalized as a result of infection with organisms acquired perinatally from their mother's vaginal flora. These can include the group B streptococcus, *Mycoplasma* species, and *Ureaplasma urealyticum*.

A recent study performed in a Canadian pediatric intensive care unit identified specific risk factors or markers associated with bacterial nosocomial pneumonia and bacterial nosocomial tracheitis (38). By multivariate analysis, the following risk factors or markers (with odds ratio) were significantly associated with nosocomial infection:

1. pneumonia—(a) neuromuscular blockade (11.4), (b) immunodeficiency (congenital or acquired) (6.9), (c) age 2 months or younger

(6.1), and (d) immunodepressant therapies (e.g., cyclosporine, aza-
thioprine, corticosteroids, high-dose barbiturates) ($\geq$ 30 mg/Kg/
day) (4.8).
2. Tracheitis—(a) head trauma (12.5) and (b) respiratory failure (8.4)
    (38).

Colinearity between factors prevented some obvious risk factors such
as mechanically assisted ventilation and intubation from reaching statistical
significance. The close association between many risk factors would likely
impact any evaluation of risk for development of nosocomial lower respiratory
tract infections in children because multiple simultaneous interventions and
therapies would be similar in critically ill children. Also, the small number
of patients in this study did not allow for identification of specific underlying
diagnosis as risk factors (e.g. severe burns, polytrauma).

The duration of mechanically assisted ventilation appears to be very
important for determining the risk of nosocomial pneumonia. In children,
nosocomial pneumonia is rare during the first 72 hours of intubation (3). The
risk increases sharply after 72 hours (3). Studies in adults suggest that, after
10 days of mechanical ventilatory support, the rate of infection declines
sharply (39). After 10 days, it is likely that some of the other risk factors
contributing to the development of nosocomial pneumonia in critically ill children (e.g., sepsis, shock, surgery, anesthesia) will have resolved.

Nosocomial LRI can have a significant impact on survival. Death and
multiple organ failure have been reported in as many as 8% of children with
bacterial nosocomial pneumonia (38). In this same group of children, no deaths
were attributed directly to nosocomial tracheitis (38). However, reintubation
was required in 24% of these patients in whom nosocomial tracheitis developed.

III. PATHOGENESIS

Most bacterial nosocomial lower respiratory tract infections occur by aspiration of bacteria that colonize the oropharynx or upper gastrointestinal tract of
the child. Both intubation and mechanical ventilation alter or circumvent some
of the patient's natural barrier defenses against infection. These interventions
allow organisms from the oropharyngeal or upper gastrointestinal tract greater
access to the lower respiratory tract. The aspiration of contaminated materials
may be obvious or, more commonly, it is subclinical. The normal respiratory
flora of children admitted to a hospital consists of both gram-positive and

gram-negative organisms with streptococci, staphylococci, and *Neisseria* species predominating. In colder months, healthy children are more likely to be colonized with organisms such as *Streptococcus pneumoniae* and *Haemophilus influenzae* (both type b and non-typeable). The presence of these normal respiratory flora seems to reduce the ability of aerobic gram-negative bacteria and other organisms to colonize in the upper respiratory tract. Studies in healthy adults have documented the failure of aerobic gram-negative bacteria such as *Escherichia coli*, *Klebsiella pneumoniae*, *Pseudomonas aeruginosa*, and *Proteus mirabilis* to colonize the oropharynx for more than a few hours (40–42). However, the physiological stresses associated with illness and hospitalization or a prior respiratory viral infection can have a strong impact on the ability of these gram-negative organisms to colonize the oropharynx (40–42). The duration of hospitalization, prior antibiotic use, and severity of the underlying illness seem to increase the likelihood of colonization with gram-negative organisms. As many as 45% of hospitalized patients in an adult medical-surgical intensive care unit were colonized with gram-negative organisms after only 96 hours of hospitalization (43). Colonization of the oropharynx with gram-negative organisms may be seen in as many as 25% of these patients within as early as the first 24 hours of hospitalization (43). Factors that appear to enhance colonization with aerobic gram-negative organisms include acidosis, endotracheal intubation, hypotension and utilization of broad-spectrum antibiotics, malnutrition, coma, immunosuppression, and viral infection (40–43). The aerobic gram-negative bacteria that ultimately colonize the upper respiratory tract of hospitalized critically ill children are acquired by the following routes: (1) fecal-oral, (2) hands of health care personnel, (3) respiratory therapy equipment, including nebulized or aerosolized medications, and (4) upper gastrointestinal tract of patient receiving therapy for gastric alkalization to prevent stress gastritis, ulcers, and bleeding. The ultimate source of the majority of these aerobic gram-negative bacteria appears to be exogenous. In one study, a policy of ''protective isolation'' delayed colonization with gram-negative bacilli by up to 5 days and increased the mean interval from admission to the onset of nosocomial LRI from 8 to 20 days (5).

The structural configuration of the nasal and oral passageways markedly restrict the access of large particles to the lower respiratory tract. Under normal circumstances, the filtration system of the upper airway and the mucociliary clearance system of the larger airways protect the lower respiratory infection from bacteria that may be present in the patient's environment or that reside in the upper respiratory tract. Nosocomial pneumonia and tracheitis may occur when the mucociliary and cellular defense mechanisms of the lower respiratory tract are evaded.

Nasotracheal, orotracheal, or tracheostomy tubes bypass these initial host barrier defense mechanisms, providing direct access of bacteria and other pathogens directly to the lower respiratory tract. Dense bacterial polysaccharide biofilms coat endotracheal tubes. Polymicrobial flora become embedded into this film. Endotracheal suctioning can dislodge these aggregates of bacteria, providing a large bacterial inoculum directly into lower airways. Viruses (e.g., influenza), hypoxia and hyperoxia, injuries from burns, or inhaled or ingested chemicals impair or damage the mucociliary clearance apparatus. Prior viral respiratory infection, particularly with influenza viruses, predisposes to the development of pneumonia in children. *S. aureus* and *S. pneumoniae* predominate as the etiological agents of these secondary bacterial pneumonias following viral infections. However, secondary bacterial pneumonia is not common following RSV infection. Primary or secondary immunodeficiency states, adult respiratory distress syndrome, and pulmonary edema significantly impact on the ability of the local cellular host defenses to clear bacteria which have reached the lower respiratory tract.

Although the exact mechanism is not established, neutropenia in low birth weight infants of hypertensive mothers increases the risk of nosocomial infection (44). Pneumonia was the most common nosocomial infection noted in this neonatal population (44).

Entry of bacteria from the upper respiratory tract or upper gastrointestinal tract into the lungs usually occurs by aspiration (obvious or subclinical). Children who have either altered swallowing mechanisms or anatomical abnormalities that prevent adequate protection of their airway are at increased risk for aspiration. Specific conditions or situations associated with an increased risk for aspiration of upper respiratory tract or upper gastrointestinal tract secretions include tracheoesophageal fistula, gastroesophageal reflux, cleft palate, anesthesia, neuromuscular blockade, primary and secondary myopathies and central or peripheral nervous system disease associated with swallowing dyscoordination, and uncuffed endotracheal tubes (seven times greater than cuffed) (45–47).

Even though bacterial pathogens usually gain access to the lungs by aspiration, there is evidence of direct inoculation of the respiratory tract with nosocomial pathogens (airborne transmission). Nosocomial respiratory infections acquired by small- or large-droplet airborne transmission have occurred with varicella-zoster virus, *Bordetella pertussis*, influenza A and B, measles, mumps, rubella, enteroviruses, adenoviruses, *Mycobacterium tuberculosis*, *Neisseria meningitidis*, *Aspergillus* species, *Nocardia asteroides*, *Yersinia pestis*, and *Chlamydia psittaci*. Outbreaks of *Pneumocystis carinii* in closed populations support the possibility of airborne transmission (48). Nebulizers, manual ventilation bags, spirometers, suctioning equipment, oxygen analyzers, ventilation tubing, and nebulized medications contaminated with bacteria may be contaminated with bacteria during use, resulting in outbreaks of nosocomial pneumonia. Nosocomial transmission from contaminated equipment is for the most part preventable through use of disposable devices and use of effective methods for decontamination of reused equipment.

On rare occasions in children, nosocomial pneumonias may occur as a result of metastatic infection secondary to a bacteremia or fungemia, or primary infection at some distant site, or from contiguous spread. Respiratory tract symptoms, such as tachypnea and increasing oxygen requirements with or without roentgenogram evidence of pneumonia, are common in infants with fungemia resulting from *Malassezia furfur*. (49).

IV. ETIOLOGICAL AGENTS

As would be expected, the agents causing nosocomial pneumonia in children are frequently the same as those seen colonizing the upper respiratory tract. As mentioned previously, hospitalized patients, particularly those who are critically ill, have alterations in their oropharyngeal flora to include a greater proportion of aerobic gram-negative bacteria. The most common bacteria causing nosocomial pneumonia in children include *P. aeruginosa*, *S. aureus*, *K. pneumoniae*, *Enterobacter* species, *Moraxella catarrhalis*, non-typeable *H. influenzae*, *Citrobacter* species, *Candida albicans*, and other *Candida* species (1,26,31). Almost any aerobic or anaerobic bacteria may be responsible for nosocomial LRI at times; but others are far less common than those previously mentioned. Frequently, nosocomial bacterial pneumonia and tracheitis in children is polymicrobial.

Viruses such as RSV, adenovirus, influenza, and parainfluenza are responsible for up to 20% of cases of nosocomial pneumonia in children (50). Whereas nosocomial viral infections occur frequently in intensive care settings, their occurrence is commonly lower in the PICU and NICU than in other parts of a pediatric hospital. Possible explanations for this reduced nosocomial transmission of respiratory viruses within intensive care settings include (1) better patient-to-nurse ratios, (2) less cross coverage of infected and potentially infected patients, (3) fewer visitors (especially young children), (4) greater use of personalized equipment, (5) minimal patient–patient direct contact, and (6) greater availability of handwashing apparatus. Less common viral agents that can cause nosocomial lower respiratory tract infections include varicella-zoster virus (VZV), herpes simplex virus (HSV), cytomegalovirus (CMV), rhinoviruses, enteroviruses, and measles. HSV, CMV, VZV are particularly troublesome for immunocompromised patients.

Agents causing nosocomial pneumonia in infants cared for in neonatal intensive care units are similar to those in older children in a pediatric intensive care unit setting. However, there is a greater frequency of infections with the group B. streptococcus and coagulase-negative *Staphylococcus* (7,51). In centers that accept children into the NICU from the community, there is an increased risk for these neonates and health care providers to be exposed to community-acquired agents, such as RSV, adenovirus, influenza, and para-influenza viruses. Once introduced into a nursery, these highly communicable agents can rapidly infect other susceptible and vulnerable infants.

U. urealyticum and possibly other genital mycoplasma species represent a unique problem for the neonate. Acquisition of *U. urealyticum* occurs by contact with contaminated maternal cervicovaginal secretions during delivery. In colonized neonates, particularly preterm infants, pneumonia or, more commonly, chronic lung disease can develop (52–55). Tracheal aspirates or blood specimens may be positive for *U. urealyticum*. In infants with pneumonia, the total white blood cell count, absolute neutrophil count, and number of band forms are increased. A role for antimicrobial therapy for the prevention or amelioration of chronic lung disease in neonates infected with *U. urealyticum* has not yet been established.

Legionnaires' disease is a multisystem illness with pneumonia caused by *Legionella* species. This infection, both community acquired and nosocomially acquired, is rarely identified in children. Although it is probably less common in children than adults, it is very likely that the true incidence of nosocomial *Legionella* infections in children is underreported. Acquisition of *Legionella* requires exposure to contaminated water. The likelihood of infection following this exposure depends on the type and intensity of the exposure and the child's underlying health status. Persons who are severely immunocompromised are at greatest risk if they are exposed to aerosols of contaminated water (e.g., showers, nebulization of tap water) (37).

Candida species and other yeasts are becoming increasingly important as causes of nosocomial infections in both PICUs and NICUs (2,26). Isolation of these fungi usually occurs in association with other bacteria and in a setting of broad-spectrum antibiotic use. Establishing causation for a nosocomial respiratory infection for an identified yeast is usually difficult. However, it is clear that yeasts are responsible for nosocomial pneumonia in some critically ill children. Endogenous spread of the yeasts from other sites on the child accounts for most of these infections. However, exogenous acquisition from health care provider hands or the environment is likely and may be responsible for initial colonization.

Ubiquitous environmental fungi, such as *Aspergillus* species, *Fusarium* species, and *Rhizopus* species may be responsible for nosocomial pneumonia in immunosuppressed patients. These fungi are commonly present in the soil, water, and decaying vegetation (56). Within the hospital, *Aspergillus* can be found in unfiltered air, ventilation systems, contaminated dust dislodged during hospital renovation and construction, dusty horizontal surfaces, food, and ornamental plants (56,57). Nosocomial infections with *Aspergillus* species and *Fusarium* species have occurred as isolated events or as hospital outbreaks. Hospital outbreaks occur primarily in neutropenic patients, particularly those who have received bone marrow transplantation. Outbreaks most commonly result when the air that patients breath is contaminated with these environmental fungi from dust that is created during renovations, outside construction, and demolition. However, the hospital air supply may also be contaminated by bird droppings in air vents, contaminated air filters or air conditioning coils, and following water damage affecting ceiling tiles, dry wall, and fireproofing and insulation materials. Laundry chutes, elevator shafts, and tube systems may create currents that bring contaminated air into patient care areas.

The meconium aspiration syndrome is a unique condition that occurs in newly born infants who have passed meconium in utero. Passage of meconium frequently occurs following antepartum or intrapartum asphyxia (58). However, many unstressed infants may pass meconium in utero as a normal maturational event (58). In any case, in utero passage of meconium coupled with aspiration (in utero gasping or postpartum) can result in significant lower respiratory tract disease in the infant (inflammatory and chemical pneumonitis; proximal airway obstruction; peripheral airway obstruction). Each year in the United States, meconium aspiration syndrome develops in nearly 5% of all live born infants (26,000), with a mortality rate of 4% (58). Although there is still considerable controversy, it appears that aggressive airway management during delivery and immediately after birth is associated with a decreased mortality rate attributable to meconium aspiration syndrome (58,59). Amnioinfusion may also provide an opportunity for obstetricians to decrease the frequency of meconium aspiration syndrome in infants by diluting the meconium-stained amniotic fluid (60).

V. DIAGNOSIS

The optimal method for establishing the presence of nosocomial pneumonia or tracheitis in children remains to be established. In children with underlying pulmonary disease, it may be difficult to differentiate between the pulmonary disease occurring as a result of the primary underlying condition as compared to the development of new respiratory symptoms referable to a nosocomial pneumonia or tracheitis. In general, the diagnosis of nosocomial pneumonia is based on clinical changes with appropriate corroboration by chest roentgenogram findings. Clinical findings that might suggest the onset of a nosocomial pneumonia include increase in respiratory rate or effort, cough (new or significant change), wheezing; change in the amount or the consistency of sputum production or tracheal secretions, alterations in requirements for assistance with oxygenation and ventilation, and fever. In neonates, apnea may also signal the onset of a nosocomial pneumonia. Unfortunately, relying on clinical changes and chest roentgenogram findings in children hospitalized in a pediatric or neonatal intensive care setting will usually overestimate the true incidence of nosocomial pneumonia. Frequently, other entities, particularly deterioration in the underlying condition, may be responsible for these changes. Children with atelectasis, underlying congenital heart disease, bronchopulmonary dysplasia, hydrocarbon ingestions, cystic fibrosis, pulmonary hemorrhage, pulmonary edema, and surgical procedures affecting the chest may have radiographical changes that are similar to changes seen with pneumonia. In addition, clinical symptoms associated with pneumonia, particularly fever, may be due to multiple causes in a child in the intensive care unit.

Laboratory tests documenting the presence of inflammation and pathogenic microorganisms in lower respiratory tract secretions may assist the clinician in establishing the presence of a nosocomial lower respiratory tract infection. However, the isolation of a bacteria or virus from respiratory secretions does not by itself necessarily establish a causal relationship.

The etiological agent of bacterial pneumonia is frequently identified by direct sampling of lower respiratory tract secretions. However, young children rarely produce a sputum specimen that is adequate for evaluation. When young children cough, they usually swallow any sputum that is produced. Older children and adolescents may be instructed on proper techniques for providing a sputum specimen. This may be enhanced by using nebulization techniques.

Obtaining samples from patients who are intubated on mechanically assisted ventilation is relatively simple. However, interpretation of the results obtained from sampling of these respiratory tract secretions through an endotracheal tube is not always straightforward. The correlation between culture results obtained from endotracheal suction specimens and those from samples obtained directly from the lung, pleural cavity, or blood is frequently poor (61,62). In most cases, the presence of bacteria in specimens obtained by suctioning the endotracheal tube represents colonization rather than an invasive infection, such as pneumonia or tracheitis. The physician caring for the child in the intensive care setting must be cognizant that colonization of the upper airway, including the endotracheal tube and trachea, is common and frequently occurs in the absence of any disease. Also, symptoms such as fever, leukocytosis, and changes in tracheobronchial secretions obtained by endotracheal suctioning may occur for reasons other than the development of a nosocomial lower respiratory tract infection. For that reason, a multipronged approach must be taken to enhance the accuracy of defining nosocomial pneumonia or tracheitis.

Clinical considerations that increase the likelihood that nosocomial bacterial pneumonia has developed in a patient who is receiving mechanically assisted ventilation include changes in the patient's respiratory status that is unexplained by other events (e.g., decreased oxygenation, increased requirement for supplemental oxygen therapy, or increased ventilator pressure requirements) and a significant increase in the quantity and quality (e.g., purulence, color) of respiratory secretions when determined by a knowledgeable health care provider. When it is likely that a nosocomial bacterial pneumonia is present, there are a number of procedures that can assist in establishing the etiological agent. A Gram's stain of the sputum or specimen obtained by suctioning through the endotracheal tube can provide evidence of an inflammatory and potentially infectious process in the lower respiratory tract (63). The presence of an abundance of polymorphonuclear neutrophils (PMNs) or a significant increase in PMNs from a prior Gram's stain of the same secretions, with or without the presence of a predominant bacterial organism, provides valuable information when trying to determine whether pneumonia or tracheitis is present (63). Since these specimens are often contaminated with upper airway flora, the cultures may or may not reflect the bacterial organisms present in the trachea or lung tissue. However, the presence of an organism obtained by culture that is consistent with an organism identified on the Gram's stain markedly improves the likelihood that this agent is causally related to the nosocomial bacterial pneumonia (63). Quantitative sputum cultures, washed sputum cultures, and microscopic screening of sputa for the presence of cells from the upper airway have been used to assist in assessing whether the sample obtained represents lower airway secretions or is significantly contaminated with upper airway secretions (64,65). However, these additional measures do not add significantly to the value of routine Gram's stains with culture (63–65).

Numerous efforts have been made to develop techniques for obtaining specimens from the lower respiratory tract that can identify the bacteria responsible for the nosocomial pneumonia without interference by upper airway contamination. Transtracheal aspiration, transthoracic needle aspiration and biopsy, and bronchoscopy have been used to obtain samples directly from the lower respiratory tract with diminished contamination by upper airway flora. Most of the information concerning the sensitivity and specificity of these techniques has been obtained in adults. Use of these approaches in children, particularly those who are critically ill, may at times be medically contraindicated (e.g., transtracheal aspiration, transthoracic needle aspiration and biopsy, and transbronchial needle aspiration and biopsy). The specificity of these sampling techniques is greatest for patients who have a definite pneumonia. For that reason, they may be associated with a high rate of false-positive results in children who have underlying pulmonary or other conditions that might be confused with pneumonia by their clinical and radiographical appearances.

Bronchoalveolar lavage (BAL) is a safe, rapid, and reliable method for obtaining lower respiratory tract secretion samples. In intubated children, tracheal aspirates usually provide similar information as that which can be obtained by BAL. However, for those children with rapidly progressing lower respiratory tract disease or in whom a diagnosis is not established with routine tracheal aspirate, a BAL is appropriate. To obtain BAL fluid, a single isolated lung segment or, at times, multiple lung segments can be sampled using a flexible fiberoptic bronchoscope. The lung segment is lavaged with nonbacteriostatic saline through the wedged fiberoptic bronchoscopy (64,66). The aspirated fluid can be centrifuged and the pellet can be examined immediately for bacteria (Gram's stain or acridine orange), *P. carinii* (Gomori's methenamine silver stain), mycobacteria (acid fast stain or polymerase chain reaction), fungi (KOH or Calcofluor), and *Legionella*. Cultures can be performed for aerobic bacteria, *Legionella*, mycobacteria, fungi, *M. pneumoniae*, *Chlamydia* species, and viruses. Cytological evaluation can be useful for documenting the presence of malignant cells, lipid- or hemosiderin-laden macrophages, or, at times, cellular inclusions consistent with herpesviruses. The differential, count of white blood cells from BAL fluid may also be helpful. Children with bacterial or fungal infections are more likely to have a high proportion of granulocytes in BAL fluid (64,67).

For intubated infants, flexible fiberoptic bronchoscopy may not always be feasible. Modifications of fiberoptic bronchoscopy techniques have been performed with moderate success. A styletted intracatheter wedged blindly by way of the endotracheal tube and blind wedging of a double catheter system through the endotracheal tube to obtain lower respiratory tract secretions have been described (68).

Rarely, a percutaneous or open lung biopsy is required to establish the presence of a bacterial pathogen in nosocomial pneumonia. However, these invasive procedures are more helpful for establishing nonbacterial agents such as *P. carinii*, *Aspergillus*, and viruses as the cause of the nosocomial pneumonia.

Isolation of a bacterial pathogen from the blood of a child who has a nosocomial pneumonia when it is identical to the bacteria isolated from the lower respiratory tract usually confirms this organism to be the agent responsible for the nosocomial pneumonia. However, only approximately 2% to 5% of patients with nosocomial bacterial pneumonia have positive blood cultures (67).

Nonculture techniques can detect the presence of bacteria, either in respiratory tract secretions or the urine. Bacterial antigen detection systems for *H. influenzae* type b, *S. pneumoniae*, and Group B streptococcus have been used for many years. With the exception of detecting *H. influenzae* type b, these antigen detection systems are hindered by significant problems with sensitivity (*S. pneumoniae*) and specificity (Group B streptococcus). In addition, none of these agents is commonly responsible for nosocomial bacterial pneumonia in children. *Legionella pneumophila*, a rare cause of nosocomial pneumonia in children, can be reliably identified using a urine latex agglutination assay (56). *L. pneumophila* (56) and *B. pertussis* can be identified from respiratory secretions of patients using a direct florescent antibody microscopy. A PCR assay can be used to identify *B. pertussis* (69) and this technology (PCR) will likely be used to a greater extent for other bacteria. Serological assays are rarely useful for a timely diagnosis. However, a four-fold increase in *L. pneumophila* antibody titer to ≥1:128 in paired acute and convalescent sera (IFA) confirms recent infection with *L. pneumophila* (56).

VI. TREATMENT

Critically ill infants and children in whom nosocomial lower respiratory tract infections (either pneumonia or tracheitis) develop usually require immediate initiation of empirical antibiotics. Because the nosocomial lower respiratory tract infection can be life threatening, it is appropriate to administer broad-spectrum antimicrobials whose therapeutic spectrum would be capable of treating potential pathogens before culture and susceptibility results are available. However, it is this very common practice of using broad-spectrum antibiotics that has played a role in the ever increasing frequency of multiresistant organisms in critical care and chronic care settings. The approach to antibiotic diagnosis of nosocomial lower respiratory tract infections should include (1) initially, use empirical broad-spectrum intravenous antibiotics, (2) switch antibiotic therapy to more narrow-spectrum antibiotics based on appropriate susceptibility studies, (3) oral antibiotics can be used as soon as the patient has shown clinical improvement and can adequately tolerate medications given by mouth or tube (nasogastric or gastrostomy tube), (4) complete a full course of antibiotic therapy (10–14 days is usually adequate; 21 days may be necessary for staphylococcal pneumonia or pneumonia with empyema, or *Legionella* pneumonia in immunosuppressed patients), and (5) discontinue antibiotics as soon as it is likely that disease is not bacterial (viral or noninfectious).

Empirical therapy for nosocomial lower respiratory tract infections in infants and children should include antibiotics adequate to treat the majority of gram-negative and gram-positive bacteria usually identified as causal agents. Numerous antibiotics or antibiotic combinations would be acceptable. A combination of nafcillin and an aminoglycoside (aminoglycoside choice based on susceptibility data from individual patient care unit) or a combination of nafcillin and ceftazidime would be appropriate as initial empirical therapy for most children with a diagnosis of a nosocomial lower respiratory tract infection. Clindamycin could be used instead of nafcillin in the penicillin-allergic child or if significant aspiration is likely. Vancomycin should not be used for empirical therapy unless the patient is known to be colonized with a methicillin-resistant *S. aureus*. Meropenem or Timentin could be used alone or in combination with an aminoglycoside in critical care settings experiencing outbreaks of multiresistant organisms. Erythromycin or azithromycin (oral or intravenous) can be included in the empirical antibiotic regimen in hospitals that have experienced nosocomial *Legionella* or in immunosuppressed patients at risk for *Legionella* infection. The initial choice of antibiotics is also affected by prior antibiotic therapy in the child who is receiving antibiotics at the time the nosocomial LRI develops.

If a bacterial pathogen is identified, antibiotic therapy can be modified to provide adequate antibiotic coverage for the offending agent (Table 5) (70). This results in less of an impact on the remainder of the patient's resident microbial flora and it should reduce pressure for the development of antibiotic resistance and secondary multiresistant infections, particularly with fungi and enterococci.

Antibiotic concentrations in respiratory secretions following systemic administration (oral or parenteral) may be inadequate for rapid treatment of airway disease such as tracheitis or bronchitis (71). Administration of antibiotics by aerosol has been used successfully and safely in children with cystic fibrosis and in infants and children who have endotracheal or tracheostomy tubes (72–74). Nebulization of antibiotic solutions allows delivery of high concentrations of antibiotics (10–40 times greater than following parenteral

Table 5 Antimicrobial Therapy for Nosocomial Bacterial Pneumonia and Tracheitis in Children

Bacterial pathogen	Drug of choice[a]	Alternative
Gram-positive organisms		
Methicillin-sensitive *Staphylococcus aureus*	Nafcillin	Cefazolin
Methicillin-resistant *S. aureus*	Vancomycin	Add rifampin or gentamicin
Group A streptococcus	Penicillin	Cefazolin or clindamycin
Group B streptococcus	Penicillin	Add gentamicin if tolerant
Streptococcus pneumoniae—penicillin-sensitive	Penicillin	Macrolide if penicillin-allergic
Streptococcus pneumoniae—penicillin-resistant	Vancomycin	Ceftriaxone[a] or clindamycin[a]
Viridans streptococcus	Penicillin	Vancomycin
Enterococcus	Ampicillin	Add gentamicin; or vancomycin
Anaerobic streptococcus	Penicillin	Clindamycin
Gram-negative organisms		
Klebsiella pneumoniae	Ceftriaxone; cefotaxime	Aminoglycoside
Pseudomonas aeruginosa	Ceftazidime	Add aminoglycoside; meropenem
Escherichia coli	Ceftriaxone; cefotaxime	Aminoglycoside
Serratia marcescens	Ceftriaxone; cefotaxime	Aminoglycoside; meropenem
Acinetobacter species	Meropenem	Ceftazidime + aminoglycoside
Burkholderia cepacia	Ceftazidime	TMP/SMX
Stenotrophomonas maltophilia	Aminoglycoside + rifampin	Ceftazidine; TMP/SMX
Moraxella catarrhalis	Ampicillin-sulbactam	Cefuroxime
Haemophilus species-β-lactamase negative	Ampicillin	Cefuroxime
Haemophilus species-β-lactamase positive	Ceftriaxone; cefotaxime	Ampicillin-sulbactam
Legionella species	Macrolide + rifampin	Ciprofloxacin
Gram-negative anaerobes	Metronidazole	Clindamycin; ticarcillin-clavulanate
Other bacteria		
Mycobacterium tuberculosis	Isoniazid; rifampin; pyrazinamide	Based on patient's or local susceptibility patterns

[a] Always dependent on susceptibility testing done on the patient's isolate.
Source: Ref. 70.

administration) directly to the airways of the lower respiratory tract, with considerably lower levels of systemic absorption (75). An enhanced efficacy of aerosolized antibiotics as compared to parenteral antibiotics is yet to be conclusively established. In addition, the amount of antibiotic that is actually delivered to an individual patient may be greatly affected by the nebulizing system (ultrasonic > jet nebulizer) and the reservoir concentration of the antibiotic (76). Adverse effects associated with aerosolized antibiotics are primarily related to bronchial hyperactivity following administration.

Ribavirin aerosol therapy may be considered for selected infants and children with nosocomial RSV infections. Infants and children at greatest risk for severe RSV disease and who deserve consideration for ribavirin aerosol therapy include infants and children with the following (77):

1. Complicated congenital heart disease (including pulmonary hypertension)
2. Bronchopulmonary dysplasia
3. Cystic fibrosis
4. History of prematurity (infants <37 weeks' gestation)
5. Age younger than 6 weeks
6. Immunosuppressive diseases or therapy
7. Severe illness requiring mechanically assisted ventilation
8. Multiple congenital anomalies
9. Certain neurological or metabolic diseases (e.g., cerebral palsy or myasthenia gravis)

The recommendation concerning the use of ribavirin for the treatment of RSV infections was softened in 1997 because reports did not corroborate earlier efficacy data (78,79). Information obtained in infants and children with RSV infections requiring mechanically assisted ventilation has led to equivocal results. Some studies have demonstrated poorer outcomes, including more prolonged hospitalizations when ribavirin was administered to mechanically ventilated children. Meticulous care of mechanical ventilators is required with ribavirin administration to avoid plugging of in-line filters. Ribavirin deposition in filters can result in dangerous elevations in positive end-expiratory pressures (PEEP). Ribavirin is administered as a small-particle aerosol using a SPAG-2 collision generator. Six grams of ribavirin are mixed with 300 mL of sterile water (final concentration of 20 mg/mL). The aerosol solution is usually administered over an 18-hour period. Intermittent aerosols with higher concentrations of ribavirin (60 mg/mL) over 2-hour intervals on an every 8-hour schedule have been given safely; efficacy has not been established (80).

Treatment with ribavirin aerosol is given for at least 3 days; 5 days is usually adequate for previously healthy infants and children. Prolonged therapy may be necessary for immunocompromised children (81).

Infants and children older than 12 months of age who acquire influenza A (but not influenza B) while hospitalized within an intensive care setting should be given rimantadine if the infection has been identified or suspected within 48 hours of the onset of symptoms. Rimantadine must be given orally or by way of a nasogastric or gastrostomy tube. The rimantadine dose is 5 mg/kg/day, up to a maximum of 150 mg, for children younger than 9 years of age, and 200 mg for children older than 9 years old (82). Rimantadine could be given as a single daily dose or as two divided doses. Rimantadine (and amantadine) may exacerbate seizures in infants and children with a prior history of seizures. Ribavirin could be used for the treatment of severe influenza B infections or for children with severe influenza A infections who have a prior history of seizures. The dose and route of administration of ribavirin for the treatment of influenza infections is the same as that for the treatment of RSV infections described previously.

In immunosuppressed infants and children, particularly those who have received a bone marrow transplant, pneumonia may develop with herpesviruses, cytomegalovirus, or herpes simplex. These infections can be rapidly progressive and antiviral therapy is indicated. Intravenous ganciclovir (70) (induction—10 mg/kg/day given every 12 hours; maintenance—5 mg/kg/day) can be given in 1- to 2-hour infusions for CMV pneumonitis. Daily infusions are required for induction and lasts at least 3 weeks. Maintenance therapy can be given as daily infusion administered three to five times per week for an additional 20 doses. Cytomegalovirus hyperimmune globulin (400 mg/kg/dose) or intravenous immunoglobulin (IVIg) (500 mg/kg/dose) should be given on days 1, 2, and 7, and then weekly for two to eight more doses (83). If ganciclovir resistance is proven or suspected, foscarnet can be added or substituted. Foscarnet infusions are given at 180 mg/kg/day divided in three daily doses for 2 to 3 weeks followed by a maintenance dose of 90 mg/kg/day in one daily dose for an additional 3 to 6 weeks (70).

Acyclovir (30–60 mg/kg/day) can be given intravenously in three divided doses infused over a minimum of 1 hour for HSV pneumonitis. Two to 3 weeks of therapy usually suffices. Longer durations may be needed for patients with a poor response or those who are severely immunosuppressed. Foscarnet can be used to treat HSV pneumonitis in patients who have proven or suspected acyclovir-resistant HSV. Two to 3 weeks of intravenous foscarnet at a dosage of 180 mg/kg/day divided in three daily doses should be adequate (70).

If opportunistic fungi are suspected or proven, therapy with an appropriate antifungal agent is required. In general, amphotericin B is used as initial therapy because of its broad antifungal spectrum. A test dose of 0.1 mg/kg (maximum, 1 mg) can be given over a 20- to 60-minute period to assess the child's febrile and hemodynamic response. If no serious adverse effects are noted with the test dose, an additional 0.4 mg/kg can be given on the same day as the test dose. The necessity of giving a test dose has been challenged recently (84). Most patients tolerate the full dose of 0.5 mg/kg on the first day of therapy. Intravenous infusions of amphotericin B are better tolerated in recent years as a result of an improved formulation of amphotericin B (84). The daily dose of amphotericin B can range from 0.1 to 1.0 mg/kg (for *Candida* species) to as high as 1.5 mg/kg for *Aspergillus*. For children with nosocomial pneumonia caused by fungi, it is prudent to increase the daily dose by 0.25 mg/kg/dose up to 1 mg/kg if tolerated. Infusions of amphotericin B can be given routinely over a 2- to 6-hour interval. However, shorter infusions of 1 hour may be acceptable in most patients with greater convenience. For children whose pneumonia is documented to be caused by *Aspergillus* or other environmental fungal pathogens, amphotericin B at higher doses (1.25–1.5 mg/kg) or amphotericin B lipid formulations (3–5 mg/kg/day) should be considered. The amphotericin B lipid formulations allow delivery of higher daily doses of amphotericin B with less nephrotoxicity (85,86). Amphotericin B lipid formulations can be used for the treatment of invasive fungal infections in infants and children who are refractory to or intolerant of amphotericin B. Adding flucytosine or rifampin for treatment of *Aspergillus* infections is controversial. There is little evidence of benefit with these combination therapies. Fluconazole, itraconazole, and ketoconazole may be used for treatment of non–life-threatening infections by susceptible fungi or for maintenance therapy of susceptible fungi after improvement with amphotericin B.

Trimethoprim-sulfamethoxazole (TMP-SMX) (20 mg/kg/day of trimethoprim) is the treatment of choice for *P. carinii* pneumonia (PCP). Oral therapy with TMP-SMX is reserved for children with mild PCP who do not have malabsorption or diarrhea. Intravenous pentamidine (4 mg/kg/day, given once a day) can be given to children with PCP who are intolerant of TMP-SMX or who have not responded after 5 days of TMP-SMX therapy. Other treatment regimens that may be considered for patients who are intolerant of or fail TMP-SMX and pentimidine are (1) atovaquone (40 mg/kg/day, in two divided doses) for mild/moderate PCP only; (2) dapsone with trimethoprim; (3) trimetrexate with leucovorin; and (4) clindamycin and primaquine. These alternate treatments have limited experience in pediatric patients.

VII. PREVENTION

Recently published guidelines from the CDC for the prevention of nosocomial pneumonia apply to pediatric patients as well as adults (56). These guidelines should be used as a framework for infection control practices within all pediatric intensive care settings. However, because of rapidly changing technologies and unique characteristics of certain pediatric populations (e.g., neonates, ECMO), it is appropriate for hospitals caring for critically ill children to periodically review these guidelines as well as their own actual policies and practices. Adaptations of guidelines or creating new infection control practices may be required to address the constantly changing needs of critically ill children. Continuous perusal of the medical literature and networking with colleagues can help with the development of pediatric-specific infection control practices that provide a safe environment in this ever-changing and cost-conscious medical climate.

The prevention of nosocomial pneumonia in pediatric intensive care settings requires attention to and modification of the patient's environment, staff behaviors, and therapies given to the child. The primary effort to reduce nosocomial pneumonia or tracheitis is to reduce exposure and subsequent acquisition of potential pathogens (viral, bacterial, fungal). Meticulous attention to handwashing, preferably with an agent with antimicrobial activity, before and after all patient contacts is extremely valuable for preventing transmission of nosocomial pathogens from patient to patient as well as from health care worker to patient. Even though the importance of this relatively simple and inexpensive infection control practice is commonly recognized, it is rarely practiced at appropriate levels (87,88); Health care workers with the greatest understanding of the impact of nosocomial infections may be the least compliant with handwashing practices. For this reason, routine use of gloves or waterless soaps have been advocated to reduce the incidence of cross contamination (89,90). If gloves are used routinely, they must be changed between patient contacts. Nosocomial pathogens can colonize gloves and can be transferred from patient to patient (91). Waterless soaps may offer an acceptable alternative when handwashing is not possible in busy units with children requiring rapid intervention (92). Alcoholic hand disinfection is rapid and may improve compliance when routine handwashing rates are not 100% (92).

Oral hygiene and mouth care should be performed when appropriate (e.g., in sedated or intubated patients). Every 2 to 4 hours, the mouth and lips should be cleansed with sterile water, saline, or disposable glycerin swabs. Saliva ejectors or adaptors used to suction a child's mouth should be changed every 8 hours and kept in a clean sheath when not in use. Lips should be coated with petroleum or similar material to prevent chapping or cracking.

Intubation associated with mechanical ventilation is the single most important risk factor for the development of nosocomial pneumonia and tracheitis. Intubation should be used only when medically indicated. Extubation should be accomplished as quickly as it is clinically feasible. It may be appropriate for individual pediatric and neonatal intensive care units to develop criteria for intubation and continued mechanical ventilation. Auditing practice versus predetermined criteria might identify opportunities to reduce patient ventilator-days.

For patients on mechanical ventilation, it is important to minimize the introduction of pathogens to the patient's respiratory tract. Medications and other materials administered by way of the endotracheal tube may reach distal airways and should be sterile. Whenever it is feasible, disposable materials should be used. If any equipment is reused, it should be disinfected or sterilized in accordance with manufacturer's instructions. Proper care and cleaning applies not only to the patient's mechanical ventilator but also to all materials that will come into contact with the upper and lower respiratory tract. This includes nebulizers, spirometers, bronchoscopes, and anesthesia equipment, among others. Gentle suctioning using aseptic technique can reduce bacterial aggregates that are present in the glycocalyx biofilm that lines the endotracheal tube. However, vigorous suctioning may dislodge these aggregates, which may embolize to the lower respiratory tract. Suctioning of artificial airways should be done gently and only as often as needed, varying from patient to patient and even at different times in the same patient.

Some simple maneuvers may significantly assist in preventing nosocomial pneumonia in intubated children. The head of the bed should be elevated (30 to 45 degrees), unless medically contraindicated. The patient should be turned frequently. Removal of respiratory secretions may be facilitated by the use of percussion and vibration on the chest well. However, small premature infants (extremely low birth weight infants) may not tolerate these activities well (e.g., decreased oxygen saturation, rib fractures, bruising). If an orogastric or nasogastric tube is present, its placement should be evaluated routinely to prevent aspiration. Enteral feedings should be withheld if the residual volume in the stomach is large or if bowel transit is impaired. Using small flexible, small-bore tubes or placing the enteral tube beyond the stomach (e.g., in the jejunum) might reduce the risk of gastroesophageal reflux and aspiration.

Gram-negative bacillary nosocomial pneumonia is usually caused by endogenous bacteria found in the patient's oropharynx, trachea, or stomach. Efforts to reduce colonization with these bacteria using prophylactic aerosolized antibiotics did not result in any improved clinical outcome and was associated with an increase in antibiotic-resistant organisms and superinfections (93,94). Topical oropharyngeal or gastric-instilled antibiotics have reduced oropharyngeal and gastric colonization with gram-negative bacilli (95,96). The clinical impact of this approach has been varied. The development of resistance has not been a problem (97). Bacterial interference with nonpathogenic bacteria (i.e., alpha-hemolytic streptococci) has been used successfully to reduce oropharyngeal colonization with aerobic gram-negative bacilli (98,99). However, the efficacy of this approach for preventing nosocomial lower respiratory tract infections needs to be established.

Antacids and H_2 blockers increase gastric pH, which enhances gastric bacterial overgrowth (100–102). Sucralfate, a cytoprotective agent, has the ability to protect against gastritis or gastric ulcers with little impact on gastric pH (101–102). Sucralfate may also have antibacterial activity (103). For these reasons, sucralfate may be preferable for prevention of erosive gastritis in intubated children. The benefit of sucralfate appears to be greatest for prevention of late-onset pneumonia (>4 days after intubation).

Patient placement within the intensive care setting is more critical for preventing nosocomial lower respiratory tract infections in children than adults. During winter months, a high proportion of hospitalized children have community-acquired respiratory viral infections. Viral infection may be present even in the absence of overt symptoms. Some institutions routinely screen patients for RSV, influenza, and other respiratory viruses. However, preventive measures should be instituted for all patients suspected of having viral respiratory tract infections regardless of laboratory diagnostic test results. Screening asymptomatic children admitted to the hospital from the community yields a low number of cases and may only be cost effective in certain high-risk closed settings (e.g., NICU, chronic care units). Patients with proven or suspected viral respiratory tract infections should be placed in appropriate isolation: (1) Contact precautions for RSV and parainfluenza and (2) contact and droplet precautions for influenza and adenovirus (Table 6) (104,105). Use of eye-nose goggles rather than masks has protected health care workers from RSV infection (106). However, the use of eye-nose goggles is not widespread because they are inconvenient to wear. Having a private room or isolation room within the intensive care setting is optimal. However, when a private room is not available, cohorting patients with similar infections is an acceptable alternative. It my be equally as important to cohort health care workers taking care of patients infected with respiratory viruses within the intensive care unit. Strict adherence to isolation precautions and handwashing should minimize cross contamination. However, because of poor compliance, it is

Table 6 Transmission-based Precautions for Hospitalized Patients

Category	Pathogen[a]	Single room	Masks	Gowns	Gloves
Airborne	*Mycobacterium tuberculosis* Measles Varicella	Yes, with negative air-pressure ventilation	Yes	No	No
Droplet	*Bordetella pertussis* Influenza[d] Group A Streptococcus[c] Adenovirus[d] Mumps Rubella Parvovirus B19	Yes[b]	Yes, for those close to patient	No	No
Contact	Respiratory syncytial virus Parainfluenza Mauti-resistant bacteria Adenovirus[d] Influenza[d]	Yes[b]	No	Yes	Yes

[a] For proven or suspected infections with these pathogens.
[b] Preferred but not required. Cohorting may be acceptable.
[c] Until 24 hours after initiation of effective therapy.
[d] Some pathogens may require more than one type of precaution.
Source: Refs. 104 and 105.

beneficial to limit contact by health care workers caring for infected children with other noninfected children at high risk for severe disease. This may be difficult in the PICU and NICU where many health care workers (especially physicians and respiratory therapists) care for many diverse patients. However, because a large amount of the most intimate care and contact is provided by nurses, nursing assignments might take into consideration the need to minimize cross contact between infected and uninfected patients. Restricting health care workers who have symptoms of upper respiratory tract symptoms from caring for uninfected children, particularly those at high risk for severe or fatal lower respiratory tract infection, is prudent. Modification of visitor policies during community outbreaks can be important in reducing the introduction of community viruses into the PICU and NICU. During peak viral activity, it may be necessary to limit visitors to intensive care units to a small number of healthy family members. Sibling visitation can be particularly problematic. Most sibling visitation programs rely on symptom screening. During community outbreaks, the frequency of asymptomatic shedding of respiratory viruses can increase dramatically in young children. This might warrant a change in sibling visitation practices or possibly temporarily discontinuing sibling visitation to high-risk patients. Elective surgery on high-risk patients should be postponed until respiratory virus infection is less common in the community and in hospitalized children.

A recent report suggested that isolation of symptomatic patients during respiratory virus season might be discontinued at 48 hours when both rapid test (enzyme immunoassay for RSV antigen) and early culture results (using shell vial technique) are negative (107). This approach is somewhat risky. Most symptomatic children during the respiratory virus season are infected with some potentially contagious virus. Viral detection sensitivity varies considerably by test method employed and by the laboratory performing the test. Maintaining isolation of antigen- or culture-negative symptomatic children is prudent, particularly in closed populations with vulnerable children, such as PICUs and NICUs. The reduction in isolation days was hardly worth the increased risk of nosocomial transmission of respiratory viruses, especially in hospital units with vulnerable patients.

The impact of nosocomial influenza in critically ill patients may be diminished by judicious use of immunoprophylaxis and chemoprophylaxis. Hopefully, targeting high-risk children (older than 6 months of age) and adolescents (Table 7) (82) for annual preseason influenza immunization will afford those at greatest risk some protection against influenza if they are hospitalized during a community outbreak. It is also appropriate that all health care workers in pediatric intensive care settings (PICU and NICU) receive their annual influenza vaccination to avoid infection and transmission of influenza to their patients.

If an outbreak of influenza A occurs in a patient population that includes those at risk for severe influenza disease, chemoprophylaxis with rimantadine or amantadine can be considered for the uninfected. Rimantadine has a better safety profile and is preferred. If either rimantadine or amantadine is used, it should be administered to susceptible patients (and staff) as early in the outbreak as possible. Use of rimantadine or amantadine for treatment in this setting may be problematic. Treatment of children with influenza A with rimantadine or amantadine frequently results in emergence of resistant virus during therapy. Transmission of resistant virus negates the benefit of chemoprophylaxis of susceptible contacts. A decision to use either rimantadine or amantadine for treatment of infected children should take into account the risk status of other exposed children and the likelihood that the infected child will receive benefit from therapy (e.g., benefit is diminished after 48 hours of symptoms).

Nosocomial Legionnaires' disease does occur in children but it is far less common than in hospitalized adults (37). The full explanation for this discrepancy has yet to be elucidated. In addition, a paucity of Legionnaires'

Table 7 Infants, Children, and Adolescents Who Are Candidates for Yearly Immunization with the Inactivated Influenza Vaccine (Children > 6 Months of Age)

1. Targeted high-risk children and adolescents
   Asthma and other chronic pulmonary diseases
   Hemodynamically significant cardiac disease
   Immunosuppressive disorders and therapy
   Infection with human immunodeficiency virus
   Sickle cell anemia and other hemoglobinopathies
   Diseases requiring long-term aspirin therapy (e.g., rheumatoid arthritis or
      Kawasaki disease)
2. Other high-risk children and adolescents (potential candidates who may benefit)
   Diabetes mellitus
   Chronic renal disease
   Chronic metabolic disease
   Pregnancy (beyond 14 weeks)
3. Close contacts of targeted high-risk patients
   Health care workers
   Household contacts
   Other primary caregivers

Source: Ref. 82.

disease cases makes it more difficult for hospitals caring for children to know to what extent *Legionella* prevention efforts should be maintained. The recent CDC guidelines (56) divide efforts into Primary Prevention (for hospitals with no identified cases) and Secondary Prevention (for hospitals with identified cases). Primary Prevention efforts should be adequate for most pediatric facilities. Key components of Primary Prevention of nosocomial legionellosis include (1) maintaining a high index of suspicion (e.g., appropriate diagnostic studies for *Legionella* for all cases of nosocomial pneumonia), (2) routinely maintaining cooling towers, (3) using only sterile water for the filling and terminal rinsing of nebulization devices, and (4) initiating an investigation for a hospital source of *Legionella* species upon identification of one definite or two possible cases of nosocomial Legionnaires' disease. The CDC guidelines do not recommend routine monitoring of water from the hospital's potable water system and from aerosol-producing devices as part of their Primary Prevention strategy. In facilities that know that they have *Legionella* species in their potable water system, it may be desirable to restrict immunocompromised patients from taking showers and to maintain heated water at $>50°C$ or $<20°C$

at the tap, even if a case of nosocomial Legionnaires' disease has not been identified.

For pediatric facilities that have experienced nosocomial legionellosis, a number of additional environmental investigations and decontamination measures may be appropriate. These are described in detail in the published CDC guidelines under Secondary Prevention.

REFERENCES

1. Horan TC, White JW, Jarvis WR, Emori TG, Culver DH, Munn VP, Thornsberry C, Olson DR, Hughes JM. Nosocomial infection surveillance 1984. MMWR CDC Surv Summ 1986; 35:17SS–29SS.
2. National Nosocomial Infections Surveillance (NNIS) System. National Nosocomial Infections Surveillance (NNIS) report, Data Summary from October 1986-April 1996, Issued May 1996. Am J Infect Control 1996; 24:380–388.
3. Milliken J, Tait CA, Mindorff CM, Ford-Jones EL, Gold R, Mullins G. Nosocomial infections in a pediatric intensive care unit. Crit Care Med 1988; 16:233–237.
4. Donowitz LG. High risk of nosocomial infection in the pediatric critical care patient. Crit Care Med 1986; 14:26–28.
5. Klein BS, Perloff WH, Maki DG. Reduction of nosocomial infection during pediatric intensive care by protective isolation. N Engl J Med 1989; 320:1714–1721.
6. Hemming VG, Overall JC, Britt MR. Nosocomial infections in a newborn intensive-care unit: results of forty-one months of surveillance. N Engl J Med 1976; 294:1310–1316.
7. Goldman DA, Freeman J, Durbin WA. Nosocomial infection and death in a neonatal intensive care unit. J Infect Dis 1983; 147:635–641.
8. The HIFI Study Group. High-frequency oscillatory ventilation compared with conventional mechanical ventilation in the treatment of respiratory failure in preterm infants. N Engl J Med 1989; 320:88–93.
9. Gonzalez F, Harris T, Black P, Richardson P. Decreased gas flow through pneumothoraces in neonates receiving high-frequency jet versus conventional ventilation. J Pediatr 1987; 110:464–466.
10. Merenstein GB, Gardner SL. Handbook of Neonatal Intensive Care. St. Louis: CV Mosby, 1989.
11. Bartlett RH, Bazzaniga AB, Huxtable RF, Schippers HC, O'Connor MJ, Jeffries MR. Extracorporeal circulation (ECMO) in neonatal respiratory failure. J Thorac Cardiovasc Surg 1977; 74:826–833.
12. Bartlett RH, Roloff DW, Cornell RG, Andrews AF, Dillon PW, Zwischen-

berger JB. Extracorporeal circulation in neonatal respiratory failure. A prospective randomized trial. Pediatrics 1985; 70:479–487.

13. Klein MD, Whittlesey GC. Extracorporeal membrane oxygenation. Pediatr Clin North Am 1994; 41:365–383.

14. Fuhrman BP. Perfluorocarbon liquid ventilation: the first human trial. J Pediatr 1990; 117(part 1 of 2):73–74.

15. Greenspan JS. Liquid ventilation: Physiology and potential neonatal applications. Proceedings of the 7th Annual Meeting of the National Association of Neonatal Nurses. New York: National Association of Neonatal Nurses, 1991.

16. Fujiwara T, Maeta H, Chida S, Morita T, Watabe Y, Abe T. Artificial surfactant therapy in hyaline membrane disease. Lancet 1980; 1:55–59.

17. Merritt TA, Hallman M, Bloom BT, Berry C, Benirschke K, Sahn D, Key T, Edwards D, Jarvenpaa AL, Pohjavuori M, Kankaapaa K, Kumas M, Paatero H, Rapole J, Jaaskelainen J. Prophylactic treatment of very premature infants with human surfactant. N Engl J Med 1986; 315:785–790.

18. Merritt TA, Hallman M, Berry C, Pohjavuori M, Edwards DK, Jaaskelainen J, Grate MR, Vaucher Y, Wozinak P, Heldt G, Rapola J. Randomized, placebo-controlled trial of human surfactant given at birth versus rescue administration in very low birth weight infants with lung immaturity. J Pediatr 1991; 118: 581–594.

19. Bloom BJ, Kattwinkel J, Hall RT, Delmore PM, Egan EA, Trout JR, Malloy MH, Brown DR, Holzman IR, Coghill CH, Waldemar AC, Pramanik AK, McCaffree MA, Toubas PL, Laudert S, Gratry LL, Weatherstone KB, Segvin JH, Willett LD, Gutcher GR, Mueller DH, Topper WH. Comparison of Infasurf (calf lung surfactant extract) to Survanta (beractant) in the treatment and prevention of respiratory distress syndrome. Pediatrics 1997; 100:31–38.

20. Coffin SE, Bell LM, Manning ML, Polin R. Nosocomial infections in neonates receiving extracorporeal membrane oxygenation. Infect Control Hosp Epidemiol 1997; 18:93–96.

21. Douglass BH, Keenan AL, Purohit DM. Bacterial and fungal infection in neonates undergoing venoarterial extracorporeal membrane oxygenation: an analysis of the registry data of the Extracorporeal Life Support Organization. Artif Organs 1996; 20:202–208.

22. Jones R, Wincott E, Elbourne D, Grant A. Controlled trial of dexamethasone in neonatal chronic lung disease: a 3-year follow-up. Pediatrics 1995; 96:897–906.

23. Durand M, Sardesai S, McEvoy C. Effects of early dexamethasone therapy on pulmonary mechanics and chronic lung disease in very low birth weight infants: a randomized, controlled trial. Pediatrics 1995; 95:584–590.

24. Mammel MC, Fiterman C, Coleman M, Boros SJ. Short-term dexamethasone therapy for bronchopulmonary dysplasia: acute effects and 1-year follow-up. Dev Pharmacol Ther 1987; 10:1–11.

25. Kazzi NJ, Brans YW, Poland RL. Dexamethasone effects on the hospital course of infants with bronchopulmonary dysplasia who are dependent on artificial ventilation. Pediatrics 1990; 86:722–727.

26. Ford-Jones EL, Mindolff CM, Langley JM, Allen U, Navas L, Patrick ML, Milner R, Gold R. Epidemiologic study of 4684 hospital-acquired infections in pediatric patients. Pediatr Infect Dis J 1989; 8:668–675.

27. Garner JS, Jarvis WR, Emori TG, Horan TC, Hughes JM. CDC definitions for nosocomial infections, 1988. Am J Infect Control 1988; 16:128–140.

28. Hughes JM. Epidemiology and prevention of nosocomial pneumonia. In: Remington JS, Schwartz MN, eds. Current Clinical Topics in Infectious Diseases. Vol. 9. New York: McGraw-Hill, 1988:241–259.

29. Centers for Disease Control and Prevention. National Nosocomial Infection Surveillance (NNIS) System. Report to participating hospitals. 1998.

30. McGlone C. NNIS Surveillance Data. Reported annually to the Infection Control Committee of Children's Hospital, Columbus. 1998.

31. Welliver RC, McLaughlin S. Unique epidemiology of nosocomial infection in a children's hospital. Am J Dis Child 1984; 138:131–135.

32. Hall CB, Powell KR, MacDonald NE, Gala CL, Menegus ME. Respiratory syncytial viral infection in infants with compromised immune function. N Engl J Med 1986; 315: 77–81.

33. MacDonald NE, Hall CB, Suffin SC, Alexson C, Harris PJ, Manning JA. Respiratory syncytial viral infection in infants with congenital heart disease. N Engl J Med 1982; 307:397–400.

34. Hall CB. Hospital-acquired pneumonia in children: the role of respiratory viruses. Semin Respir Infect 1987; 2:48–56.

35. Frank AL, Taber LH, Wells CR, Wells JM, Glezen WP, Paredes A. Patterns of shedding of myxoviruses and paramyxoviruses in children. J Infect Dis 1981; 144:433–441.

36. Graman PS, Hall CB. Epidemiology and control of nosocomial viral infections. Infect Dis Clin North Am 1989; 3:815–841.

37. Brady MT. Nosocomial Legionnaires disease in a children's Hospital. J Pediatr 1989; 115:46–50.

38. John M, Tucci M, Lacroix J, Farrell CA, Gauthier M, Lafleur L, Nadeau D. Nosocomial pneumonia and tracheitis in a pediatric intensive care unit. Am J Respir Crit Care Med 1997; 155:162–169.

39. Langer M, Mosconi P, Cigada M, Mandelli M. Long-term respiratory support and risk of pneumonia in critically ill patients. Intensive Care Unit Group of Infection Control. Am Rev Respir Dis 1989; 140:302–305.

40. Johanson WG Jr, Woods DE, Chanduri T. Association of respiratory tract colonization with adherence of gram-negative bacilli to epithelial cells. J Infect Dis 1979; 139:667–673.

41. Niederman MS, Merrill WM, Ferranti RD, Pagano KM, Palmer LB, Reynolds HY. Nutritional status and bacterial binding in the lower respiratory tract

in patients with chronic tracheostomy. Ann Intern Med 1984; 100:795–800.

42. Ramphal R, Small PM, Shands JW Jr, Fischlschwieger W, Small PA Jr. Adherence of *Pseudomonas aeruginosa* to tracheal cells injured by influenza infection or by endotracheal intubation. Infect Immun 1980; 27:614–619.

43. Johanson WG Jr, Pierce AK, Sanford JP, Thomas GD. Nosocomial respiratory infections with gram-negative bacilli: the significance of colonization of the respiratory tract. Ann Intern Med 1972; 77:701–706.

44. Cadnapaphornchai M, Faix RG. Increased nosocomial infection in neutropenic low birth weight (2000 grams or less) infants of hypertensive mothers. J Pediatr 1992; 121:956–961.

45. Huxley EJ, Viroslav J, Gray WR, Pierce AK. Pharyngeal aspiration in normal adults and patients with depressed consciousness. Am J Med 1978; 64:564–568.

46. Goodwin SR, Graves SA, Haberkern CM. Aspiration in intubated premature infants. Pediatrics 1985; 75:85–88.

47. Browning DH, Graves SA. Incidence of aspiration with endotracheal tubes in children. J Pediatr 1983; 102:582–584.

48. Fenelon LE, Keane CT, Bakir M, Temperley IG. A cluster of *Pneumocystis carinii* infections in children. BMJ [Clin Res] 1985; 291:1683–1685.

49. Powell DA, Aungst J, Snedden S, Hansen N, Brady M. Broviac catheter-related *Malassezia furfur* sepsis in five infants receiving intravenous fat emulsions. J Pediatr 1984; 105:987–990.

50. Valenti WM, Menegus MA, Hall CB, Pincus PH, Douglas RG Jr. Nosocomial viral infections: epidemiology and significance. Infect Control 1980; 1:33–37.

51. Drews MB, Ludwig AC, Leititis JU, Daschner FD. Low birth weight and nosocomial infection of neonates in a neonatal intensive care unit. J Hosp Infect 1995; 30:65–72.

52. Waites KB, Crouse DT, Cassell, GH. Antibiotic susceptibilities and therapeutic options for *Ureaplasma urealyticum* infection in neonates. Pediatr Infect Dis J 1992; 11:23–29.

53. Walsh WF, Stanley S, Lally KP, Stribley RG, Treece DP, McCloskey F, Mull DM. *Ureaplasma urealyticum* demonstrated by open lung biopsy in newborns with chronic lung disease. Pediatr Infect Dis J 1991; 10:823–827.

54. Garland SM, Bowman ED. Role of *Ureaplasma urealyticum* and *Chlamydia trachomatis* in lung disease in low birth weight infants. Pathology 1996; 28:266–269.

55. Cassell GH, Waites KB, Crouse DT, Rudd PT, Canupp KC, Stagnos, Cutter GR. Association of *Ureaplasma urealyticum* infection of the lower respiratory tract with chronic lung disease and death in very low birth weight infants. Lancet 1988; 2:240–245.

56. Centers for Disease Control and Prevention. Guidelines for prevention of nosocomial pneumonia. MMWR 1997; 46(No. RR-1).

57. Walsh TJ, Dixon DM. Nosocomial aspergillosis: environmental microbiology, hospital epidemiology, diagnosis and treatment. Eur J Epidemiol 1989; 5:131–142.

58. Wiswell TE, Bent RC. Meconium staining and the meconium aspiration syndrome: unresolved issues. Pediatr Clin North Am 1993; 40:955–981.

59. Wiswell TE, Tuggle JM, Turner BS. Meconium aspiration syndrome: have we made a difference? Pediatrics 1990; 85:715–721.

60. Dye T, Aubry R, Gross S, Artal R. Amniotransfusion and the intrauterine prevention of meconium aspiration. Am J Obstet Gynecol 1994; 171:1601–1605.

61. Berger R, Arango L. Etiologic diagnosis of bacterial nosocomial pneumonia in seriously ill patients. Crit Care Med 1985; 13:833–836.

62. Hill JD, Ratliff JL, Parrott JCW, Lamy M, Fallat RJ, Koeniger E, Yaeger EM, Whitmer G. Pulmonary pathology in acute respiratory insufficiency: lung biopsy as a diagnostic tool. J Thorac Cardiovasc Surg 1976; 71:64–71.

63. Salata RA, Lederman MM, Shales DM, Jacobs MR, Eckstein E, Tweardy D, Toosi Z, Chmielewski R, Marino J, King CH. Diagnosis of nosocomial pneumonia in intubated, intensive care unit patients. Am Rev Respir Dis 1987; 135:426–432.

64. Griffin JJ, Meduri GU. New approaches in the diagnosis of nosocomial pneumonia. Med Clin North Am 1994; 78:1091–1122.

65. Jourdain B, Novara A, Joly-Guillou ML, Dombret MC, Calvat S, Trouillet JL, Gilbert C, Chastre J. Role of quantitative cultures of endotracheal aspirates in the diagnosis of nosocomial pneumonia. Am J Respir Crit Care Med 1995; 152:241–246.

66. Wimberly N, Faling LJ, Bartlett JG. A fiberoptic bronchoscopy technique to obtain uncontaminated lower airway secretions for bacterial culture. Am Rev Respir Dis 1979; 119:336–346.

67. Scheld WM, Mandell GL. Nosocomial pneumonia: pathogenesis and recent advances in diagnosis and therapy. J Infect Dis 1991; 13(suppl 9):S743–S751.

68. Barzilay Z, Mandel M, Keren G, Davidson S. Nosocomial bacterial pneumonia in ventilated children: clinical significance of culture-positive peripheral bronchial aspirates. J Pediatr 1988; 112:421–424.

69. He Q, Mertsola J, Soini H, Viljanen MK. Sensitive and specific polymerase chain reaction assays for detection of *Bordetella pertussis* in nasopharyngeal specimens. J Pediatr 1994; 124:421–426.

70. Nelson JD. Pocket Book of Pediatric Antimicrobial Therapy. 12th ed. Baltimore: Williams & Wilkins, 1966.

71. Pennington JE. Penetration of antibiotics into respiratory secretions. Rev Infect Dis 1981; 3:67–73.

72. Fiel SB. Aerosol delivery of antibiotics to the lower airways of patients with cystic fibrosis. Chest 1995; 107:615–645.

73. Smith AL, Ramsey B. Aerosol administration of antibiotics. Pediatr Pulmonol Suppl 1995; 11:68–69.

74. Steinkamp G, Tummler B, Gappa M, Albus A, Potel J, Doring G, Von der

Hardt H. Long-term tobramycin aerosol therapy in cystic fibrosis. Pediatr Pulmonol 1989; 6:91–98.

75. Pascal S, Diot P, Lemaire E. Antibiotics in aerosols. Rev Mal Respir 1992; 9: 145–153.

76. Hung JCC, Hambelton G, Super M. Evaluation of two commercial jet nebulizers and three compressors for the nebulization of antibiotics. Arch Dis Child 1994; 71:335–338.

77. American Academy of Pediatrics. In: Peter G, ed. 1997 Red Book: Report of the Committee on Infectious Diseases. 24th ed. Elk Grove Village, IL: American Academy of Pediatrics, 1997:443–447.

78. Law BJ, Wang EEL, MacDonald N, McDonald J, Dobson S, Boucher F, Langley J, Robinson J, Mitchell I, Stephens D. Does ribavirin impact on the hospital course of children with respiratory syncytial virus (RSV) infection? An analysis using the Pediatric Investigators Collaborative Network or Infections in Canada (PICNIC) RSV database. Pediatrics 1997; 99:E7.

79. Ohmit SE, Moler FW, Monto AS, Khan AS. Ribavirin utilization and clinical effectiveness in children hospitalized with respiratory syncytial virus infection. J Clin Epidemiol 1996; 49:963–967.

80. Englund JA, Piedra PA, Ahn YM, Gilbert BE, Hiatt P. High-dose, short duration ribavirin aerosol therapy compared with standard ribavirin therapy in children with suspected respiratory virus infection. J Pediatr 1994; 125:635–641.

81. McIntosh K, Kurachek SG, Cairns LM, Burns JC, Goodspeed B. Treatment of respiratory viral infection in an immunodeficient infant with ribavirin aerosol. Am J Dis Child 1984; 138:305–308.

82. American Academy of Pediatrics. In: Peter G, ed. 1997 Red Book: Report of the Committee on Infectious Diseases. 24th ed. Elk Grove Village, IL: American Academy of Pediatrics, 1997:307–315.

83. Syndman DR. Cytomegalovirus immunoglobulins in the prevention and treatment of cytomegalovirus disease. Rev Infect Dis 1990; 12(suppl 7):5839–5848.

84. American Academy of Pediatrics. In: Peter G, Ed. 1997 Red Book: Report of the Committee on Infectious Diseases. 24th ed. Elk Grove Village, IL: American Academy of Pediatrics, 1997:630–631.

85. Janknegi R, Marie de S, Bakker-Woldenberg J, Crommelin JA. Liposomal and lipid formulations of amphotericin B: clinical pharmacokinetics. Clin Pharmacokinet 1992; 23:279–291.

86. Rapp RP, Gubbins PO, Evans ME. Amphotericin B lipid complex. Ann Phamacother 1997; 31:1174–1186.

87. Grahm M. Frequency and duration of handwashing in an intensive care unit. Am J Infect Control 1990; 18:77–81.

88. Albert RK, Condie F. Handwashing patterns in medical intensive-care units. N Engl J Med 1981; 304:1465–1466.

89. Garner JS, Simmons BP. Guideline for handwashing and environmental control. Infect Control 1986; 7:231–242.

90. Garner JS, HICPAC. Draft guideline for isolation precautions in hospitals. Fed Reg 1994; 59(part V):55552–55570.
91. Doebbeling BN, Pfaller MA, Houston AK, Wenzel RP. Removal of nosocomial pathogens from the contaminated glove. Ann Intern Med 1988; 109:394–398.
92. Voss A, Widmer AF. No time for handwashing!? Handwashing versus alcoholic rub: can we afford 100% compliance? Infect Control Hosp Epidemiol 1997; 18:205–208.
93. Feely TW, Du Moulin GC, Hedley-Whyte J. Aerosol polymyxin and pneumonia in seriously ill patients. N Engl J Med 1975; 293:471–475.
94. Klastersky J, Huysmans E, Weerts D, Hensgens C, Daneau D. Endotracheally administered gentamicin for the prevention of infections of the respiratory tract in patients with tracheostomy: a double-blind study. Chest 1974; 6:650–654.
95. Johanson WG Jr, Seidenfeld JJ, de los Santos R, Coalson JJ, Gomez P. Prevention of nosocomial pneumonia using topical and parenteral antimicrobial agents. Am Rev Respir Dis 1988; 137:265–272.
96. Van Uffelen R, Rommes JH, van Saene HK. Preventing lower airway colonization and infection in mechanically ventilated patients. Crit Care Med 1987; 15: 99–102.
97. Stoutenbeek CP, van Saene HK, Zandstra DF. The effect of oral non-absorbable antibiotics on the emergence of resistant bacteria in patients in an intensive care unit. J Antimicrob Chemother 1987; 19:513–520.
98. Sprunt K, Redman W. Evidence suggesting importance of role of enterobacterial inhibition in maintaining balance of normal flora. Ann Intern Med 1968; 68:579–590.
99. Sprunt K, Leidy G, Redman W. Abnormal colonization of neonates in an ICU: conversion to normal colonization by pharyngeal implantation of alpha hemolytic streptococcus strain 215. Pediatr Res 1980; 14:308–313.
100. Craven DE, Kunches LM, Killinsky V, Lichtenberg DA, Make BJ, McCabe WR. Risk factors for pneumonia and fatality in patients receiving continuous mechanical ventilation. Am Rev Respir Dis 1986; 133:792–793.
101. Kappstein I, Friedric T, Hellinger P. Incidence of pneumonia in mechanically-ventilated patients treated with sucralfate or cimetidine as prophylaxis for stress bleeding: bacterial colonization of the stomach. Am J Med 1991; 91:125–131.
102. Prodhom G, Leunberger PH, Koerfer J, Blum A, Chiolero R, Schaller MD, Perret C, Spinnler O, Blondel J, Siegrist H. Nosocomial pneumonia in mechanically ventilated patients receiving antacid, ranitidine or sucralfate as prophylaxis for stress ulcer. Ann Intern Med 1994; 120:653–662.
103. Tryba M, Mantey-Stiers F. Antibacterial activity of sucralfate in human gastric juice. Am J Med 1987; 83:125–127.
104. Garner JS. Hospital Infection Control Practices Advisory Committee. Guidelines for isolation precautions in hospitals. Infect Control Hosp Epidemiol 1996; 17:53–80.
105. American Academy of Pediatrics. In: Peter G, ed. 1997 Red Book: Report of the

Committee on Infectious Diseases. 24th ed. Elk Grove Village, IL: American Academy of Pediatrics, 1997:100–107.

106. Gala CL, Hall CB, Schnabel KC, Pincus PH, Blossom P, Hildreth SW, Betts RF, Douglas RG Jr. The use of eye-nose goggles to control nosocomial respiratory syncytial virus infection. JAMA 1986; 256:2706–2708.

107. Beekmann SE, Engler HD, Collins AS, Canosa J, Henderson DK, Friefeld A. Rapid identification of respiratory viruses: impact on isolation practices and transmission among immunocompromised pediatric patients. Infect Control Hosp Epidemiol 1996; 17:581–586.

9

The Operating Room

ARNOLD J. BERRY

Emory University School of Medicine
Atlanta, Georgia

I. INTRODUCTION

During the perioperative period, patients undergo many interventions and have significant physiological alterations that may be associated with an increased risk of nosocomial pneumonia. The complex interplay of the physiological stresses resulting from anesthesia and surgery along with concomitant medical conditions present significant opportunities for pulmonary infection. The current rate of postoperative nosocomial pneumonia has undoubtedly been affected by the multiple changes that have occurred in health care recently. Many surgical procedures are performed on an outpatient basis, and, for patients who will remain in the hospital postoperatively, presurgical workups are routinely conducted outside the hospital with admission occurring only a short time before surgery. When patients must be admitted to the hospital after major surgical procedures or for coexisting complex medical conditions, the length of hospital stay associated with most surgeries has decreased as a result of changes in the economics of health care. Countering these trends is an increase in the number of immunosuppressed patients undergoing solid organ transplantation or major, aggressive operations for cancer. These alterations of both the surgical patient population and the duration of hospitalization associated with surgery make it difficult to compare data obtained in current studies from those conducted in the era with long preoperative and postoperative hospital stays.

For thoracic and upper abdominal surgical procedures, general anesthesia with intubation of the trachea is usually required. Postoperative mechanical ventilation may be necessary when surgery is prolonged, after procedures with massive blood loss or large fluid shifts, or for patients who are debilitated or have significant cardiac or pulmonary impairment. Therefore, in many circumstances, the operative setting merges into that of the intensive care unit because this subset of postoperative patients requires prolonged endotracheal intubation and mechanical ventilation, placing them at risk for ventilator-associated pneumonia (1,2). Although some of the risk factors and causes of postoperative nosocomial pneumonia are similar to those of ventilator-associated pneumonia, the latter is specifically considered in other chapters.

II. INCIDENCE OF POSTOPERATIVE PNEUMONIA

There is a great deal of data on the incidence of nosocomial pneumonia from the National Nosocomial Infection Surveillance System (NNIS) and other investigations, but rates of postoperative pneumonia in nonmechanically ventilated postoperative patients is more limited. Jarvis et. al. pointed out that mechanical ventilation was a risk factor for pneumonia using NNIS data collected from 1986 to 1990. They demonstrated a range of ventilator-associated pneumonia rates from 4.7 cases in pediatric intensive care units (ICUs) to 34.4 in burn ICUs per 1000 ventilator-days compared to the range of medians for nonventilator-associated pneumonia rates of 0 (pediatric and respiratory ICUs) to 3.2 (trauma ICUs) pneumonias per 1000 ICU-days (3). Therefore, the proportion of patients requiring mechanical ventilation and the ventilator-days must be stated when reporting postoperative nosocomial pneumonia rates to permit comparisons between patient populations. The published NNIS data do not include surgery as a confounder so that rates of postoperative pneumonia cannot be ascertained from this national surveillance system (4).

The Study on the Efficacy of Nosocomial Infection Control (SENIC Project) published in 1981 demonstrated an association between surgery and nosocomial pneumonia (5). In this survey, pneumonias constituted 14% of all nosocomial infections detected among surgical patients, but 74% of all pneumonias occurred in surgical patients (40% of the total study population) (5).

When comparing data from multiple studies, the specific surgical population and the criteria used to diagnose pneumonia have a great effect on the reported incidence of postoperative pneumonia (Table 1). Data collected from 1972 through 1975 at a university hospital demonstrated an overall rate of nosocomial pneumonia of 0.4 per 100 general anesthetics, but the rate was greater (2.1 per 100 patients) on the thoracic and cardiovascular surgery service and for those requiring mechanical ventilation (3.4 per 100 patients) (6). In one series of 520 patients undergoing either elective thoracic or upper or lower abdominal surgeries, postoperative pneumonia developed in 17.5% (7). When microbiological confirmation of pneumonia was required in a population of patients having a mix of surgical procedures, the incidence of postoperative pneumonia was 1.3% (8). The incidence of postoperative pneumonia ranges from 0% to 63% depending on the specific surgical population (see Table 1).

III. MORTALITY RATE

Several investigators have demonstrated that postoperative pneumonia is associated with an increased mortality rate. In one surgical series, pneumonia developed in 1.3% of all patients (136 patients) after surgery, but postoperative pneumonia was diagnosed in 10% of the patients who died (8). The role of pneumonia in the causality of death was unclear from the study. Factors associated with death included gram-negative pneumonitis, emergent surgical procedures, ventilator-associated pneumonia, postoperative peritonitis, and multiple organ failure (8). In a prospective study of 140 surgical patients, postoperative pneumonia occurred in 18.6% with a mortality rate of 19.2% compared to 1.7% among those without pneumonia (9). Significant morbidity including prolonged stay in the intensive care unit (6.2 versus 2.6 days), increased duration of intubation (2.7 versus 0.6 days), and overall increased duration of postoperative hospital stay (15.3 versus 8.4 days) was also associated with pneumonia (9).

IV. RISK FACTORS AND PATHOGENESIS

Conditions required for postoperative pneumonia include a source of bacteria in the oropharynx, a mechanism to allow bacteria to enter the lower airway, and altered pulmonary host defenses to permit infection. Factors associated with postoperative pneumonia are listed in Tables 1 and 2. Risk for pneumonia is associated with preoperative, intraoperative, and postoperative factors: tho-

Table 1 Incidence of Postoperative Pneumonia

Author	Incidence of pneumonia % (proportion)	Surgical site or type of surgery	Risk factors
Garabaldi[7]	17.5 (91/520)	T, UA, LA	ASA physical status ≥ 2 Smoking Longer preoperative stay Longer operative procedure T or UA
Martin[8]	1.3 (136/10,154)	All	
Ephgrave[9]	18.6 (26/140)	All (all had postoperative nasogastric tube)	COPD
Dauch[11]	20.8 (60/289)	NS	Age Tumor type Cardiac failure Preoperative mental status Preoperative corticosteroids
Mermel[97] (pneumonia within 1 month of transplant)	13 50 57 63	Renal transplant Heart transplant Liver transplant Heart-lung transplant	
Zickmann[13]	10.8 (23/213)	Cardiac	Male COPD Lower respiratory tract colonization
Ejlertsen[98]	8.5 (11/130)	UA	
Argov[15]	15 (23/150) vs 1.5 (2/150)	UA	NG tube
Carrel[12]	30.7 (8/26) vs 1.4 (1/72)	Cardiac	Positive tracheal culture at time of surgery Other: smoking, COPD
Windsor[16]	50 (8/16) vs 15 (3/20)	UA	Protein depletion with atelectasis
Lehot[14]	15 (6/40) vs 0 (0/20)	Cardiac	Preoperative use of gastric acid (H_2) inhibitors

Abbreviations: ASA, American Society of Anesthesiologists; COPD, chronic obstructive pulmonary disease; LA, lower abdominal surgery; NS, neurosurgery; NG, nasogastric; T, thoracic surgery; UA, upper abdominal surgery.

Table 2   Factors Associated with Nosocomial Postoperative Pneumonia

Factors	Possible methods to reduce pneumonia
Fixed factors:	
Age >65 years	Incentive spirometry and deep breathing exercises, early ambulation after surgery, effective pain control, avoid supine position
Sex, male	Incentive spirometry and deep breathing exercises, early ambulation after surgery, effective pain control, avoid supine position
American Society of Anesthesiologists physical status classification ≥ 2	Incentive spirometry and deep breathing exercises, early ambulation after surgery, effective pain control, avoid supine position
Emergency surgery	Delay surgery if possible, preoperative use of nonparticulate antacid to reduce gastric acidity
Anatomical site of surgery (thoracic, upper abdominal)	Postoperative epidural for pain control, ambulate as soon as possible
Immunosuppressive therapy	Decrease duration of immunosuppression if clinically feasible
Chronic obstuctive pulmonary disease	Use of bronchodilators, good pulmonary toilet, incentive spirometry, preoperative antibiotics to clear infectious bronchitis
Neuromuscular disease	Protect airway when indicated
Factors that might be modified:	
Length of preoperative stay	Minimize duration of hospitalization prior to surgery, outpatient workup
Length of hospitalization	Minimize hospitalization after surgery
Duration of surgery	Minimize duration of surgery
Tracheal intubation	Use an endotracheal tube with a subglottic suction port when prolonged intubation is anticipated, use oral route for endotracheal tube placement, optimize pressure in endotracheal tube cuff, remove endotracheal tube as soon as no longer necessary
Mechanical ventilation	Optimize selection of anesthetic agents and postoperative pain control to reduce duration of intubation and ventilation, optimize pressure in endotracheal tube cuff

Table 2 Continued

Factors	Possible methods to reduce pneumonia
Intensive care unit stay	Minimize stay in intensive care unit after surgery
Depressed level of consciousness	Protect airway in patients with depressed level of consciousness, minimize use of sedating narcotics, use nonsedating analgesic drugs or pain control techniques
Aspiration	Minimize use of sedating narcotics, ensure full reversal of neuromuscular blocking agents, appropriate positioning of at risk patients, use an endotracheal tube with a subglottic suction port when prolonged intubation is anticipated
Smoking	Smoking cessation for at least 5 weeks preoperatively
Poor nutrition	Supplement nutrition with enteral or intravenous alimentation before and after surgery
Pre- or postoperative use of gastric acid (H_2) blockers	Administer preoperative H_2 blockers only when indicated or use nonparticulate neutralizing agents preoperatively and use nonalkalinizing gastric protecting agents for postoperative ulcer prophylaxis
Pharyngeal colonization with gram negative bacteria	Avoid use of agents that block gastric acid production, possible role for pharyngeal and gut sterilization protocols
Premature extubation	Secure endotracheal tube to avoid inadvertent extubation, assess adequacy of pulmonary mechanics and gas exchange before planned extubation
Nasogastric tube	Avoid use of nasogastric tube or remove as soon as indicated, semirecumbent position
Contaminated anesthesia breathing circuit	Appropriate disinfection of nondisposable items or single patient use devices
Contaminated humidifiers on anesthesia breathing circuit	Use single patient heat–moisture exchanger, adequate disinfection of heated humidifier between patients

Source: Refs. 5, 6, 86, 99.

racic or upper abdominal surgery (7), longer operative procedures (7), advanced age (8,10,11), depressed mental status (11), longer preoperative or postoperative stay (7,10), chronic obstructive pulmonary disease (COPD), lower respiratory tract (12,13) or gastric (9,14) bacterial colonization at the time of surgery, use of a nasogastric tube (15), protein depletion (7,16), smoking history (7,12), American Society of Anesthesiologists physical status classification greater than 2 (7), use of large doses of corticosteroids (11,17), preoperative use of gastric acid inhibitors (H_2-receptor antagonist) (14), contaminated anesthesia equipment (18,19,20) or mechanical ventilator (21), and requirement for postoperative intubation and mechanical ventilation (22,23).

The mechanisms responsible for postoperative pneumonia are similar to the etiologies of other types of nosocomial pneumonia. The most frequent mechanism for bacteria to enter the lower respiratory tract is via aspiration of contaminated oropharyngeal or gastric fluids. Less commonly, organisms can be transmitted via contaminated anesthesia or respiratory therapy equipment or may spread hematogenously from a distant site of infection. As described later, both general anesthesia and postoperative alterations in pulmonary mechanics may increase the likelihood of infection after bacterial contamination of the lower respiratory tract.

Regurgitation and aspiration of small volumes of gastric contents is not infrequent during surgery under general or regional anesthesia (24). In one study using dye as a marker of gastric contents, 8% of patients regurgitated dye; of these, 9% had evidence of pulmonary aspiration of the material. Regurgitation was more frequent during upper abdominal operations and among patients with nasogastric tubes. This subclinical or ''silent'' regurgitation and aspiration during anesthesia and surgery is in contrast to aspiration pneumonitis produced after pulmonary soilage by a large volume of unneutralized gastric contents of pH less than 2.5 (25). Pulmonary injury in this situation (Mendelson's syndrome) results from a chemical pneumonitis from the effect of gastric acid on the lung tissue. Bacterial infection can occur in addition to the acid-induced injury when bacteria from the pharynx or proximal small bowel enter the lower respiratory tract with the gastric material. In one retrospective study of 172,334 adult patients undergoing 215,488 general anesthetics at one institution, the overall rate of clinically apparent pulmonary aspiration was 1 in 3216 anesthetics (26). Emergency surgery was associated with a significantly higher rate of aspiration than elective procedures (1:895 versus 1:3,886) (26). Patients particularly at risk for aspiration pneumonitis during the perioperative period include pregnant women, primarily during the second and third trimesters; individuals with gastric outlet or small bowel obstruction, ileus, or achalasia; and those undergoing emergency surgery after recent ingestion of food or liquids. These high-risk patients who require general anesthesia are usually treated with the rapid induction of anesthesia using an intravenously administered anesthetic agent and a rapidly acting neuromuscular blocking agent followed immediately by placement of an orotracheal tube to secure the airway. During this induction sequence, firm manual pressure is placed on the cricoid cartilage to occlude the esophagus in an attempt to prevent regurgitation of gastric contents (27). Other modalities to reduce the risk of aspiration of gastric contents include inhibition of gastric acid secretion (28), use of orally administered, nonparticulate neutralizing agents such as sodium citrate, or reduction of gastric volume with metoclopramide (29) or by suctioning via a nasogastric tube.

Hospitalized or chronically ill patients frequently have altered resident oropharyngeal flora and/or colonization of the normally sterile upper gastrointestinal tract (30), which may subsequently lead to lower respiratory tract infection when aspiration occurs. Johanson was among the first to demonstrate that the composition of oropharyngeal flora changes in hospitalized patients with an increased prevalence of gram-negative bacilli (30). Multiple factors have been found to promote this change in colonization of the pharynx (31,32), and the mechanisms whereby the bacterial flora of the oropharynx are altered in hospitalized patients has been reviewed (1).

Although samples of gastric fluid are usually sterile when the contents are at a low pH, bacteria may proliferate when the acid environment is altered. Administration of an H_2-receptor antagonist, ranitidine, on the evening before cardiac surgery and on the morning of surgery, 1 hour before induction of anesthesia, resulted in an increase in intragastric pH when measured intraoperatively and a concomitant increased rate of bacteria being recovered from gastric juice (75% versus 8%) (14). H_2-receptor antagonists are commonly administered preoperatively to patients who are suspected of having a greater risk of low gastric pH in an attempt to prevent aspiration pneumonitis. This practice may have an overall detrimental effect because it appears to increase the incidence of postoperative pneumonia while the risk of aspiration pneumonitis in the overall surgical population, especially for nonemergent procedures, appears to be quite low (23,26). Additional studies on the routine preoperative use of H_2-receptor antagonists in elective surgical patients appear warranted to determine whether there are adequate benefits for prevention of aspiration pneumonitis compared to the risk of nosocomial pneumonia.

A tracheal aspirate positive for bacteria at the time of surgery is associated with an increased risk of postoperative pneumonia (12,13). In a prospective study of 100 patients undergoing cardiac surgery, a culture was obtained by endotracheal tube immediately after induction of anesthesia and tracheal intubation (12). Lower respiratory tract infection later developed in 8 of 26 patients (30.7%) with a positive culture at the beginning of surgery compared to 1.4% of those with a negative culture (sensitivity of 30.8% and specificity of 98.6% for early postoperative pneumonia). Neither of these reports controlled for other risk factors such as prolonged hospitalization before surgery, a factor likely to change oropharyngeal bacterial flora, or the requirement for intubation and mechanical ventilation in the postoperative period.

Prolonged placement of an endotracheal tube having a low-volume, high-pressure cuff is associated with a high risk of damage to the tracheal mucosa and subsequent tracheal stenosis; therefore, the cuffs have been redesigned to reduce ischemia of the underlying tracheal mucosa (34). The large-volume, low-pressure cuffs currently used on endotracheal and tracheostomy tubes produce less ischemia of tracheal mucosa but do not completely prevent aspiration of fluids that accumulate in the oropharynx above the cuff (35). Studies in patients undergoing prolonged intubation and mechanical ventilation have demonstrated that the risk of nosocomial pneumonia can be decreased by about 50% with aspiration of subglottic secretions by way of an endotracheal tube constructed with an additional lumen having the distal aperture above the cuff (36–38). This suggests that leakage of contaminated secretions around low-pressure endotracheal tube cuffs is responsible for some cases of postoperative pneumonia. For patients likely to have oropharyngeal or gastric bacterial colonization or for those likely to require postoperative mechanical ventilation, endotracheal tubes with subglottic aspiration channels should be used to permit intraoperative and postoperative secretion removal. Endotracheal tubes with this additional channel are not widely available in the United States, however. Because an endotracheal tube with the suction channel is likely to be more expensive than a standard tube and would not be necessary for all patients, further research should be directed toward defining when it would be most beneficial. In the interim, attention to appropriate intracuff pressure may be adequate to prevent contamination of the lower respiratory tract with subglottic fluid in some patients (39). Leakage is more likely around thicker walled, large-diameter cuffs, which permit channeling of liquids through cuff folds, especially when intracuff pressure is low. Controlling the intracuff pressure between 25 and 34 cm H_2O in high-compliance, thin-wall cuffs appears to prevent significant aspiration (39). Therefore, careful attention to intracuff pressure appears to be warranted.

Clinicians prefer orotracheal intubation in most patients, but some situations such as facial or oral trauma require that the tube be inserted through the nasopharynx. Although long-term nasotracheal intubation is associated with fewer mechanical problems (biting on tube, self-extubation) compared with the orotracheal route (40), nasotracheal intubation may produce local edema, which impairs maxillary sinus drainage. When nasotracheal intubation persists for more than 4 days, there is an increased rate of sinusitis (41). A prospective, randomized study has demonstrated that the incidence of pulmonary infection with prolonged oral intubation was half of that in nasally intubated patients, although this result did not reach statistical significance (42). It was presumed that sinusitis was the origin of bacteria that entered the lower respiratory tract. The risk of postoperative pneumonia associated with short-term nasotracheal intubation used only for the duration of a surgical procedure has not been determined.

When postoperative intubation is required to protect the airway or to facilitate mechanical ventilation, the endotracheal tube can inadvertently be removed prematurely or must be changed because of a cuff leak or other mechanical complication. A case-contol study demonstrated that the need for reintubation was associated with an increased likelihood of pneumonia (OR: 5.9; 95% CI: 1.3–22.7) (43). Patients who were kept in a semirecumbent position (45 degrees) during the unintubated period were at greater risk for development of pneumonia than those who were supine (73% versus 16%). Factors present after the initial extubation that may contribute to aspiration include the competency of glottic function, level of consciousness, and body position. The need for reintubation may not be a primary risk factor but may represent a marker of patients with more complex medical problems. These data would suggest that, after inadvertent extubation or with patients who fail to have adequate ventilation after planned extubation, efforts should be made to keep the patient supine and to ensure that the pharynx is clear of secretions. After it is decided that reintubation is required, it should be accomplished without delay to prevent aspiration and to reduce the possibility of subsequent pneumonia.

Other sources of pathogenic organisms that may be responsible for postoperative pneumonia are contaminated anesthesia machines (18), respiratory therapy equipment, or monitoring devices (19,20,23). The anesthesia machine mixes oxygen with volatile and gaseous anesthetic agents for delivery to the lungs for absorption. The anesthesia machine has a high-pressure source of oxygen, nitrous oxide, and air (either bulk supplies or compressed gas cylinders) with reducing valves to decrease the driving pressure of the gases before they enter calibrated flow meters and pass into the patient breathing circuit. The most commonly used anesthetic breathing circuit for adults and older children is a circle system, which contains the following components: two one-way valves, inspiratory and expiratory tubing, oxygen and carbon dioxide monitors, reservoir bag, carbon dioxide absorber, mechanical ventilator and circuit, pressure release valve, and Y-connector to join the circuit to the face mask or endotracheal tube. Although bacteriological studies have demonstrated that all portions of the anesthesia breathing circuit may become contaminated during patient use (44,45), with implementation of proper infection control techniques, including single-use items or disinfection between patients (46–48), the anesthesia breathing circuit is not a source for transmission of organisms to the airway (49). Self-inflating resuscitation bags are used to ventilate intubated patients during transport to the operating room or when positive pressure ventilation is required in locations without an anesthesia machine or mechanical ventilator. There are many reports in which improperly disinfected resuscitation bags have served as a source of organisms for contamination of patients' respiratory tract (50,51). Devices used on the respiratory tract are considered "semicritial items" and should be sterilized or undergo high-level disinfection before reuse (46,52). These include inspiratory and expiratory tubing, Y-piece, and reservoir bag on the breathing circuit, face mask, endotracheal tube, humidifier, laryngoscope blades, bronchoscopes, monitoring devices (e.g., spirometers, oxygen analyzer), oral and nasal airways, resuscitation bags, stylets, suction catheters, and temperature sensors. Contamination of the internal components of the anesthesia machine and the valves and carbon dioxide absorber canister of the breathing circuit has not been associated with pulmonary infection. Therefore, these portions of the anesthesia machine and breathing circuit do not require disinfection after each use. Use of either sterile anesthesia breathing circuits (53) or placement of bacterial filters on the inspiratory and expiratory limbs of the breathing circuit (54) were not associated with a decrease in the rate of postoperative pneumonia in prospective, randomized studies.

Because dry anesthesia gases are frequently delivered by way of an endotracheal tube, which bypasses the humidifying portions of the airway, heated water-filled humidifiers were commonly used on the inspiratory portion of the anesthesia breathing circuit during long surgical procedures to provide moisture to the lower respiratory tract and to prevent heat loss. These devices frequently became contaminated by organisms carried from the patient's airway in condensate and which drained back into the humidifier (21). Because of their convenience, single-use heat and moisture exchangers (55) have largely replaced heated water-filled humidifying devices in anesthesia breathing circuits.

Prophylactic antibiotics are administered intravenously to most patients immediately before surgery to reduce the rate of surgical site infection (56–58). This therapy has been shown to be effective with many types of surgery, but its effect on the rate of postoperative nosocomial pneumonia is unknown.

V. EFFECTS OF ANESTHESIA AND SURGERY ON PULMONARY MECHANICS

The alteration in respiratory function resulting from anesthesia and surgery can be divided into early and late effects, with early changes being related to the effects of anesthetic agents and neuromuscular blockers, endotracheal intubation, and mechanical ventilation, and the late changes being affected by the site of operation, physical status of the patient, and postoperative pain. Compared with lower abdominal procedures, thoracic surgery is associated with an eight-fold greater rate of postoperative pneumonia and an upper abdominal operation is associated with a three times greater rate (7).

It has been known for many years that arterial oxygen tension is decreased after surgery, especially in patients undergoing thoracic and upper abdominal procedures (59). When nonabdominal operations lasting more than 30 minutes are performed under general anesthesia, there is a decrease in arterial oxygen tension that is greatest immediately after anesthesia and progressively returns toward normal by the end of the first postoperative day. For abdominal operations under general anesthesia, the reduction in arterial oxygen tension persists for several days before returning to normal. In contrast, when abdominal surgery is performed with regional anesthesia (spinal or epidural), the arterial oxygen tension remains normal for several hours after completion of the procedure but then decreases to levels comparable to those after general anesthesia and subsequently follows a similar pattern (60).

The effect of the type of anesthesia on postoperative pulmonary function has been extensively investigated. During general anesthesia there is a significant reduction of functional residual capacity regardless of whether spontaneous or controlled ventilation is used (61). Other pulmonary changes associated with general anesthesia include an increase in dead space ventilation, airway closure, and alveolar collapse. Atelectasis in dependent areas of the lung is a major cause of impaired gas exchange and shunting during general anesthesia (62). Alveolar collapse can be attributed to multiple factors, one of which is absorption atelectasis that results from replacement of alveolar nitrogen with oxygen and anesthetic gases (63,64). During surgery, atelectatic lung segments can be reexpanded with manual hyperinflation to an airway pressure of 40 cm H_2O (64). Although manual hyperinflation using an inspired oxygen concentration of 0.4 eliminates atelectasis for at least 40 minutes, atelectasis recurs within 5 minutes when an inspired oxygen fraction of 1.0 is administered. After 45 minutes, the amount of atelectasis does not differ, suggesting that manual hyperinflation results in only temporary recruitment of atelectatic alveoli during general anesthesia.

Computerized tomography (CT) has demonstrated that, in supine patients breathing spontaneously or mechanically ventilated during general anesthesia, crest-shaped densities (approximately 3% of lung volume) develop in the caudal (basal) segments of the lung within 5 to 10 minutes (65). The densities persisted for more than an hour postoperatively in most patients and were present in half on examination at 24 hours after anesthesia. Additional studies confirmed that these densities were areas of atelectasis (66). General anesthesia produces changes in diaphragmatic position and movement patterns during respiration that are associated with the formation of basilar atelectasis. In anesthetized, supine adults, there is a cephalad shift of the diaphragm in the end-expiratory position, which is greatest in dependent areas (67). During spontaneous ventilation, diaphragmatic movement is greatest in the dependent portion. With use of neuromuscular blocking agents during general anesthesia, there is also a cephalad shift, but with positive pressure ventilation, the majority of diaphragmatic displacement occurs in nondependent areas.

More recent work has challenged the proposal that the change in diaphragmatic position during general anesthesia is responsible for producing atelectasis. Three-dimensional fast CT was used to determine lung volumes in awake and anesthetized supine volunteers (68). There was no correlation between the degree of cephalad displacement of the diaphragm and the amount of atelectasis. The investigators concluded that changes in the position of the diaphragm or chest wall structures were not responsible for atelectasis under anesthesia and they attributed it to interaction of unidentified factors.

Use of cardiopulmonary bypass is associated with a greater amount of atelectasis than either anesthesia or sternotomy alone (69). The etiology of the atelectasis after cardiopulmonary bypass has not been elucidated but may be related to the period during bypass when the lungs are not ventilated. The increase in atelectasis after cardiopulmonary bypass may contribute to postoperative pneumonia in patients undergoing cardiac surgical procedures.

Other causes of atelectasis and pulmonary complications during general anesthesia and surgery include endobronchial intubation, which may result from an improperly placed endotracheal tube, or plugging of airways from secretions or blood (70). Excessive sputum production in patients who smoke likely contributes to pulmonary sequelae. In a retrospective study in patients undergoing coronary artery bypass surgery, compared to current smokers, there was a three-fold decrease in postoperative pulmonary complications in individuals who had stopped smoking for more than 5 weeks (71). Although the etiology for this improved outcome was not confirmed, a decrease in sputum production after stopping cigarette smoking may have contributed.

Anesthetic gases administered through an endotracheal tube bypass the humidifying portions of the patient's upper airway, dry the tracheobronchial mucosa, and produce diminished ciliary activity and increased mucous viscosity (72). Ciliated epithelial cells of the tracheobronchial tree undergo significant morphological changes when exposed to dry anesthetic gases, but these changes do not occur when the humidity of the gas is at least 60% (73). This suggests that humidifying devices such as heat and moisture exchangers should be used to reduce injury to ciliated epithelium and prevent drying of secretions, which may lead to bronchial plugging.

Regional anesthesia is not associated with the same intraoperative pulmonary changes that occur during general anesthesia. Spinal anesthesia resulting in analgesia to the mid-thoracic level produces a slight decrease in vital capacity, an increase in dead space ventilation, and minimal effect on tidal volume and inspiratory function (74). Therefore, spinal anesthesia has been advocated for patients with COPD because oxygenation and pulmonary function are not adversely affected (75). Epidural anesthesia with sensory blockade to T1 in healthy volunteers has been shown to slightly decrease total lung capacity, vital capacity, and inspiratory capacity through motor block of the intercostal muscles (76). During surgery under regional anesthesia, patients continue to breathe spontaneously, thereby avoiding atelectasis and the decrease in functional residual capacity that routinely accompanies general anesthesia. More recent studies have demonstrated that high epidural anesthesia (T1 sensory level with paralysis of the muscles of the rib cage) increases functional residual capacity as a result of a caudal motion of the end-expiratory position of the diaphragm (77). The diminished displacement of the rib cage during inspiration produced no adverse effects on pulmonary expansion, but the beneficial pulmonary effects of regional anesthesia do not persist postoperatively after cessation of the neurological blockade.

In addition to the direct effects of anesthesia and surgery, other factors such as pain, use of systemic narcotic analgesics, site of incision, and preexisting pulmonary disease appear to contribute to postoperative atelectasis and risk of pneumonia. Immediately after surgery, as the patient awakens from general anesthesia, depressed consciousness from residual anesthetic agents or partial neuromuscular blockade from inadequately reversed relaxants may result in hypoventilation, a weakened cough that is inadequate to clear secretions from the airway, and an increased risk of aspiration. Neuromuscular blocking agents are commonly administered during general anesthesia to facilitate surgery by providing muscle paralysis. When a group of adult patients were assessed in the recovery room more than 40% had residual neuromuscular blockade attributable to inadequate reversal of muscle relaxants (78). This residual weakness of the striated muscles of the oropharynx accompanied by sedation from anesthetic agents and narcotic analgesics in the immediate postoperative period make aspiration of oropharyngeal secretions more likely. Several developments, including better intraoperative monitoring of neuromuscular function, more widespread use of agents to antagonize neuromuscular blockade, and the introduction of short-acting, nondepolarizing, neuromuscular-blocking drugs have decreased the likelihood of postoperative residual skeletal muscle weakness.

VI. MODALITIES TO REDUCE THE RISK OF POSTOPERATIVE PNEUMONIA

Many factors associated with postoperative pneumonia have been identified, and some of these may be altered to decrease the risk for this complication (see Table 2). Intermittent positive pressure breathing was used in postoperative patients to prevent atelectasis and pulmonary complications, but when it was found to be ineffective (79) it was replaced with incentive spirometry and postoperative chest physical therapy to clear respiratory secretions (80,81). A controlled trial in elderly patients undergoing high-risk surgical procedures demonstrated that addition of preoperative chest physical therapy reduced the rate of atelectasis but not pneumonia (82). Furthermore, use of postoperative incentive spirometry offered no benefit in decreasing postoperative pulmonary complications compared with unstructured deep breathing exercises in low-risk patients (83). In a group of patients having open heart surgery, one preoperative teaching session and treatment with breathing exercises twice a day after surgery significantly decreased the incidence of pulmonary complications (84).

Although narcotic analgesics produce hypoventilation by sedation and reducing the respiratory response to carbon dioxide, prudent use of narcotics reduces postoperative pain, which facilitates coughing and maximizes vital capacity, especially after thoracic or abdominal surgery. Parenteral narcotics administered by nurses on a fixed-time basis are likely to produce an initial period of sedation followed by inadequate analgesia (85). When used in an episodic manner in doses that adequately control postoperative pain, narcotic analgesics may reduce the patient's level of consciousness and, in a postoperative patient with an unprotected airway, may be associated with silent aspiration and nosocomial pneumonia (86). As an alternative, patient-controlled analgesia (PCA) permits the patient to self-administer small doses of narcotic analgesics on a frequent, preset basis (87). With the use of PCA, the patient can better titrate the timing and dosage of narcotic to produce effective analgesia by maintaining opioid blood levels in a therapeutic range (88). Because the patient must be awake to activate the PCA and because incremental small doses of narcotics are administered, profound sedation is unlikely. Although it would seem that postoperative PCA use would be associated with earlier patient mobilization and improved respiratory function, well-controlled outcome studies are lacking.

Postoperative pain can be effectively managed with regional anesthetic techniques, which may have advantages over the use of parenteral opioids. Epidural analgesia using either a local anesthetic agent, an opioid, or a combination of the two provides excellent postoperative pain relief after thoracic, abdominal, or lower extremity surgery (88). A group of high-risk surgical patients having intrathoracic, intraabdominal, or major vascular surgical procedures was studied to assess whether there were outcome differences when epidural analgesia with local anesthetics was combined with a light level of general anesthesia during surgery and continued postoperatively for pain control. Compared with patients having a standard general anesthetic and intermittent parenteral narcotics for postoperative pain control, the rate of postoperative complications, including major infections, was reduced with the use of the epidural (89). Two patients in the epidural analgesia group had a nonfunctioning epidural catheter, and if they were excluded from the analysis, the rate of postoperative respiratory failure would have been decreased significantly compared with patients receiving parenteral narcotics. This is one of the only studies demonstrating a reduction in the rate of postoperative respiratory complications with the use of epidural analgesia, but because of the study design, it cannot be determined whether the improved outcome was attributable to the difference in intraoperative anesthetic technique or the use of postoperative epidural analgesia. Cuschieri compared the amount of pain relief and rate of postoperative pulmonary complications in patients who received either parenteral morphine or epidural bupivacaine after open cholecystectomy (90). Use of epidural analgesia was associated with better postoperative pain relief, higher postoperative arterial oxygen tension, and a significant decrease in the incidence of pulmonary complications, defined as atelectasis and chest infection. Although epidural analgesia was used for the first 12 hours after the conclusion of surgery, it provided good pain relief and was associated with an improved pulmonary status, which persisted through the fourth postoperative day. In another study demonstrating the benefits of epidural narcotics for postoperative analgesia, morbidly obese patients undergoing gastroplasty for weight reduction were able to be mobilized more quickly and had earlier postoperative recovery of peak expiratory flow compared with patients receiving intramuscular morphine (91). Although there were no statistical differences in vital capacity between treatment groups, pulmonary complications, including atelectasis or infiltrate on chest radiograph, occurred in 40% of patients receiving intramuscular morphine compared with 13% in the epidural group. These studies suggest that postoperative epidural analgesia may be effective in reducing the risk of pulmonary complications but the beneficial effects may be greatest in high-risk patients.

Because multiple variables may affect postoperative outcome, it is difficult to assess the benefits of techniques available to manage postoperative analgesia. Factors that must be considered include the specific narcotic analgesic and its route of administration as well as patient-related variables such as the surgical procedure and coexisting medical conditions. For agents administered epidurally, the site of the epidural catheter placement, use of opioid analgesic versus local anesthetic, and intraoperative or postoperative epidural use (92) must be considered. For example, epidural morphine provides greater pain relief than administration of the drug intravenously through PCA (90,93) but has a slow onset of action because its passage into cerebrospinal fluid is delayed as a result of its lipophilicity. As a result of the long time to absorption, epidural morphine often produces pruritus, nausea, vomiting, and late respiratory depression from rostral spread of drug to the brainstem (94). More lipophilic narcotics (e.g., fentanyl) are rapidly absorbed from the epidural space, which results in plasma concentrations that do not differ from that observed when the drug is administered intravenously by PCA (95). Much of the analgesic effect of epidural fentanyl is produced from systemic absorption; therefore, studies assessing the efficacy of epidural fentanyl must include a control group receiving the drug by way of PCA. In contrast to the use of epidurally administered local anesthetics, epidural narcotics provide analgesia by blocking opiate receptors in the spinal cord without producing sympathetic blockade, thus permitting patient ambulation without the risk of orthostatic hypotension. Clonidine, an α_2-adrenergic agonist, produces analgesia without significant respiratory depression when administered in the epidural space (96). Side effects of clonidine include hypotension and bradycardia, but the improved duration and intensity of analgesia may be associated with improved outcome. Although epidural analgesia produces more complete relief of postoperative pain, few studies demonstrate an improved pulmonary outcome. Because placement and management of epidural analgesia requires additional costs to the health care system, the benefits to postsurgical patients should be established before more widespread application of the technique.

REFERENCES

1. Estes RJ, Meduri GU. The pathogenesis of ventilator-associated pneumonia: I. Mechanisms of bacterial transcolonization and airway inoculation. Intensive Care Med 1995; 21:365–383.
2. Meduri GU, Estes RJ. The pathogenesis of ventilator-associated pneumonia: II. The lower respiratory tract. Intensive Care Med 1995; 21:452–461.
3. Jarvis WR, Edwards JR, Culver DH, et al. Nosocomial infection rates in adult and pediatric intensive care units in the United States. Am J Med 1991; 91 (suppl 3B):185S–191S.
4. Emori TG, Culver DH, Horan TC, et al. National nosocomial infections surveillance system (NNIS): description of surveillance methods. Am J Infect Control 1991; 19:19–35.
5. Haley RW, Hooton TM, Culver DH, et al. Nosocomial infections in U.S. hospitals, 1975–1976: estimated frequency by selected characteristics of patients. Am J Med 1981; 70:947–959.
6. Wenzel RP, Osterman CA, Hunting KJ. Hospital-acquired infections: II. Infection rates by site, service and common procedures in a university hospital. Am J Epidemiol 1976; 104:645–651.
7. Garibaldi RA, Britt MR, Coleman ML, Reading JC, Pace NL. Risk factors for postoperative pneumonia. Am J Med 1981; 70:677–680.
8. Martin LF, Asher EF, Casey JM, Fry DE. Postoperative pneumonia: determinants of mortality. Arch Surg 1984; 119:379–383.
9. Ephgrave KS, Leiman-Wexler R, Pfaller M, Booth B, Werkmeister L, Young S. Postoperative pneumonia: a prospective study of risk factors and morbidity. Surgery 1993; 114:815–821.
10. Warren CPW, Grimwood M. Pulmonary disorders and physiotherapy in patients who undergo cholecystectomy. Can J Surg 1980; 23:384–386.
11. Dauch WA, Landau G, Krex D. Prognostic factors for lower respiratory tract infections after brain-tumor surgery. J Neurosurg 1989; 70:862–868.
12. Carrel T, Schmid ER, von Segesser L, Vogt M, Turina M. Preoperative assessment of the likelihood of infection of the lower respiratory tract after cardiac surgery. Thorac Cardiovasc Surg 1991; 39:85–88.
13. Zickmann B, Sabblotzki A, Fussle R, Gorlach G, Hempelmann G. Perioperative microbiologic monitoring of tracheal aspirates as a predictor of pulmonary complications after cardiac operations. J Thorac Cardiovasc Surg 1996; 111:1213–1218.

14. Lehot JJ, Deleat-Besson R, Bastien O, Brun Y, Adeleine P, Robin J, Estanove S. Should we inhibit gastric acid secretion before cardiac surgery? Anesth Analg 1990; 70:185–190.
15. Argov S, Goldstein I, Barzilai A. Is routine use of the nasogastric tube justified in upper abdominal surgery? Am J Surg 1980; 139:849–850.
16. Windsor JA, Hill GL. Risk factors for postoperative pneumonia: The importance of protein depletion. Ann Surg 1988; 208:209–214.
17. Gorensek MJ, Stewart RW, Keys TF, Mehta AC, McHenry MC, Goormastic M. A multivariate analysis of risk factors for pneumonia following cardiac transplantation. Transplantation 1987; 46:860–865.
18. Olds JW, Kisch AL, Eberle BJ, Wilson JN. *Pseudomonas aeruginosa* respiratory tract infection acquired from a contaminated anesthesia machine. Am Rev Respir Dis 1972; 105:628–632.
19. Ahmed J, Brutus A, D'Amato RF, Glatt AE. *Acinetobacter calcoaceticus anitratus* outbreak in the intensive care unit traced to a peak flow meter. Am J Infect Control 1994; 22:319–321.
20. Klick JM, du Moulin GC. An oxygen analyzer as a source of *Pseudomonas*. Anesthesiology 1978; 49:293–294.
21. Craven DE, Goularte TA, Make BJ. Contaminated condensate in mechanical ventilator circuit: a risk factor for nosocomial pneumonia? Am Rev Respir Dis 1984; 129:625–628.
22. Langer M, Mosconi P, Cigada M, et al. Long-term respiratory support and risk of pneumonia in critically ill patients. Am Rev Respir Dis 1989; 140:302–305.
23. Cross AS, Roupe B. Role of respiratory assistance devices in endemic nosocomial pneumonia. Am J Med 1981; 70:681–685.
24. Blitt CD, Gutman HL, Cohen DD, Weisman H, Dillon JB. "Silent" regurgitation and aspiration during general anesthesia. Anesth Analg 1970; 49:707–712.
25. Wynne JW, Modell JH. Respiratory aspiration of stomach contents. Ann Intern Med 1977; 87:466–474.
26. Warner MA, Warner ME, Weber JG. Clinical significance of pulmonary aspiration during the perioperative period. Anesthesiology 1993; 78:56–62.
27. Fanning GL. The efficacy of cricoid pressure in preventing regurgitation of gastric contents. Anesthesiology 1970; 32:553–555.
28. Toung T, Cameron JL. Cimetadine as a preoperative medication to reduce the complications of aspiration of gastric contents. Surgery 1980; 87:205–208.
29. Manchikanti L, Grow JB, Colliver JA, Hadley CH, Hohlbein LJ. Bicitra (sodium citrate) and metoclopramide in outpatient anesthesia for prophylaxis against aspiration pneumonitits. Anesthesiology 1985; 63:378–384.
30. Johanson WG, Pierce AK, Sanford JP. Changing pharyngeal bacterial flora of hospitalized patients: emergence of gram-negative bacilli. N Engl J Med 1969; 281:1137–1140.
31. Mackowiak PA, Martin RM, Jones SR. Pharyngeal colonization by gram-negative bacilli in aspiration-prone persons. Arch Intern Med 1978; 138:1224–1227.
32. Valenti WM, Trudell RG, Bentley DW. Factors predisposing to oropharyngeal

colonization with gram-negative bacilli in the aged. N Engl J Med 1978; 298: 1108–1111.

33. Manchikanti L, Canella MG, Hohlbein LJ, Colliver JA. Assessment of effect of various modes of premedication on acid aspiration risk factors in outpatient surgery. Anesth Analg 1987; 66:81–84.

34. Geffen B, Pontoppidan H. Reduction of tracheal damage by the prestretching of inflatable cuffs. Anesthesiology 1969; 31:462–463.

35. Pavlin EG, VanNimwegan D, Hornbein TF. Failure of a high-compliance low-pressure cuff to prevent aspiration. Anesthesiology 1975; 42:216–219.

36. Mahul P, Auboyer C, Jospe R, et al. Prevention of nosocomial pneumonia in intubated patients: respective role of mechanical subglottic secretions drainage and stress ulcer prophylaxis. Intensive Care Med 1992; 18:20–25.

37. Valles J, Artigas A, Rello J, et al. Continuous aspiration of subglottic secretions in preventing ventilator-associated pneumonia. Ann Intern Med 1995; 122:179–186.

38. Cook D, De Jonghe B, Brochard L, Brun-Buisson C. Influence of airway management on ventilator-associated pneumonia: evidence from randomized trials. JAMA 1998; 279:781–787.

39. Bernhard WN, Cottrell JE, Sivakumaran C, Patel K, Yost L, Turndorf H. Adjustment of intracuff pressure to prevent aspiration. Anesthesiology 1979; 50:363–366.

40. Salord F, Gaussorgues P, Marti-Flich J, Sirodot M, Allimant C, Lyonnet D, Robert D. Nosocomial maxillary sinusitits during mechanical ventilation: a prospective comparison of orotracheal versus the nasotracheal route for intubation. Intensive Care Med 1990; 16:390–393.

41. Bach A, Boehrer H, Schmidt H, Geiss HK. Nosocomial sinusitis in ventilated patients: nosotracheal versus orotracheal intubation. Anaesthesia 1992; 47:335–339.

42. Holzapfel L, Chevret S, Madinier G, et al. Influence of long-term oro- or nasotracheal intubation on nosocomial maxillary sinusitis and pneumonia: results of a prospective randomized clinical trial. Crit Care Med 1993; 21:1132–1138.

43. Torres A, Gatell JM, Aznar E, El-Ebiary M, de la Bellacasa JP, Gonzales J, Ferrer M, Rodriguez-Roisin R. Re-intubation increases the risk of nosocomial pneumonia in patients needing mechanical ventilation. Am J Respir Crit Care Med 1995; 152:137–141.

44. Hovig B. Lower respiratory tract infections associated with respiratory therapy and anaesthesia equipment. J Hosp Infect 1981; 2:301–305.

45. Winge-Hedén K. Bacteriologic studies on anaesthetic apparatus. Acta Chir Scand 1962; 124:294–303.

46. American Society of Anesthesiologists. Prevention of nosomial infections in patients. In: Recommendations for Infection Control for the Practice of Anesthesiology. Park Ridge, IL: American Society of Anesthesiologists, 1998:6–8.

47. Spaulding EH. Chemical sterilization of surgical instruments. Surg Gynecol Obstet 1939; 69:738–744.

48. Favero MS. Principles of sterilization and disinfection. Anesth Clin North Am 1989; 7:941–949.
49. du Moulin GC, Saubermann AJ. The anesthesia machine and circle system are not likely to be sources of bacterial contamination. Anesthesiology 1977; 47: 353–358.
50. Weber DJ, Wilson MB, Rutala WA, Thomann CA. Manual ventilation bags as a source for bacterial colonization of intubated patients. Am Rev Respir Dis 1990; 142:892–894.
51. Hartstein AI, Rashad AL, Liebler JM, et al. Multiple intensive care unit outbreak of *Acinetobacter calcoaceticus* subspecies *anitratus* respiratory infection and colonization associated with contaminated, reusable ventilator circuits and resuscitation bags. Am J Med 1988; 85:624–631.
52. Centers for Disease Control and Prevention and the Hospital Infection Control Practices Committee. Guideline for prevention of nosocomial pneumonia. Respir Care 1994; 39:1191–1236.
53. Feeley TW, Hamilton WK, Xavier B, Moyers J, Eger EI. Sterile anesthesia breathing circuits do not prevent postoperative pulmonary infection. Anesthesiology 1981; 54:369–372.
54. Garibaldi RA, Britt MR, Webster C, Pace NL. Failure of bacterial filters to reduce the incidence of pneumonia after inhalation anesthesia. Anesthesiology 1981; 54:364–368.
55. Chalon J, Markham JP, Ali MM, Ramanathan S, Turndorf H. The Pall Ultipor breathing circuit filter—an efficient heat and moisture exchanger. Anesth Anal 1984; 63:566–570.
56. Bernard HR, Cole WR. The prophylaxis of surgical infection: the effect of prophylactic antimicrobial drugs on the incidence of infection following potentially contaminated operations. Surgery 1964; 156:151–157.
57. Platt R, Zaleznik DF, Hopkins CC, et al. Perioperative antibiotic prophylaxis for herniorrhaphy and breast surgery. N Engl J Med 1990; 322:153–160.
58. Classen DC, Evans RS, Pestotnik SL, Horn SD, Menlove RL, Burke JP. The timing of prophylactic administration of antibiotics and the risk of surgical-wound infection. N Engl J Med 1992; 326:281–286.
59. Marshall BE, Wyche MQ. Hypoxemia during and after anesthesia. Anesthesiology 1972; 37:178–209.
60. Boutros AR, Weisel M. Comparison of effects of three anaesthetic techniques on patients with severe pulmonary obstructive disease. Can Anaesth Soc J 1971; 18:286–292.
61. Laws AK. Effects of induction of anaesthesia and muscle paralysis on functional residual capacity of the lungs. Can Anaesth Soc J 1968; 15:325–331.
62. Hedenstierna G, Tokics L, Strandberg A, Lundquist H, Brismar B. Correlation of gas exchange impairment to development of atelectasis during anaesthesia and muscle paralysis. Acta Anaesthesiol Scand 1986; 30:183–191.
63. Dery R, Pelletier J, Jacques A, et al. Alveolar collapse induced by denitrogenation. Can Anaesth Soc J 1965; 12:531–544.

64. Rothen HU, Sporre B, Engberg G, Wegenius G, Hogman M, Hedenstierna G. Influence of gas composition on recurrence of atelectasis after a reexpansion maneuver during general anesthesia. Anesthesiology 1995; 82:832–842.

65. Strandberg A, Tokics L, Brismar B, Lundquist H, Hedenstierna G. Atelectasis during anaesthesia and in the postoperative period. Acta Anaesthesiol Scand 1986; 30:154–158.

66. Strandberg A, Hedenstierna G, Tokics L, Lundquist H, Brismar B. Densities in dependent lung regions during anaesthesia: atelectasis or fluid accumulation? Acta Anaesthesiol Scand 1986; 30:256–259.

67. Froese AB, Bryan AC. Effects of anesthesia and paralysis on diaphragmatic mechanics in man. Anesthesiology 1974; 41:242–255.

68. Warner DO, Warner MA, Ritman EL. Atelectasis and chest wall shape during halothane anesthesia. Anesthesiology 1996; 85:49–59.

69. Magnusson L, Zemgulis V, Wicky S, Tyden H, Thelin S, Hedenstierna G. Atelectasis is a major cause of hypoxemia and shunt after cardiopulmonary bypass: an experimental study. Anesthesiology 1997; 87:1153–1163.

70. Ding Y, White PF. Lung collapse after induction of anesthesia in a healthy outpatient. Anesthesiology 1994; 80:689–690.

71. Warner MA, Divertie MB, Tinker JH. Preoperative cessation of smoking and pulmonary complications in coronary artery bypass patients. Anesthesiology 1984; 60:380–383.

72. Gray TD, Benson DW. Systemic and pulmonary changes with inhaled humid atmosphere: clinical applications. Anesthesiology 1969; 30:199–207.

73. Chalon J, Loew DAY, Malebranche J. Effects of dry anesthetic gases on tracheobronchial ciliated epithelium. Anesthesiology 1972; 37:338–343.

74. Askrog VF, Smith TC, Eckenhoff JE. Changes in pulmonary ventilation during spinal anesthesia. Surg Gynecol Obstet 1964; 119:563–567.

75. Paskin S, Rodman T, Smith TC. The effect of spinal anesthesia on the pulmonary function of patients with chronic obstructive pulmonary disease. Ann Surg 1969; 169:35–41.

76. Sundberg A, Wattwil M, Arvill A. Respiratory effects of high thoracic epidural anaesthesia. Acta Anasthesiol Scand 1986; 30:215–217.

77. Warner DO, Warner MA, Ritman EL. Human chest wall function during epidural anesthesia. Anesthesiology 1996; 85:761–773.

78. Viby-Mogensen J, Jørgensen BC, Ørding H. Residual curarization in the recovery room. Anesthesiology 1979; 50:539–541.

79. Baxter WD, Levine RS. An evaluation of intermittent positive pressure breathing in the prevention of postoperative pulmonary complications. Arch Surg 1969; 98:795–798.

80. Byrd RB, Burns JR. Cough dynamics in post-thoracotomy state. Chest 1975; 67: 654–657.

81. Gale CD, Sanders DE. Incentive spirometry: its value after cardiac surgery. Can Anaesth Soc J 1980; 27:475–480.

82. Castillo R, Haas A. Chest physical therapy: comparative efficacy of preoperative and postoperative in the elderly. Arch Phys Med Rehabil 1985; 66:376–379.

83. Davies BL, MacLeod JP, Ogilvie HMJ. The efficacy of incentive spirometers in post-operative protocols for low-risk patients. Can J Nursing Res 1990; 22:19–36.

84. Vraciu JK, Vraciu RA. Effectiveness of breathing exercises in preventing pulmonary complications following open heart surgery. Phys Ther 1977; 57:1367–1371.

85. Marks RM, Sachar EJ. Undertreatment of medical inpatients with narcotic analgesics. Ann Intern Med 1973; 78:173–181.

86. Celis R, Torres A, Gatell JM, Almela M, Rodriguez-Roisin R, Agusti-Vidal A. Nosocomial pneumonia: a multivariate analysis of risk and prognosis. Chest 1988; 93:318–324.

87. Graves DA, Foster TS, Batenhorst RL, Bennett RL, Baumann TJ. Patient-controlled analgesia. Ann Intern Med 1983; 99:360–366.

88. Lutz LJ, Lamer TJ. Management of postoperative pain: review of current techniques and methods. Mayo Clin Proc 1990; 65:584–596.

89. Yeager MP, Glass DD, Neff RK, Brinck-Johnsen T. Epidural anesthesia and analgesia in high-risk surgical patients. Anesthesiology 1987; 66:729–736.

90. Cuschieri RJ, Morran CG, Howie JC, McArdle CS. Postoperative pain and pulmonary complications: comparison of three analgesic regimens. Br J Surg 1985; 72:495–498.

91. Rawal N, Sjöstrand U, Christoffersson E, Dahlström B, Arvill A, Rydman H. Comparison of intramuscular and epidural morphine for postoperative analgesia in the grossly obese: influence of postoperative ambulation and pulmonary function. Anesth Analg 1984; 63:583–592.

92. Gottschalk A, Smith DS, Jobes DR, et al. Preemptive epidural analgesia and recovery from radical prostatectomy: a randomized controlled trial. JAMA 1998; 279:1076–1082.

93. Loper KA, Ready LB, Nessly M, Rapp SE. Epidural morphine provides greater pain relief than patient-controlled intravenous morphine following cholecystectomy. Anesth Analg 1989; 69:826–828.

94. Gourlay GK, Cherry DA, Cousins MJ. Cephalad migration of morphine in CSF following lumbar epidural administration in patients with cancer pain. Pain 1985; 23:317–326.

95. Glass PSA, Estok P, Ginsberg B, Goldberg JS, Sladen RN. Use of patient-controlled analgesia to compare the efficacy of epidural to intravenous fentanyl administration. Anesth Analg 1992; 74:345–351.

96. Eisenach J, Detweiler D, Hood D. Hemodynamic and analgesic actions of epidurally administered clonidine. Anesthesiology 1993; 78:277–287.

97. Mermel LA, Maki DG. Bacterial pneumonia in solid organ transplantation. Semin Respir Infect 1990; 5:10–29.

98. Ejlertsen T, Nielsen PH, Jepsen S, Olsen A. Early diagnosis of postoperative pneumonia following upper abdominal surgery. Acta Chir Scand 1989; 155:93–98.

99. Hanson LC, Weber DJ, Rutala WA. Risk factors for nosocomial pneumonia in the elderly. Am J Med 1992; 92:161–166.

·

AUTHOR INDEX

Italic numbers give the page on which the complete reference is listed.

SUBJECT INDEX